ACTIVE LEARNING MANUAL

EMT-B

BRADY

ACTIVE LEARNING MANUAL

EMT-B

- DANIEL LIMMER, AS, EMT-P
- CHRISTOPHER J. LE BAUDOUR, MS ED, NREMT

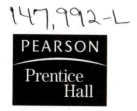

PEARSON

Prentice
Hall

Upper Saddle River, NJ 07458

Library of Congress Cataloging-in-Publication Data

Limmer, Daniel.
 Active learning manual / Daniel Limmer, Chris Le Baudour.
  p. ; cm.
 "... the Active learning manual for Brady's Emergency care 10th ed.
textbook ..."–Pref.
 Includes bibliographical references and index.
 ISBN 0-13-113629-1
 1. Emergency medicine. 2. First aid in illness and injury. 3. Rescue
work. 4. Emergency medical personnel.
  [DNLM: 1. Emergency Medical Services–methods. 2. Emergencies.
3. Emergency Medical Technicians. 4. First Aid–methods. WX 215 L734a 2005]
 I. Le Baudour, Chris. II. Emergency care. III. Title.

 RC86.7.B68 2005 Suppl.
 616.02'5--dc22   2004013994

Publisher: Julie Levin Alexander
Publisher's Assistant: Regina Bruno
Executive Editor: Marlene McHugh Pratt
Senior Managing Editor for Development: Lois Berlowitz
Development Editor: Andrea Edwards, Triple SSS Press Media
        Development
Assistant Editor: Monica Moosang
Senior Marketing Manager: Katrin Beacom
Channel Marketing Manager: Rachele Strober
Marketing Coordinator: Michael Sirinides
Director of Production and Manufacturing: Bruce Johnson
Managing Production Editor: Patrick Walsh
Production Liaison: Faye Gemmellaro
Production Editor: Mark Corsey/nSight, Inc.
Manufacturing Manager: Ilene Sanford
Manufacturing Buyer: Pat Brown
Creative Director: Cheryl Asherman
Senior Design Coordinator: Christopher Weigand
Cover Designer: Christopher Weigand
Interior Designer: Amanda Kavanaugh
Composition: Laserwords
Printing and Binding: Banta-Harrisonburg
Cover Printer: Phoenix Color

Pearson Education LTD.
Pearson Education Australia PTY, Limited
Pearson Education Singapore, Pte. Ltd
Pearson Education North Asia Ltd
Pearson Education Canada, Ltd
Pearson Educacion de Mexico, S.A. de C.V.
Pearson Education—Japan
Pearson Education Malaysia, Pte. Ltd
Pearson Education Upper Saddle River, NJ

NOTICE ON CARE PROCEDURES

This workbook reflects current EMS practices based on the 1994 U.S. Department of Transportation's EMT-Basic National Standard Curriculum. It is the intent of the authors and publisher that this workbook be used as part of a formal Emergency Medical Technician education program taught by qualified instructors and supervised by a licensed physician. The procedures described in this workbook are based upon consultation with EMS and medical authorities. The authors and publisher have taken care to make certain that these procedures reflect currently accepted clinical practice; however, they cannot be considered absolute recommendations.

The material in this workbook contains the most current information available at the time of publication. However, federal, state, and local guidelines concerning clinical practices, including, without limitation, those governing infection control and universal precautions, change rapidly. The reader should note, therefore, that new regulations may require changes in some procedures.

It is the responsibility of the reader to familiarize himself or herself with the policies and procedures set by federal, state, and local agencies as well as the institution or agency where the reader may be employed. The author and the publisher of this workbook disclaim any liability, loss, or risk resulting directly or indirectly from the suggested procedures and theory, from any undetected errors, or from the reader's misunderstanding of the text. It is the reader's responsibility to stay informed of any new changes or recommendations made by any federal, state, and local agency as well as by his or her employing institution or agency.

If when reading this workbook you find an error, have an idea for how to improve it, or simply want to share your comments with us, please send your letter to the address below.

Managing Editor
Brady/Prentice Hall Health
Pearson Education
One Lake Street
Upper Saddle River, New Jersey 07458

NOTICE ON BCLS PROCEDURES

The national standards for BCLS are reviewed and revised on a regular basis and may change slightly after this book is printed. It is important that you know the most current procedures for CPR, both for the classroom and your patients. The most current information may always be downloaded from www.bradybooks.com or obtained from your instructor.

Studentaid.ed.gov, the U.S. Department of Education's website on college planning assistance, is a valuable tool for anyone intending to pursue higher education. Designed to help students at all stages of schooling, including international students, returning students, and parents, it is a guide to the financial aid process. The website presents information on applying to and attending college as well as on funding your education and repaying loans. It also provides links to useful resources, such as state education agency contact information, assistance in filling out financial aid forms, and an introduction to various forms of student aid.

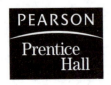

Contents

Preface

▶ A ONE-OF-A-KIND RESOURCE FOR EMT STUDENTS

You now hold in your hands the *Active Learning Manual* for Brady's *Emergency Care* 10th edition textbook. Not to be mistaken for "just another workbook," the *Active Learning Manual* (ALM) is a "first of its kind" resource for serious EMT-B students and instructors alike.

The ALM began as the brainchild of well-known EMS author and educator Dan Limmer. Dan has teamed up with Christopher Le Baudour, another Brady author and career EMS educator, who together share over 40 years of combined experience in this valuable student resource.

First and foremost, the ALM is *not* a workbook. Most workbooks today are comprised mainly of test questions that prepare students for both in-class and national written exams. The ALM does this and a whole lot more! It is just what its name implies, an accumulation of active learning exercises that expand the walls of the classroom and encourage students to develop a deeper understanding of both the knowledge and skills necessary to become an excellent EMT-B.

While the ALM table of contents does follow Brady's *Emergency Care* 10th edition chapter for chapter, the activities for the most part are not textbook specific but instead are curriculum specific. What this means is that no matter which primary textbook you may be using for your EMT-Basic program, you will still benefit immensely from the addition of the ALM to your study program.

▶ WHAT IS ACTIVE LEARNING?

Active: *adjective.* To participate (take an active role)

Learning: *noun.* To acquire wisdom, knowledge, or skill

Active Learning: To take an active role in the acquisition of knowledge and skills

As you will see from the definition we have provided above, active learning is a process whereby you, the student, must take an active part in the learning process. Of course, you are probably thinking that you already take part in the learning process, and to some extent this is true. You take notes during lectures, ask questions of the instructor, and participate in skills practice sessions. While all these do require some level of action on your part, they for the most part place the instructor at the center of the learning. Research suggests that, as students, you must do more than simply listen. Active learning involves reading, writing, discussing, and being involved in solving problems. Simply stated, active learning means getting you, the student, involved in doing things and thinking about the things you are doing.

> *Most ideas about teaching are not new,*
> *but not everyone knows the old ideas.*
> *Euclid, c. 300 B.C.*

The concept of active learning is not new. Socrates encouraged active learning by using open-ended questions to stimulate discussion and critical thinking among his students. Active learning can also take many forms such as reading, discussion, writing, exploration, and reflection. For that reason, we have assembled a variety of tools within each chapter that encourage you to become more active in your own learning, both in and out of the classroom.

▶ DO YOU KNOW HOW YOU LEARN?

One of the best ways you can affect the learning process is to have an understanding of how you as an individual learn. There are several ways people take in information from their environment and transform that information into learning. Some of those styles of learning include visual (seeing), aural listening), and kinesthetic (doing), as well as reading and writing. Everyone has learning preferences where one or more learning styles are used for the majority of the learning.

Here is a link to a website that will provide a glimpse into your learning preferences. You may be surprised to discover that your learning preference is not what you thought it was. Once at the VARK site, begin by clicking the FAQ link to learn more about the assessment. Once you are ready to complete the assessment, click on the questionnaire link.

VARK—A guide to learning styles http://www.vark-learn.com/

In addition to discovering more about your preferred learning style, you may discover a little more about how others around you process information as well. What style does your instructor emphasize in the classroom? Does his style match your style according to the VARK assessment?

▶ MAKING ACTIVE LEARNING WORK FOR YOU

As we stated earlier in the introduction, this ALM is for the serious student who wishes to develop a deeper understanding of what it takes to become an excellent EMT-B. That deeper understanding comes at a cost. You must be willing to extend your EMT-B training beyond the classroom and engage in the recommended activities and exercises both in and out of the classroom.

In many cases, we ask that you partner with a fellow student or students to complete the exercise together. While your partner does not always have to be a fellow student, it would help tremendously if he were participating in the same class as you are. Finding one or more fellow students early on who are willing to meet before class and outside of class to work through the exercises will make the learning much more valuable and enjoyable.

▶ ANATOMY OF THE ACTIVE LEARNING MANUAL

We have assembled a variety of activities that place you at the center of the learning process. In addition, we have strived to create activities that address as many learning styles as possible. What follows is a brief description of each of the chapter elements and how to best take full advantage of the learning opportunities they provide.

Chapter Summary

The ALM summary is a much more expanded summary than the one at the end of the chapter in the textbook. For this reason, it works especially well as a study tool prior to any in-class or national certification exams you may be taking.

Med Minute

The Med Minute feature is only contained in those chapters dealing specifically with patient emergency care, or, as we will call them, the clinical chapters. It is designed to provide a general overview of commonly prescribed medications likely to be encountered by the EMT-B while treating a patient. This feature will help develop the EMT-B's medication vocabulary and knowledge, which can be especially helpful when the patient is not able to provide a detailed history.

Pathophysiology Pearls

The Pathophysiology Pearl feature is contained in all clinical chapters and is designed to provide enhancement information relating to specific medical conditions and/or disease processes. This information will build upon the foundation started by the EC textbook. As your understanding of disease processes increases, so will your ability to anticipate and appropriately treat the patient's condition.

Pearls from the Podium

In those chapters deemed nonclinical, we have included the feature we call Pearls from the Podium. These are simple but valuable insights shared by the authors covering such topics as study tips, patient emergency care, and career tips.

Review Questions

Along with becoming an EMT-B is the opportunity to take a multitude of written exams. You will encounter many of these exams during your initial training as well as for many state and national certification processes. Like so many other things in life, more practice makes for better scores.

In an effort to provide you with as much experience as possible with written exams, we have included a variety of exam questions that resemble those you are likely to encounter in your quest to become an EMT-B and maintain your certification. Question types included in the ALM include:

- Short answer
- Multiple choice
- Scenario

Detailed answers to all review questions are provided and can be found in Appendix A at the end of this manual.

Case Studies

Here is where you will really begin using your critical-thinking skills and applying the knowledge you have gained from the textbook. We have included two case studies in each chapter. Each case study presents a slightly different problem or set of problems for you to solve. Following the case study, a series of questions are asked to stimulate critical thinking. In some case studies, you will be provided additional information and presented with additional questions before completing the exercise.

Detailed answers to all case studies are provided and can be found in Appendix A at the end of this manual.

Active Exploration

Are you having fun yet? Because here is where the fun really begins! Each chapter contains two Active Exploration exercises. Many of these involve getting out and actively exploring the information and concepts presented in the textbook. Some of these can be completed by yourself while others require that you recruit others to assist you. For exercises that require additional help, we encourage you to arrange to meet with fellow students from your class so that all of you can learn together. Of course if this is not possible, you may use any available person.

You will get out of the Active Exploration exactly what you put into it. We recommend taking time to prepare thoroughly before jumping into the activities. The Active Exploration exercises will engage you in ways the classroom simply cannot. By completing each exercise, you will gain insight and develop skills that simply cannot be obtained in the classroom setting. Much of the experience gained through these activities will prove extremely valuable to your job as an EMT-B.

Retro Review

One of the difficulties of being an EMT-B student and taking in so much new information is that what you learned two weeks ago can easily be forgotten if you do not constantly go back and refresh. This becomes a big challenge when trying to prepare for a final written exam that addresses everything you learned during your course.

The Retro Review feature helps you stay on top of key concepts and information that has already been presented. This feature provides a minimum of three multiple-choice questions from previous chapters, keeping the cobwebs from forming on information presented earlier in the course.

Thinking and Linking

As instructors, we understand that learning to be an EMT-B can appear as many unrelated pieces to a huge puzzle. To help with tying the loose pieces together, we have created the Thinking and Linking table. This table is a quick reference guide for relating current chapter information to other chapters in the textbook. Here you will learn the connection and importance of related information that will help you begin to put your puzzle together.

Our Challenge to You...

Now that we have shared how this Active Learning Manual can work for you, it is up to you to make it happen! We, as the authors of this manual and as EMS educators, challenge you to take a more active role in your EMS education and to encourage your fellow students to do the same. We promise that if you work through the exercises in this manual along with the reading in your EMT textbook, you will know more about your EMS system and be more confident when treating patients than you ever thought possible!

Acknowledgments

▶ CONTRIBUTORS

We wish to acknowledge the remarkable talents and efforts of the following people who contributed to the development of the Active Learning Manual.

Brian Bricker, NREMT
Bricker Professional Education, Inc.
Norman, Oklahoma

Tony Crystal
Director, Emergency Medical Services
Lake Land College
Mattoon, Illinois

Lieutenant Alyson Emery, EMT-P
Kennebunk Fire Rescue
Kennebunk, Maine

William S. Krost
Program Manager, Division of EMS
Clinical Coordinator of Prehospital Research
University of Cincinnati College of Medicine
Cincinnati, Ohio

▶ REVIEWERS

The reviewers of the Active Learning Manual have provided many excellent suggestions and ideas for improving the text. The quality of the reviews has been outstanding, and the reviews have been a major aid in the preparation of the manuscript. The assistance provided by these experts is deeply appreciated.

Robert Hawkes
Southern Maine Community College
South Portland, Maine

Stanley Johnson
Northern Virginia Community College
Alexandria, Virginia

Eric T. Mayhew
EMS Instructor/Coordinator
Gaston College
Department of Emergency Medical Science
Dallas, North Carolina

Denise Schultz
Colonie EMS
Colonie, New York

Francis Stewart-Dore
Instructor and Clinical Coordinator
Paramedic Program
Southern Maine Community College
South Portland, Maine

About the Authors

▶ DANIEL LIMMER

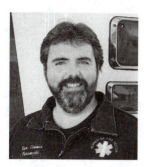

Dan Limmer, EMT-P, has been involved in EMS for more than 25 years. He remains active as a paramedic with Kennebunk Fire Rescue in Kennebunk, Maine, and the Kennebunkport EMS (KEMS) in Kennebunkport, Maine. A passionate educator, Dan teaches EMT and paramedic courses at the Southern Maine Community College in South Portland, Maine, and has taught at the George Washington University in Washington, D.C. and the Hudson Valley Community College in Troy, New York. He is a charter member of the National Association of EMS Educators and a member of the National Association of EMTs (NAEMT), for which he serves on the Advanced Medical Life Support Committee.

Dan was formerly involved in law enforcement, beginning as a dispatcher and retiring as a police officer in Colonie, New York, where he received three command recognition awards as well as the distinguished service award (Officer of the Year) in 1987. During his 20-year-law-enforcement career, he served in the communications, patrol, juvenile, narcotics, and training units.

In addition to authoring several EMS journal articles, Dan is coauthor of a number of EMS textbooks for Brady including *First Responder: A Skills Approach, Essentials of Emergency Care, Advanced Medical Life Support,* the military and fire service editions of *Emergency Care,* and others. He speaks frequently at regional, state, and national EMS conferences.

▶ CHRISTOPHER J. LE BAUDOUR

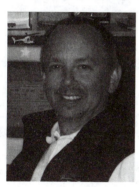

Christopher Le Baudour has been involved in EMS since 1978. He has worked as an EMT-I and an EMT-II in both the field and clinical settings. In 1984, Christopher began his teaching career in the Department of Public Safety—EMS Division at Santa Rosa Junior College in Santa Rosa, California.

In addition to Christopher's numerous certifications, he holds a master's degree in Education, with an emphasis on on-line teaching and learning, from California State University at Hayward. Christopher has spent the past 20 years perfecting the art of experiential learning in EMS and is well known for his innovative classroom techniques and his passion for both teaching and learning in both the traditional and on-line classrooms.

Christopher is very involved in EMS education at the national level as a member of the Distributed Learning subcommittee of the National Association of EMS Educators. He has been a presenter at both state and national conferences and is currently working on several EMS publications.

ACTIVE LEARNING MANUAL

EMT-B

Introduction to Emergency Medical Care

CHAPTER SUMMARY

The Emergency Medical Services (EMS) system was developed to assist people where most illnesses and injuries occur—*outside* of the hospital. It is designed to bring highly trained personnel directly to the scene of a crash or illness in order to initiate emergency care. The intention is to minimize patient deterioration between the onset of the injury or illness and arrival at the hospital. The Emergency Medical Technician-Basic (EMT-B) is a very important component of this system.

The first known EMS system began in the 1790s when wounded French soldiers were taken from the battlefield and cared for by physicians elsewhere. The concept was as simple then as it is now—carry the patient from the location of the injury or illness to where advanced medical help is available. This model was carried through and developed during other wars and armed conflicts.

Major American cities saw the creation of nonmilitary ambulance services around the turn of the twentieth century, and smaller communities followed that lead in the late 1940s. The first ambulance services, however, were strictly for transport and usually utilized a hearse from the local funeral home.

The development of the modern EMS system, the one you now recognize, began in the 1960s. Governmental actions spanning from 1966 to 1973 provided momentum for the improvement and standardization of EMS systems nationwide.

The National Highway Traffic Safety Administration (NHTSA) Technical Assistance Program developed a set of standards covering such areas of the EMS system as Regulation and Policy, Resource Management, Human Resources and Training, Transportation, Communication, Medical Direction, and so on.

The evolution of the EMS system did away with the image of the unskilled, strong-backed ambulance driver and replaced it with the reality of a highly trained Emergency Medical Technician, as an extension of the hospital emergency department.

In most cases, accessing the EMS system begins with the telephone. A person contacts an emergency dispatcher who sends the appropriate personnel to the scene. The ambulance personnel provide the needed emergency care at the scene and transport the patient to the hospital emergency department (ED) where he receives various diagnostic services and advanced treatment. Some hospitals are equipped and staffed to specialize in the treatment of certain types of emergency cases such as trauma, burns, or pediatrics.

Most communities now have a 911 system whereby those in need of assistance can simply dial 911 from any phone and are connected to the appropriate agency (medical, police, fire, and so on). Some agencies even have an enhanced version of the 911 system, whereby the caller's phone number and location are displayed on the dispatcher's computer screen.

In general, there are four levels of EMS training: First Responder, EMT-Basic, EMT-Intermediate (EMT-I), and, most advanced, EMT-Paramedic (EMT-P). EMT-Basic is usually the minimum level of training you will require to work on an ambulance.

As an EMT-B, you will have a wide range of responsibilities, including personal safety; crew, patient, and bystander safety; patient assessment; patient emergency care; lifting and moving; transportation; transfer of care; documentation; and patient advocacy.

As an EMT-B, you should be in relatively good physical condition. Carrying patients and equipment (sometimes over extended distances) is an important aspect of your job. Good observation, listening, and communication skills (verbal and written) are also essential to your success.

You should have a pleasant manner as well as be sincere and empathetic to the patient's situation and immediate needs. EMT-Bs must be resourceful, self-starting, emotionally stable, able to lead, neat, respectful, of good moral character, and demonstrate excellent self-control under pressure.

You must maintain up-to-date knowledge and continually practice your skills. Reading industry periodicals and attending refresher and continuing-education courses are all good ways to maintain a current knowledge base. You should see the EMT-Basic course as just the beginning of your EMS education.

In order to help establish and maintain national EMS standards, the National Registry of Emergency Medical Technicians (NREMT) provides testing and registration for First Responders, EMT-Bs, EMT-Is, and EMT-Ps. Being registered with the NREMT may also make it easier to transfer your EMT-B certification to another state or region.

The EMS system undergoes a constant self-review called Quality Improvement (QI). The goal of QI is to pinpoint areas where the system needs to be improved in order to provide the highest quality of prehospital care. Your role in the QI process includes ensuring proper documentation and seeking feedback from patients and hospital staff regarding your patient emergency care.

Medical direction, or medical oversight, is essential to the operation of every EMS system. The physician ultimately responsible for the patient-care aspects of your EMS system is called the Medical Director. The Medical Director develops protocols that direct the actions of EMS personnel in each type of situation. As an EMT-B, you will be acting as the Medical Director's designated agent. You will actually be providing emergency care under his license to practice medicine.

There are two sides to medical direction, on line and off line. Off-line medical direction, often called standing orders, allows EMS personnel to follow preexisting and documented instructions while treating patients in certain situations. On-line direction, used for situations not covered by protocol, requires the EMT-B to contact the on-duty physician via radio or phone prior to performing a particular skill or task.

Protocols vary from system to system, so become familiar with yours.

PEARLS FROM THE PODIUM

- Keeping up with class work (reading and workbook assignments) is essential for success in your EMT training.

- You can find additional practice test questions on the CD-ROM that accompanies your book and at www.bradybooks.com/emergencycare and www.prenhall.com/limmer.

  Take every opportunity to learn more about the EMS system you are about to become a part of. Find out by asking those you know who may be currently working in the EMS system what resources are available in your system and how one can best access those resources.

- The EMT course you are taking is the beginning of your EMS education. The learning you receive after you finish the class and begin providing emergency care in the field is critical and ongoing—for the length of your service in the EMS.

REVIEW QUESTIONS

SHORT ANSWER

1. Explain "patient advocacy."

2. What is the difference between a basic and an enhanced 911 system?

MULTIPLE CHOICE

1. The individual who assumes ultimate responsibility for the patient-care aspects of the EMS system is the _____.
   A. Designated Agent
   B. Medical Director
   C. EMT-P
   D. Quality Improvement (QI) Officer

2. An EMT-B with color vision problems may have difficulty _____.

    A. assessing a patient's skin

    B. correctly sizing a C-spine collar

    C. operating an AED (Automated External Defibrillator)

    D. selecting an appropriate airway adjunct

3. Continuing education is an important element in the EMT-B's involvement in the _____ process.

    A. chain-of-survival   **B.** standing-order

    C. resource-management   **D.** quality-improvement

4. In order to help maintain national standards, the _____ provides testing and certification for First Responders, EMT-Bs, EMT-Is, and EMT-Ps.

    A. DOT   **B.** EMSAA

    C. NREMT   **D.** NHSA

5. The EMS system, as we know it today, began _____.

    A. in eighteenth-century France

    B. with an act of Congress in 1977

    C. during World War II

    D. in the 1960s

SCENARIO QUESTIONS

A man dials 911 from the phone in his kitchen and is only able to say, "Help me," before dropping the phone. Emergency personnel are dispatched to the scene where the distressed patient explains that he is diabetic and forgot to eat breakfast. Upon hearing this, an EMT-B immediately administers oral glucose and the patient begins to recover.

1. The EMT in the above scenario is able to provide care based on _____.

    A. transfer of care   **B.** on-line medical direction

    C. a standing order   **D.** reciprocity

2. This patient benefited from _____.

    A. the Americans with Disabilities Act (ADA)

    B. an enhanced 911 system

    C. nationally registered emergency personnel

    D. an effective trauma assessment

You are dispatched to a construction site where a worker has been electrocuted. As you are pulling up in the ambulance, you observe a man lying motionless on the ground. Several of his coworkers have gathered around him and one of them is waving you over.

1. Your first priority in this situation is to _____.

    A. make sure that the patient has a patent airway and is breathing

    B. move the coworkers away from the scene

    C. contact on-line medical direction

    D. ensure that you are not in any danger

2. The emergency care that you provide this patient is based on standards first developed by _____.

    A. the Department of Transportation

    B. the National Association of Medical Directors

    C. the Federal Emergency Management Agency

    D. the American Association of Emergency Medical Technicians

CASE STUDIES

A woman calls 911 because her husband is having difficulty breathing. An ambulance is dispatched along with a neighborhood engine company. The dispatcher gives medical instructions to the wife until the ambulance arrives. On the way, the ambulance develops mechanical problems and cannot continue to the call. An ambulance from the adjoining town is dispatched in its place. The second ambulance arrives and receives a report from the engine company crew. After evaluating the patient, the EMT-B is able to assist the patient with his medication, but it does not provide relief, and the EMT-B decides that ALS is necessary. To prevent the delay in getting advanced-level care to the patient, the ambulance crew arranges to meet a solo paramedic in a quick-response vehicle on the way to the hospital. The paramedic climbs on board with her equipment and begins advanced-level care. When transferred to the care of hospital personnel, the patient has decreased breathing difficulty, thanks to the efforts of the EMT and paramedic.

1. The term used to describe when ambulances are called from adjoining regions, cities, or towns is _____.
2. The dispatcher providing medical instructions is known as a(n) _____.
3. The fire engine crew members responding to the scene first are acting as _____.
4. The concept of a paramedic meeting the ambulance en route to the hospital is called

_____

You are dispatched to a street corner in a bad part of town for a subject who has been injured in a fight. The dispatcher advises your ambulance to stay clear of the area until the police have arrived and secured the scene. Shortly after the police arrive, the dispatcher advises you that there is one patient with a stab wound to the chest and that the police have advised you to proceed in.

You observe one patient lying on the ground in a fetal position. There are three to four people around him and a police officer is motioning you over. One of the bystanders is yelling for you to hurry up and seems quite anxious. Another seems intoxicated. You ask the police to clear the crowd away from the patient.

You introduce yourself to the patient and begin your assessment. You ensure that his airway is clear and that his breathing and circulation are normal and you start him on oxygen by nonrebreather mask. You cover the wound with a dressing and confirm there are no further injuries before you lift him to the stretcher and move him to the ambulance. You decide to take him to the trauma center because of the seriousness of his wound. En route to the hospital, you find the patient quite anxious and worried that his mother will not be notified. You take down the number and assure him that you will see to it that his mother is notified.

Upon arrival at the trauma center, you give the nurse the details of the patient, including the nature of his injuries, his vital signs, and history and that he would like his mother contacted. The staff is very busy and a nurse asks you to make the call. You call his mother and ask her to come to the hospital and to drive safely—you reassure her that her son is in good hands.

Circle and number the areas in the paragraphs above that demonstrate each of the following roles and responsibilities. There may be more than one role and responsibility for any given area.

1. Personal safety
2. Safety of the crew, patient, and bystanders
3. Patient assessment
4. Patient emergency care
5. Lifting and moving
6. Transport
7. Transfer of care
8. Patient advocacy

Active Exploration

As an EMT-B, you will become an important part of a complex system known as the Emergency Medical Services system. As a part of the EMS system, you should be well aware of the other components that make up the EMS system in your area. The following exercises are designed to increase your awareness of the EMS system of which you are a part.

Activity 1: Inventory Time

Call a local fire department or ambulance company in your area and ask to speak to one of the EMT-Bs, paramedics, or firefighters on duty. Explain that you are an EMT student doing research on the local EMS system and the resources that make up the system. Ask the following questions and get as much detail as you can for each question:

1. What levels of care are currently available in your EMS system—First Responder, EMT-B, EMT-I, EMT-P, or nurse?

2. Where do each of these levels typically work—fire department, ambulance, rescue squad, helicopter?

3. How many ambulances are currently serving the EMS system in your area? Where are they located? Do they have permanent stations or do they roam? What kinds of shifts do they work?

4. What additional specialty resources are available in your system—Jaws of Life, helicopters, HazMat teams, confined-space rescue, high-angle rescue?

Activity 2: Accessing Your System

Accessing the EMS system is not as easy as you might think. While most of the United States is served by the 911 emergency access number, many areas are not. The following activity will help you discover how to best access your EMS system.

Contact someone who is currently working in the EMS system in your area and ask him the following questions. Be advised that just because he may be working in the system, it does not mean he always knows exactly how it works.

1. Is your area served by the 911 access number? If not, what number does someone call for emergency help?

2. If so, is it an enhanced 911 system?

3. Where are emergency calls answered in your area and what kind of training do the dispatchers have?

4. Are there separate dispatchers for fire, medical, and law enforcement calls?

▌RETRO REVIEW

As you progress through the chapters of the book, this section will help you to link this chapter's contents with other chapters and topics in the book. This is done in two ways. First through the use of multiple-choice questions on topics from chapters you have previously covered. This will help you retain information you will need for your final and certification examinations. Second, each chapter will end with a "Thinking and Linking" table that shows how you will apply the topics learned in the chapter to other places in the book—and after you complete the class.

THINKING AND LINKING

CHAPTER TOPIC	HOW IT RELATES TO YOU AND OTHER COURSE AREAS
History of the EMS	The EMS you practice today and learn about in this course is a result of years of experience and research. Your practice of EMS today as an EMT-B creates history for future generations of EMTs.
Roles and responsibilities	Is this not the same as saying "I'll treat my patients the way I would want myself or one of my family members to be treated"?
Components of the EMS system	You will find yourself interacting with other members of the system, from bystanders to advanced-level providers to hospital staff.
Medical direction	Because EMT-Bs are provided more responsibility with medications and other decisions, interaction with medical direction will be frequent and important.

2

The Well-being of the EMT-Basic

CHAPTER SUMMARY

You will learn how to provide emergency care for patients with a variety of injuries and illnesses during the course of your EMT-Basic class. It is just as important to learn how to take care of yourself and fellow workers. You will accomplish this by using proper body substance isolation (BSI) precautions, learning to deal with expected and unexpected stresses from intense situations, and always making sure that the scene is safe before entering.

BSI precautions, when used appropriately, protect you from bodily fluids that may contain pathogens. You can be exposed to blood-borne or airborne pathogens. You should suspect all bodily fluids such as blood, urine, saliva, tears, and so on of being infectious and take appropriate precautions.

EXAMPLES OF PERSONAL PROTECTIVE EQUIPMENT/PRACTICES

Protective gloves—be alert for latex allergies
Hand washing—according to the CDC, the single most effective means of preventing the spread of infection
Eye protection
Masks—surgical type or N-95
Gowns

There are several immunizations and vaccinations available to EMS providers. Most EMS employers are required to offer employees a hepatitis B vaccine along with an annual purified protein derivative (PPD) to screen for exposure to tuberculosis. You may also receive immunizations against certain strains of flu and pneumonia.

STRESS

As an EMT-B, you will be exposed to stress on a daily basis. This stress will have a variety of causes, including dealing with other people, environmental conditions, lack of sleep, and self-expectations.

Stress has three phases: alarm reaction (also known as the "fight or flight" response), resistance (when the person becomes acclimated to the stressor), and exhaustion (when the normal coping mechanisms fail). There are also three types of stress reactions.

- Acute stress reaction—occurs simultaneously or shortly after an incident
- Delayed stress reaction—occurs at any time, from days to years, after the critical incident; also known as posttraumatic stress disorder (PTSD)
- Cumulative stress reaction—also known as "burnout"

Most reactions to stress are normal and expected, but some require immediate intervention.

CAUSES OF STRESS

- Multiple-casualty incidents
- Emergencies involving infants and children
- Severe traumatic injuries
- Incidents of abuse and neglect
- Death of a coworker

SIGNS AND SYMPTOMS OF STRESS

- Indecisiveness
- Guilt
- Loss of appetite
- Irritability
- Lack of concentration
- Anxiety
- Difficulty sleeping and/or nightmares
- Lack of interest in sexual activity
- Isolation
- Loss of interest in work

There are several lifestyle changes that can help you manage your stress level. These are healthy eating habits, adequate exercise, and faithfully designating time for relaxation.

Critical incident stress management (CISM) is a defined program that can be utilized to help EMTs deal with job-related stress. There are two techniques commonly used to manage the stress of a critical incident; these are defusing and debriefing. A "defusing session" should occur between 1 and 4 hours following an incident, with only those care providers directly involved in the incident. A "debriefing session" is usually held 24 to 72 hours after the incident and is open to all emergency care workers. Trained peer counselors and/or mental health professionals typically conduct both types of sessions. All sessions are confidential and are not meant to be investigative.

The concepts of debriefing and other CISM techniques are currently being questioned by some. Your instructor and EMS journals will provide additional information on this debate.

Stress is a normal reaction to critical incidents. It is important to recognize the signs and symptoms in yourself and in coworkers. You should be aware of where to seek help in your system.

UNDERSTANDING REACTIONS TO DEATH AND DYING

When a person learns that he is dying, he, as well as his family members, goes through several stages. They are:

- Denial
- Anger

- Bargaining
- Depression
- Acceptance

It is important to recognize the patient's needs. Try to:

- Listen empathetically
- Be understanding of the anger from the patient and family
- Not falsely reassure
- Comfort as much as is realistically possible

SCENE SAFETY

A *hazardous-material incident* is an event that involves harmful chemicals that could cause injury or death if you are exposed to them. Remember that you as an EMT-B will not be able to help anyone else if you are injured. You must approach this type of incident with extreme caution. The number one rule is to remain at a safe distance from the hazardous material.

Your main function as an EMT-B is to ensure your safety and the safety of others. You will need to notify the specially trained hazardous-material response teams to manage the scene before you can provide patient emergency care.

You will also need to rely on specially trained teams when patients need to be extricated from vehicles, fires, and other hazardous situations. Do not perform rescues that you have not been trained to execute. Appropriate personal protective equipment must be utilized if you are involved in any aspect of a rescue operation.

Before you can administer patient emergency care, the scene must be safe for you to enter. It is not the EMT-B's responsibility to secure a scene. Police or other trained personnel will inform you when it is safe to approach. You must plan, observe, and react when responding to a dangerous situation.

- Wear appropriate clothing.
- Make sure your equipment is easy to carry.
- Always carry a portable radio.
- Be observant.

The following should heighten your suspicion of a dangerous situation:

- Unusual silence
- Evidence of violence
- Crime scenes
- Evidence of alcohol or drug use
- The presence of weapons
- Agitated family members
- Aggressive animals
- Agitated bystanders
- Other perpetrators

If you find yourself in a dangerous scene, attempt the following:

- Retreat (flee) to a position of safety, leaving equipment behind if necessary
- Take cover
- Radio for help
- Constantly reevaluate the scene for hazards

Your first step in becoming a great EMT-B with a long and healthy career is to take good care of yourself.

PEARLS FROM THE PODIUM

- Hand washing is a key element in preventing the spread of diseases. Alcohol-based hand-washing solutions are available in the field and can be used in between calls.

- Many EMT-Bs believe that infection-control procedures are largely to prevent HIV/AIDS. In fact, hepatitis B and C are much easier to transmit and also cause serious illness and death.

- Eye and face protection are important infection-control practices. Spattering fluids can cause infection when they come into contact with the eyes, nose, and mouth.

- Scene safety is your ultimate concern. Hazards can come from a wide variety of sources including violence, fire, downed wires, dangerous pets, terrorism, environmental conditions, uneven terrain, and more.

- Working in EMS can be a stressful experience. You can experience stress from a single call or cumulatively from events over a period of time.

REVIEW QUESTIONS

SHORT ANSWER

1. Explain the difference between eustress and distress.

2. What is a pathogen?

MULTIPLE CHOICE

1. Rescuers most directly involved in the stressful aspects of a critical incident are encouraged to attend a(n) _____ within a few hours of the incident.
   A. defusing session
   B. procedural review
   C. critical incident stress debriefing
   D. individual counseling session

2. What should your first step be when confronted with a possible hazardous-material incident?
   A. Look for container labels or shipping documents to determine the nature of the hazard.
   B. Quickly move patients to a safer location.
   C. Maintain a safe distance from the scene.
   D. Begin assembling a decontamination and treatment area.

3. It is not necessary to wear (a) _____ when treating a patient with arterial bleeding.
   A. gown
   B. protective eyewear
   C. heavyweight, tear-resistant gloves
   D. face mask

4. A dying patient who says, "Look, I know what's happening to me, but first I really need to call my husband," is most likely in the _____ stage of death and dying.
   A. depression
   B. bargaining
   C. recognition
   D. acceptance

5. What are the "three Rs" of reacting to danger at a scene?
   A. Run, Range, and Rationale
   B. Reconsider, Radio, and Ready
   C. Realize, Retreat, and Reason
   D. Retreat, Radio, and Reevaluate

SCENARIO QUESTIONS

You arrive at the scene of a late-night house fire. As your partner begins treating the only apparent patient, a young woman who is coughing severely, you notice a firefighter walking slowly away from the scene. As you approach the firefighter, who is singing softly, you see that he is carrying a badly burned and unresponsive infant. "There's a convenience store up around that corner," he says with a distant gaze. "Do you think they have diapers? I've looked everywhere and I just can't find any. That's what I should do, right? I'm really not sure what babies need."

1. This firefighter is exhibiting the signs of a(n) _____.
   A. cumulative stress breakdown
   B. acute stress reaction
   C. associative crisis
   D. posttraumatic stress disorder

2. You can deal with the stress from situations like this by developing healthy eating habits, exercising regularly, and _____.
   A. drinking a glass of wine after each shift
   B. setting aside time to do nothing but relax
   C. using mild sedatives such as sleeping pills
   D. having sugar-free soft drinks instead of coffee

3. The firefighter's reaction in this situation should be considered _____.
   A. an indication of mental illness
   B. a threat to his safety and well-being
   C. a sign of weakness
   D. a normal response to an abnormal situation

You are dispatched to deal with a possible drug overdose. As you pull up in the ambulance, you see a "regular" sprawled on the sidewalk. Steven lives on the streets and is an intravenous drug abuser who requires EMS assistance at least once a week. You and your partner get out, grab your equipment and, as you approach, he greets you groggily. You know from past experience that he is HIV positive and usually has open abscesses on his forearms and hands.

1. What personal protective equipment should you use during your assessment of Steven?
   A. Latex or vinyl exam gloves, goggles, and a gown.
   B. A turnout coat, face shield, and heavyweight gloves.
   C. Latex or vinyl exam gloves only.
   D. A surgical mask, long sleeves, and exam gloves.

2. What organization's guidelines require your agency to have a written policy in place in the event that you accidentally stick yourself with one of Steven's syringes?
   A. Occupational Safety and Health Administration
   B. World Health Organization
   C. National Registry of Emergency Medical Technicians
   D. Federal Emergency Medical Services Standards and Training

3. At what point in the above scenario should you put gloves on?
   A. En route to the scene.
   B. Prior to exiting the ambulance.
   C. Just before examining the patient.
   D. Once you find out whether he still has abscesses.

CASE STUDIES

CASE STUDY 1   SLIP, TRIP, AND BLEED

You have been dispatched to an assisted-living facility for a patient who is having difficulty breathing. Upon your arrival, you are greeted by a nurse's aide who directs you to room 211. Upon entering the room, you find an approximately 70-year-old man being helped into a chair by another nurse's aide. You are told that the patient is new to the facility and has only been there for a couple of days. He came in with a mild cough that has been getting worse each day. Just before your arrival, the patient slipped next to his bed, cutting his arm on the metal frame of the bed. The aide is holding a bloodied towel over the wound in an attempt to control the bleeding.

1. What precautions do you feel are most appropriate to take before treating this patient?

2. Is there any additional history that you will want to get from the staff before leaving with this patient?

The staff at the facility has very little history on the patient as the chart was lost when the patient was brought to the facility a couple of days ago. You are told that the patient has tested positive for hepatitis B and that he has been coughing nonstop since the day before.

1. Given the known history of hepatitis B, will you change anything with regard to the BSI precautions that you have already taken? If so, what will you change?

2. Is there anything else about how the patient is presenting and the recent history that concerns you? What and why? How will you manage this patient, given your concerns?

For each of the following potential hazards describe any dangers that may exist and what you would do (if anything) to prevent harm to yourself, other members of your crew, and bystanders.

- A patient holding a pencil and looking "angry"

- A large dog standing just inside the door of a home with a person lying apparently unresponsive inside

- A tractor-trailer (tanker) overturned on the roadway

- A house from which a 911 call was received, but no one answers the door

- A person who is lethargic, with alcohol and marijuana visible

- A three-car collision on a four-lane interstate highway

Active Exploration

Regardless of the fact that you are becoming an EMT in order to help others in their time of need, you are not obligated to do so if it puts you at unreasonable risk. The key word here is "unreasonable." Many of the major risks that you as an EMT-B will encounter are simply identified as such and the resources trained and equipped to manage those risks are called in. Such is the case with major extrication and hazardous-materials incidents.

There are, however, many risks that are simply a part of the job of the EMT-B and, for the most part, are unavoidable. It is important for you as an EMT-B to be able to identify and address each of these risks appropriately. One of the biggest risks you will be exposed to on nearly every call is exposure to bodily fluids. The following activities will help address some of these risks and reinforce the importance of taking the necessary precautions to minimize exposure to bodily fluids.

Activity 1: Slip Sliding Away

Being able to don (put on) and doff (take off) protective gloves is a skill that the EMT-B must master early on. The following exercise will test your ability to remove contaminated latex gloves without spreading the germs more. You will need a pair of latex or nonlatex gloves and a can of shaving cream.

1. Select and don an appropriate size pair of latex or nonlatex gloves. Be sure that the gloves fit snugly and are not too loose.
2. Squirt a half-dollar-size portion of shaving cream into the palm of one gloved hand and spread thoroughly over both gloved hands.
3. Now attempt to remove the gloves without getting any of the shaving cream on you or splattering it off the gloves.

   While this exercise takes the task of removing contaminated gloves to a new level, it does illustrate the point that it is a skill that takes practice and should not be taken lightly.

Activity 2: Join the Team

The world of EMS can be a stressful one, both physically and emotionally. There are stressors that affect the EMT-B that are not present in most other jobs. For that reason, it is essential that you become familiar with the signs and symptoms of stress and learn to recognize them in yourself and those you work with. Much of the stress that EMTs encounter on the job can be managed by staying healthy and talking things out with others.

   Sometimes, though, you will be exposed to a level of stress that is too strong to be easily managed in this way. In these instances, you may need the assistance of trained professionals who know how to help you cope with and manage major stress. These individuals are often part of a CISM team and receive formal training on assisting individuals and groups in dealing with stress and stressful events.

   Answering the following questions will help you identify the availability of a CISM team in your area.

1. Where is the nearest CISM team in your area?

2. How does one contact or activate the team?

3. Can anyone activate the team or must it be only certain people?

4. What kinds of people comprise a CISM team?

5. What does their training consist of?

6. What are the qualifications for joining the team in your area?

Knowing what resources are available and how to access them is an important part of being a good EMT-B. This activity will help prepare you in the event such a team is needed.

These questions review topics from previous chapters to help you maintain your knowledge throughout the course.

1. Having a standing order that allows you to assist a patient with his medication without speaking to a base station physician is known as:

   A. on-line medical direction.

   B. off-line medical direction.

   C. specific medical direction.

   D. noninvasive medical direction.

2. Which of the following is NOT a part of Quality Improvement?

   A. Performing quality documentation.

   B. Continuing your education.

   C. Obtaining liability insurance.

   D. Obtaining feedback from patients and hospital staff.

THINKING AND LINKING

CHAPTER TOPIC	HOW IT RELATES TO YOU AND OTHER COURSE AREAS
Body substance isolation (BSI)	You will make decisions regarding the use of BSI on every call. You will make it initially during the scene size-up and again if the patient's condition changes (e.g. requires suction) during the call.
Scene-safety issues	Again, during the size-up you will assess for scene safety. You will also maintain constant vigilance for safety issues developing after you arrive.
Stress	EMS can be stressful. Some calls cause more stress than others or stress may be cumulative. People feel this differently. Watch for signs that stress may be affecting you or your loved ones.
Death and dying	You may deal with family members after a patient has died suddenly and unexpectedly. Other times, you may be transporting a terminally ill patient to the hospital due to a worsening of his condition. In either case, the stages of death and dying may give you insight into the patient's and family's reactions and behavior.

3

Medical/Legal and Ethical Issues

CHAPTER SUMMARY

To some degree, medical/legal and ethical issues will be present in every call that you are dispatched to. From obtaining a patient's approval for treatment to maneuvering through a crime scene, you as the EMT-B must be knowledgeable about the legal and ethical aspects of the EMS system. When are you required to help an injured person? Do you always have to obey a do-not-resuscitate (DNR) order? Can you be sued if a patient's condition deteriorates after you have treated him? This chapter provides an essential overview of these and other issues so that you, as an EMT-B, can make sound decisions in the fast-paced world of EMS.

EMT-Bs must follow many medical, legal, and ethical guidelines. Together these guidelines form what is commonly referred to as the "scope of practice"; this scope of practice defines the limits of an EMT-B's job. The actual medical interventions and skills performed by the EMT-B may vary from state to state or even region to region. Your responsibility to the patient is to provide all necessary and legally allowed emergency care as defined under the scope of practice in your area.

An EMT-B's primary ethical consideration is to make the patient's emergency care and well-being a priority—even if it requires some personal sacrifice. This can range from adjusting the temperature in the ambulance to accommodate a patient to completing continuing education courses in order to maintain the best skill and knowledge levels possible.

Obtaining consent, or permission to treat, from a patient should be the first step an EMT-B takes when initiating emergency care. There are three types of consent recognized in the EMS system: expressed consent, implied consent, and consent for children and mentally incompetent adults. You may treat seriously injured children and mentally incompetent adults on the basis of implied consent if no parent or guardian is available.

Some patients will refuse emergency care due to denial, fear, intoxication, or failure to understand the seriousness of their situation. It is your responsibility to fully inform the patient of his situation and the consequences of refusing emergency care. In order to refuse emergency care, a patient must meet several conditions. He must be legally able to consent, mentally competent and oriented, and fully informed of the consequences of his decision. He must then sign a "release" form, releasing the ambulance squad, and all individuals involved, from any liability resulting from his refusal.

Even with signed releases, lawsuits are still filed against ambulance crews who "legally" leave a patient who has refused emergency care. With this in mind, it is imperative that you take every possible step to treat every patient. These steps may include speaking with the patient to determine his objection, clearly telling the patient the consequences of refusing medical emergency care, contacting medical direction, contacting family members, and contacting law enforcement. If all of these tactics fail, you must remember that forcing treatment or transportation on a competent patient can actually be viewed as assault and/or battery.

It is not uncommon to encounter terminally ill patients with DNR orders. These legal documents state to what extent the patient wishes resuscitative efforts to be undertaken. A DNR order can range from "absolutely no resuscitative efforts" to more detailed instructions outlining exactly which efforts may be initiated and why. Make sure that you become familiar with the accepted forms of DNR documentation in your area. Remember, oral DNR requests or family members' assurance that one exists (although they are unable to produce it at the time) should not prevent you from beginning resuscitation.

If an EMT-B has a duty to provide emergency care for a patient but does not provide the required standard of care and, as a result, the patient is harmed (either physically or psychologically), that EMT-B can be found to be negligent. Many lawsuits against prehospital emergency-care personnel claim that the rescuer acted negligently. If found to be a negligent EMT-B, you can be required to pay for the patient's medical expenses, lost wages (including future earnings), pain and suffering, and any other damages as determined by the court.

The other major cause of lawsuits against EMT-Bs is ambulance collisions. Although dangerous in any vehicle, collisions in ambulances are more serious due to their size, weight, and number of passengers (including patients). Most collisions are preventable, which is why they are no longer called "accidents."

While liability and negligence are important to keep in mind, do not work in fear of being sued. Lawsuits against EMT-Bs are actually very rare when compared to the number of calls they are dispatched to each day.

If an EMT-B has an obligation to provide emergency care to a patient, he is said to have a "duty to act." For example, if an EMT-B on an ambulance is dispatched to a call, he clearly has a duty to act. An EMT-B who initiates emergency care and then leaves the patient before ensuring that someone with equal or greater medical training has assumed care may be accused of committing abandonment.

Good Samaritan laws, which are present in all states, limit the liability of individuals trying to help others in emergencies. As long as you are acting in good faith and providing emergency care to the best of your ability and to the level of your training, you will be covered under most Good Samaritan laws. Acts of gross negligence or criminal behavior will not be protected under Good Samaritan laws.

EMT-Bs are allowed into patients' homes and have access to a considerable amount of personal information about each patient. Any information you as an EMT-B gather or any observations you make should be kept strictly confidential. You may only share patient information with other health-care professionals who will also be treating the patient, or when subpoenaed and in a court of law, or with a written release signed by the patient. The new Health Insurance Portability and Accountability Act (HIPAA) has brought significant changes to the record keeping, storage, accessing, and sharing of patient-specific medical information.

Some patients may wear medical identification devices (e.g. necklaces, bracelets, cards, and so on) that inform rescuers and health-care professionals of a particular medical condition. You will commonly see these devices on individuals with heart conditions, allergies, diabetes, and epilepsy.

Some patients whom you encounter will be organ donors. This is usually determined in the prehospital setting by looking at the front or back of the patient's driver's license for the presence of a donor's card, indicating that the patient has completed a legal process that allows his organs and/or tissues to be donated upon death. Do not treat an organ donor differently than any other patient. Medical direction should be contacted if you encounter a patient with critical injuries who is an organ donor.

You will occasionally be dispatched to provide emergency care at a crime scene. This presents special challenges to both EMS and law enforcement. The police are present to preserve the evidence and solve the crime, whereas you will be there to provide emergency care to individuals involved in the crime. Although the patient is your first priority, you should also be aware of and make every reasonable attempt to preserve evidence. As you enter the crime scene, make mental notes of (and try not to affect) the general condition of the scene, the position and condition of the patient, and any fingerprints or footprints.

To further assist law enforcement while at the crime scene, remember what you touch, minimize your impact on the scene, and try to work with law enforcement—all the while keeping your patient as the top priority.

Many states require EMT-Bs to report certain types of incidents to law enforcement, including child, elder, and domestic abuse; trauma from violence; and sexual assaults. Check your local regulations for reporting requirements and procedures.

PEARLS FROM THE PODIUM

This chapter is potentially scary. It says that you will encounter crime scenes, that you may respond to people who are near death, and that you could be sued for what you do or do not do while caring for a patient. In addition, you cannot legally discuss any of this with friends and family. Remember:

- Lawsuits against EMS providers are rare. The biggest causes of liability (ambulance collisions and patient refusals) are preventable.
- Know your local and state laws regarding DNR orders and advance directives. Although the situations are emotional, if you know the rules before you walk in, act confidently, and treat the patient and family members with compassion, it will be okay.
- A rule not always taught: if you treat people with compassion and consideration (some call this treating people the way you would want to be treated) the situation usually goes well.

REVIEW QUESTIONS

SHORT ANSWER

1. What circumstances must be present in order to prove that an EMT-B acted negligently?

2. Why is a DNR order called an advance directive?

MULTIPLE CHOICE

1. What legislation brought significant changes to record keeping, accessing, and sharing of patient-specific medical information?
   A. The Ryan White Care Act (RWCA).
   B. The American Medical Documentation Act (AMDA).
   C. The Health Insurance Portability and Accountability Act (HIPAA).
   D. The Hospital Information Systems Act (HISA).

2. In a situation where an adult patient is refusing emergency care, a(n) _____ may be able to force the patient to go to the hospital anyway.
   A. EMT-Paramedic   B. on-line physician
   C. police officer   D. on-scene physician

3. You are treating an unresponsive 17-year-old patient who may have experienced an overdose of medications. Which of the following statements is most correct regarding this situation?
   A. You may provide emergency care based on expressed consent.
   B. You must contact the parents before providing emergency care.
   C. You must wait for him to become responsive before providing emergency care.
   D. You may provide emergency care based on implied consent.

4. An EMT-B's obligation to provide emergency care is known as a(n) _____.
   A. duty to act   B. EMS code
   C. Good-Samaritan initiative   D. reciprocity provision

5. There are three types of consent: expressed, implied, and _____.
   A. consent to treat minors or incompetent adults
   B. advanced
   C. legal
   D. consent to provide emergency care for unresponsive adults

SCENARIO QUESTIONS

You are called to the scene of a two-vehicle collision. The driver of one vehicle is dead and his passenger, a 13-year-old girl, has an obviously fractured arm but declines help. In the other vehicle, you find a 32-year-old female who is bleeding profusely from a wound on her forehead. The windshield in front of the woman has been shattered, and you notice that she is not wearing a seat belt.

1. If the woman with the head injury refuses your offer for treatment, you should then _____.
   A. begin emergency care, assuming that her injury has caused her to become incompetent or disoriented
   B. have her sign your agency's Release of Liability and turn your attention to the patient in the other vehicle
   C. explain to her that, based on the seriousness of the collision, if she does not accept your help, her condition may worsen
   D. respect her wishes as a competent adult and check back with her occasionally as you assist the other patient

2. The above scenario is an example of a(n) _____.
   A. multiple-casualty incident (MCI)
   B. no-fault accident (NFA)
   C. directed-fatality incident (DFI)
   D. comprehensive-injury collision (CIC)

3. The 13-year-old informs you that the deceased driver had been her only surviving parent. Does she now have the legal right to refuse emergency care?
   A. Yes, until a guardian is appointed by the court, she would be considered temporarily emancipated.
   B. No, but you would need to assume temporary guardianship in order to treat her.
   C. Yes, implied consent for minors is only valid when parents or guardians are available but in another location.
   D. No, an unemancipated individual under the age of majority is not allowed to make emergency-care decisions.

You are transporting a 45-year-old woman with terminal cancer, and she has a legal DNR requesting no interventions. Her son is riding in the back of the ambulance also. During the trip, she becomes noticeably slower in answering your questions and is soon completely unresponsive. As her respirations slow and become shallow, her son begins shouting at you to "do something!"

1. In this situation, you should _____.
   A. begin resuscitative efforts based on the son's expressed consent
   B. maintain the patient's airway
   C. ask the son to sign a statement voiding the DNR order
   D. use a bag-valve mask (BVM) to ease her respiratory effort

2. If this patient dies, would her family be able to successfully sue you for negligence?
   A. Yes, inaction is not the required standard of care for an EMT-B.
   B. No, lack of action is a tort, not a component of negligence.
   C. Yes, your inaction caused tremendous harm to the patient.
   D. No, the DNR released you from your duty to act.

3. Since you did not get an EMS job to just sit and allow patients to die, how would you be able to legally disregard this woman's DNR?
   A. Ask the son to change the form, initial all changes, and sign the bottom.
   B. Obtain verbal dissent from two or more family members.
   C. There is no legal way to ignore a valid DNR.
   D. Use the authority of implied consent once she is unresponsive.

CASE STUDIES

It is 1600 hours and you and your senior partner are just about to begin eating your first meal of a very busy day when you receive a call from dispatch regarding a difficulty in breathing at 1730 Melbrook Way. Both you and your partner recognize the address as that of Mr. Jones, who is affectionately referred to as a "Frequent Flyer." You have been there a couple of times already this week and there is never anything wrong with him. You set your food aside and start the vehicle when your partner reaches over and pulls the keys from the ignition. He states, "Mr. Jones can wait, now relax and eat your food. You know there is never anything wrong with him."

1. **How would you respond to your partner in this situation?**

2. **What are the legal ramifications if you agree to delay your response?**

You decide to drive and let your partner finish his meal on the way to the call. Your partner waits in the rig while you go inside to find out what is wrong with Mr. Jones. Once inside, you are met by Mr. Jones's daughter who is insisting that you take her father to the hospital. When you ask Mr. Jones whether he wants to go, he says he would rather stay at home. He states that his breathing is getting better and he will be fine if he can just rest. The daughter insists that her father is having difficulty breathing and is demanding that you take him to the hospital.

1. **Who has the appropriate authority in this situation? Must you listen to and obey the orders of the daughter?**

2. **What are the ramifications of Mr. Jones's refusal of emergency care? What obligation do you have to Mr. Jones if you agree not to transport?**

Your ambulance is dispatched to a patient with severe chest pain. You arrive at a safe scene and find a 68-year-old male patient with a history of high blood pressure who developed chest pain while roller blading. He returned home where you find him in the kitchen.

He states that the pain is severe and crushing. He holds his fist to his chest in the classic sign of distress. He tells you, "I have these here nitro pills." His signs and symptoms match the criteria; his vital signs are adequate. Your medical director has issued you standing orders to use nitroglycerin in cases such as this.

You administer the nitro, which provides considerable relief to the patient. The patient does not have a recurrence of the chest pain, and his vitals remain stable en route to the hospital.

When you arrive at the hospital and the driver begins to back into the emergency department your patient says, "Thank you for letting me take my wife's nitro. It sure helped. You guys are the best!"

Your heart sinks as you realize that you are allowed to only administer the patient's own nitroglycerin. What you did was a breach of protocol. However, the patient did not seem to be negatively affected.

1. Do you tell the hospital physician about the nitroglycerin?

2. What will happen if you tell his physician? What if you do not tell the physician?

3. Do you document the fact that you gave the patient someone else's nitroglycerin on your prehospital report?

Active Exploration

As an EMT-B treating someone with an injury or illness, you must be aware of the specific legal aspects that affect how and what you do for a patient. While lawsuits involving prehospital care providers are relatively rare, you must have an awareness and understanding of the laws in order to minimize exposure to a law suit.

Activity 1: Mandatory Reporter

It is probably safe to say that all states have what are known as "Mandatory Reporting" laws that specifically name people and professions that are required by law to report such things as child abuse and neglect. Using the Internet, do a search for mandatory reporting laws in your state and make a list of those people and professions that are specifically named "Mandatory Reporters."

Are you surprised by the types of people and professions that are on the list? Are there any people or professions not on the list that you think should be?

Activity 2: Analyze the Case

As mentioned earlier, lawsuits involving prehospital care providers are relatively rare, but they do occur. Using the Internet or a local library, conduct a little research and try and find a lawsuit involving prehospital care. If that proves too difficult, find any medical lawsuit and identify the following elements in the details of the case:

- Duty
- Breach of duty

- Damages
- Causation

It is important to understand each of these terms in the context of an actual court case. This understanding combined with just the right amount of common sense will keep you out of court.

RETRO REVIEW

1. Which of the following statements about infection control is correct?
   A. The amount of protection I will use depends on the diseases my patient has.
   B. My doctor doesn't use gloves for my physical exam every year when he touches my skin. I don't need protection either.
   C. Most patients know whether they have an infectious disease. BSI is based on the medical history.
   D. The BSI precautions used are based on preventing exposure to blood and other potentially infectious materials.

2. The organization that directed the creation of the EMT-Basic curriculum in place for your class is the _____.
   A. Federal Emergency Management Agency
   B. American Heart Association
   C. National Highway Traffic Safety Administration
   D. National Association of EMS Educators

THINKING AND LINKING

CHAPTER TOPIC	HOW IT RELATES TO YOU AND OTHER COURSE AREAS
Consent and refusal	Every adult patient you treat will have a right to refuse emergency care. Most will accept your emergency care willingly. Every call you go on will involve consent.
DNR orders/advance directives	In Chapter 17 ("Cardiac Emergencies"), you will be taught how to treat patients in cardiac arrest. Some of these patients may have some sort of advance directive in place that may order you not to resuscitate.
Negligence and liability	You do not have to think about liability on every call if you treat people well and provide quality emergency care. Deviating from either of these could cause problems.
Crime scenes	If you are called to a crime scene, you will not only be called upon to carry out patient emergency care of a potentially critical patient, you will also have to preserve evidence. You may be subpoenaed to testify in court later.

CHAPTER 4

The Human Body

CHAPTER SUMMARY

In order to provide thorough emergency care, you must have an understanding of the body's anatomy and physiology. This understanding will help you during the assessment of your patient and allow you to give an accurate report to the hospital staff to whom you will transfer care. The emergency-care workforce spans many professions; therefore, a standardized method for referring to places on the body was developed.

DIRECTIONAL TERMS

Anatomical position—standing, facing forward, arms down at side with palms forward

Midline—a line drawn down the center of the body from between the eyes through the umbilicus

Medial—closer to the midline

Lateral—farther from the midline

Bilateral—both sides

Midaxillary—a line drawn from mid-armpit to the ankle

Anterior—front

Posterior—back

Superior—above

Inferior—below

Proximal—closer to the torso

Distal—farther from the torso

Midclavicular—a line drawn from the center of the clavicle down through the nipple below

Abdominal quadrants—the abdomen divided into four quadrants by perpendicular lines through the navel (right upper, left upper, right lower, left lower)

POSITIONAL TERMS

Supine—patient lying on his back

Prone—patient lying on his abdomen

Recovery position—patient lying on his side, usually the left

Fowler's position—patient in a seated position

Trendelenburg—patient lying flat with feet slightly higher than the head

MUSCULOSKELETAL SYSTEMS

The musculoskeletal system is made up of the muscles and bones. This system provides shape to the body, allows it to move, and offers protection for internal organs. The skull sits on top of the spinal column, which consists of 33 vertebrae. These vertebrae house the spinal cord. An injured spinal column can cause damage to the spinal cord, resulting in paralysis and/or death.

The thorax is the chest cavity and contains the heart, lungs, and major blood vessels. The thorax is formed by the 12 pairs of ribs, the spinal column, and the sternum.

The major bones of the pelvis are the ilium and ischium. The ilium is the superior portion, while the ischium is the inferior portion.

The large, long bone of the thigh is the femur. The patella, or kneecap, sits superior to the tibia and fibula of the lower leg. The ankle bones and bones of the foot are tarsals, metatarsals, calcaneus (heel), and phalanges (toes).

The shoulder consists of the clavicle and scapula. The humerus is the long bone of the upper arm. The ulna and radius make up the lower arm. The carpals, metacarpals, and phalanges are the bones of the wrist, hand, and fingers.

Joints are where two bones meet and are held together by ligaments. Tendons are the connective tissues that connect muscle to bone. There are three types of muscle:

- Voluntary—skeletal
- Involuntary—smooth
- Cardiac—heart muscle

"Automaticity" is the ability of the cardiac muscle to create an electrical impulse on its own.

RESPIRATORY SYSTEM

Air enters the body through the nose and/or the mouth. It then passes through the nasopharynx and oropharynx. It proceeds down the trachea, into the bronchi, to the bronchioles, and finally to the alveoli of the lungs. The alveoli are the small sacs where oxygen and carbon dioxide are exchanged. The act of inhalation is considered an "active" process because muscles (intercostals and the diaphragm) need to contract for inhalation to occur. Exhalation is considered a "passive" process because no energy is involved; the muscles simply relax. It is important to remember that the airway structures of infants and children are smaller and more easily obstructed by a foreign body or disease.

CARDIOVASCULAR SYSTEM

The cardiovascular system consists of the heart and blood vessels. The heart is divided into four chambers. The two chambers at the top of the heart are called atria and receive blood returning from the body or the lungs. The lower two chambers are called ventricles and pump blood either to the lungs (right ventricle) or out to the body (left ventricle).

Blood vessels that carry blood away from the heart are called arteries. The coronary arteries branch off the aorta and supply the heart muscle with blood. There are many major arteries in the body, the largest being the aorta. Veins are vessels that carry blood back to the heart. The blood is made up of plasma, red blood cells, white blood cells, and platelets.

A pulse is created when the left ventricle contracts, pushing a wave of blood through the arteries. A pulse can be palpated by pressing on an artery where it lies close to the skin and passes over a bone. Pulses felt at the carotid and femoral arteries are central pulses. All other pulse points are considered peripheral pulses. The force of the blood exerted on the vessel walls is called blood pressure. The systolic pressure is the pressure created when the left ventricle is contracting. The diastolic pressure is the existing pressure in the vessels when the left ventricle is at rest and refilling.

Perfusion is the adequate delivery and exchange of oxygen, nutrients, and waste products in the organs and tissues of the body. Hypoperfusion occurs when any part of the body is not getting enough oxygenated blood circulating through it. Hypoperfusion is also known as "shock" and is a very serious condition that can lead to death.

OTHER BODY SYSTEMS

The nervous system is composed of the brain, spinal cord, and nerves. The central nervous system is the brain and spinal cord. The peripheral nervous system has two types of nerves: sensory and motor. The sensory nerves send messages from the body back to the brain. The motor nerves send messages from the brain to the body. The autonomic nervous system controls involuntary actions such as heart rate and digestion.

The digestive system allows the body to ingest food and break it down into forms it can utilize. The digestive system begins at the mouth and continues through the stomach, small intestine, and large intestine. Several other organs assist with the process of digestion. These are the liver, gall bladder, pancreas, and spleen.

The skin supports the body with the following functions:

- Protection
- Water balance
- Temperature regulation
- Excretion
- Impact absorption

It consists of three layers: epidermis, dermis, and subcutaneous.

Several hormones, which regulate body function, are excreted by the endocrine system. Insulin aids the body's ability to utilize glucose, a form of sugar that is the main fuel source for the body. Epinephrine is a hormone that helps us react during stressful situations.

Your knowledge of anatomy and physiology will assist you as an EMT-B to assess and treat your patients.

PEARLS FROM THE PODIUM

- The language of medicine involves the use of terms of position and direction. The concepts of this chapter may seem unimportant to you now but will be used in every chapter—and on every call you go on.

- Describe the terms, body regions, and structures accurately when you document your patient's condition and the treatment you perform.

- A practical point: Accuracy and use of proper anatomical terms is important—but do not write with so many terms and abbreviations that your point is lost. Terms should help but not overcomplicate your documentation or make it more confusing.

REVIEW QUESTIONS

SHORT ANSWER

1. Name the three types of muscle and give an example of where you would find each.

2. What is the midaxillary line?

MULTIPLE CHOICE

1. A patient sitting with his upper body at a 40° angle is in the _____ position.
   - **A.** semi-Fowler's
   - **B.** prone
   - **C.** Fowler's
   - **D.** supine

2. The peripheral nervous system consists of both sensory and _____ nerves.
   - **A.** reactionary
   - **B.** illusory
   - **C.** autonomic
   - **D.** motor

3. The _____ is the only vein in the human body that carries oxygen-rich blood.
   - **A.** pulmonary vein
   - **B.** inferior venae cavae
   - **C.** ascending aorta
   - **D.** superior venae cavae

4. Skin pigmentation granules are found in the _____.
   - **A.** dermis
   - **B.** subdural layer
   - **C.** sebaceous glands
   - **D.** epidermis

5. The xiphoid process is inferior to the _____.
   - **A.** acetabulum
   - **B.** manubrium
   - **C.** iliac arteries
   - **D.** calcaneus

SCENARIO QUESTIONS

You and your partner are treating a patient who fell from the roof of his one-story home. There is a bone protruding from his left leg just proximal to the knee, and his right arm is bent at an 80°–90° angle, distal to the elbow.

1. Which bones do you suspect might have been broken?
   - **A.** Ulna, humerus, and fibula.
   - **B.** Ilium, scapula, and femur.
   - **C.** Femur, radius, and ulna.
   - **D.** Medial malleolus, radius, and metatarsal.

2. Which pulse could you check to make sure that the patient's suspected leg fracture did not interrupt circulation to the rest of the leg?
   - **A.** Dorsalis pedis
   - **B.** Carotid
   - **C.** Femoralis
   - **D.** Radial

You and your partner are restocking the ambulance after the last call. As your partner struggles with one of the cabinet slides, his hand slips and an edge slices deeply into his palm. His hand begins to bleed profusely and you can see that the injury extends into the dermis, if not deeper. As you apply pressure to control the bleeding, you notice that he has started sweating and his skin is getting cooler.

1. Recognizing that your partner is going into shock, you have him lie on the gurney and place him in the _____ position.
   - **A.** Fowler's
   - **B.** Trendelenburg
   - **C.** recovery
   - **D.** semi-Fowler's

2. Which of the following terms best describes the location of the injury?
   - **A.** On the posterior side of the hand.
   - **B.** On the superior side of the hand.
   - **C.** On the distal aspect of the hand.
   - **D.** On the anterior side of the hand.

3. If you are unable to control the bleeding with direct pressure and elevation, you would then apply pressure to the _____ artery.
   - **A.** brachial
   - **B.** carotid
   - **C.** femoral
   - **D.** carpal

CASE STUDIES

CASE STUDY 1	HEAD OVER HEELS

You are dispatched to a residence for a patient who has had a fall. Upon your arrival, a bystander leads you around to the back of the house where you find an approximately 30-year-old male lying on his back on the concrete patio. He is moaning in pain, and the bystander states that the patient was working on the roof and fell backwards onto the ground. He was unresponsive for about five minutes, then he started waking up.

Your assessment reveals pain and deformity above the right knee, above the left ankle, and in the upper right quadrant of his abdomen.

1. **What is the name for the position that this man is found in?**

2. **How would you best describe the location of his two suspected fractures?**

3. **What part of the anatomy lies within the upper right quadrant of the abdomen?**

CASE STUDY 2	MOTORCYCLE CRASH

Your ambulance is dispatched to a motorcycle crash on the interstate. You arrive to find a male patient who is laying facedown on the side of the road. The man appears badly injured.

You begin your assessment and emergency care. While completing a physical examination, you notice a deformity in his right lower leg, just above the ankle. He also has a deformity in his right arm, just above the elbow.

1. What position is the patient found in?

2. What bone(s) are involved in the lower leg? Is the deformity distal or proximal to the ankle?

3. What bone(s) are involved in the upper arm? Is the deformity distal or proximal to the elbow?

You move the patient to the ambulance on a backboard. Because you suspect shock, you raise the foot end of the board during transport.

1. What position is the patient now in?

Active Exploration

The human body is a highly sophisticated and complex collection of systems that are dynamic and ever changing. For some, the study of anatomy is a lifelong endeavor. For the student wishing to become an EMT-B, it does not need to be so overwhelming. You do, however, need to develop a solid understanding of basic anatomy to provide the best possible emergency care for your patients. Much of anatomy is like learning to read a map: You must know where all the big cities are and how they are connected to one another. The following activities are designed to further develop your understanding of basic anatomy while applying it to patient emergency care.

Activity 1: Do and Say

For this first activity, you will need two fellow students and your Emergency Care textbook. One student will lie supine on the floor and play the role of patient while the other student uses the Emergency Care textbook and turns to Chapter 4.

With the patient lying on the floor, perform a detailed physical exam while wearing latex (or nonlatex) gloves. The use of gloves will help you become acquainted with performing an assessment in the field on real patients. While you perform your examination, you must verbalize as much of the anatomy as possible using the correct terminology.

As you progress through your exam, the student with the textbook should follow along using the textbook and verify that you are properly identifying the anatomy. Use as much detail as you can and stop when necessary to learn the parts of the anatomy you are not familiar with. Name as many bones as possible including sections of the spine and skull. Discuss specific anatomy in each of the four quadrants of the abdomen as well as in the chest.

Activity 2: Tape it to Me Baby

This exercise is just as meaningful for two students working together as it is for the whole class. Here you will put into practice the skill of describing in anatomical terms the specific location of various injuries on the human body.

You can do this either as a one-on-one exercise or divide into groups of three to five students.
1. Have one person from each group step into another room and, using either a red dry erase marker or colored tape, place several marks to represent injuries in various locations on his body. Tape

works the best because it can be placed right over clothing. Be sure to place these marks in different locations and at different angles relative to the body. Vary the length of the marks as well.

2. Now have the "patient" reenter the room with the marks in place and stand before you or the group, in the "anatomical position," while students in the group write detailed descriptions of each of the "injuries." Descriptions must be in appropriate anatomical terms.

3. Now hand your descriptions to another group, and they must apply marks to another student using your descriptions as a guide. If all goes well, both "patients" should end up with the same "injuries."

RETRO REVIEW

1. Depression, anger, denial, and bargaining are common reactions to
_____.

    A. critical incidents   **B.** death and dying

    C. occupational stress   **D.** violent crime scenes

2. There are _____ general levels of EMS training and certification.

    A. six   **B.** three

    C. two   **D.** four

3. _____ is a leading cause of lawsuits against EMS personnel.

    A. Acting beyond the scope of practice

    B. Ignoring advanced directives

    C. Leaving competent and oriented patients who refuse emergency care

    D. Neglecting to consult with medical direction

THINKING AND LINKING

CHAPTER TOPIC	HOW IT RELATES TO YOU AND OTHER COURSE AREAS
Anatomical terms	One of the quickest ways to confuse an EMS situation is to use anatomical terms incorrectly. You will find that all advanced-care providers (paramedics, nurses, and doctors) use anatomical and directional terms almost as a second language—make sure that you speak it.

Remember that almost all verbal reports (covered in depth in Chapter 13) and written reports (Chapter 14) will make extensive use of anatomical and directional terms. They are necessary when "painting a mental picture" for someone who was either not at the scene or is not currently with the patient. |
| Nervous system | When treating patients with severe trauma or upper-body injuries, you will need to take steps to safeguard their central nervous systems (detailed in Chapter 29). You will find that no other type of injury can be so easy to suffer and yet have such catastrophic and long-lasting (or permanent) consequences.

Keep in mind that recognizing (Chapter 10) and responding to potential nervous system injuries might mean the difference between life and death for your patient. |

Skin

Since your patient's skin is his first line of defense against trauma (explained in Chapters 26 and 27), you might find yourself focusing attention on some very visible—yet superficial—injuries. Do not get distracted and forget the basics! The ABCs (Chapters 6 and 8) are going to play a much bigger role in your patient's survival than some avulsed flesh.

Skin is also a great external indicator of internal events—so examining skin for color, temperature, and moisture (Chapter 9) can tell you, in a glance, quite a bit about your patient's condition (shock—Chapter 26, hyperthermia—Chapter 22).

CHAPTER 5

Lifting and Moving Patients

CHAPTER SUMMARY

Improperly lifting and moving a patient is the quickest way to end your EMS career. Back and shoulder injuries, caused by speed and carelessness, can sideline even the most physically fit and dedicated rescue worker. This chapter covers the concepts, tips, and equipment necessary for you to actively, and safely, go about the business of helping others.

Following the laws of proper *body mechanics* when moving or lifting is essential for your health and safety. First, you must consider the object to be moved. In most cases, that object is going to be a patient, but not always. How much does that patient weigh? Can you safely move that patient by yourself? Answering those questions will require you to know your own physical limitations. Do you have any weaknesses or impairments? It is important that both you and your partner know each others' limitations. That is why good communication before, during, and after the move is very important.

The basic rules of lifting are very simple and will, when followed, minimize the chances of injury. Remember to position your feet properly, use your legs to lift, never turn or twist while lifting, do not lean to either side, keep the weight close to your body, and use a stair chair when moving a patient on stairs. Whenever possible, use wheeled devices (e.g. wheeled stretchers, wheel chairs, and so on) when moving a patient over long distances.

It is always a good idea to use an even number of people when utilizing carrying devices and when picking them up; use the *power grip* and the *power lift*. The power grip makes sure that as much palm and finger surface area as possible is in contact with the object, with all fingers bent at the same angle. The power lift requires you to squat, lock your back, and lift with your legs.

Some other basics to remember are avoid twisting while reaching, do not reach more than 15 to 20 inches in front of your body, avoid prolonged reaching, push rather than pull, kneel if the weight is below your waist, and keep your elbows bent and arms close to your sides.

There are three classifications of patient moves: emergency, urgent, and nonurgent. Use an emergency move when the situation is so dangerous that you cannot properly prepare the patient for movement. Urgent moves allow you to provide basic immobilization prior to movement, and a nonurgent situation will allow you to leave patients where they are until transportation is ready.

There are several different emergency moves, including one-person moves (the clothes drag, the incline drag, the cradle carry, the piggyback carry, and the firefighter's carry) and, if you have a partner, the two-rescuer assist and the firefighter's carry with assist.

The most common carrying devices are the wheeled stretcher, the stair chair, and the spine board. There are also portable stretchers, scoop stretchers, and flexible stretchers, among others.

When preparing to move a patient with a suspected spinal injury, the patient's head, neck, and spine must be immobilized first. Do this with a long spine board or a short spine board if he is seated in a vehicle. If no spinal injury is suspected, you can use the extremity lift, direct-ground lift, draw-sheet method, or simple-direct carry to get the patient onto the stretcher.

Unresponsive patients with no spinal injuries should be transported in the recovery position while patients showing signs of shock should be transported in the Trendelenburg position (feet raised 8 to 12 inches). Most other patients will prefer the semisitting position.

Upon your arrival at the hospital, you will be expected to move the patient to a hospital stretcher—which can be accomplished, in most cases, with the simple draw-sheet method.

PEARLS FROM THE PODIUM

- It cannot be said enough: Back injuries can cause lifelong disability. Be careful.
- Your choice of transportation device will have a profound effect on you and your patient's outcome and safety. Not only will you choose patient-carrying devices because of terrain and logistics but also for patient comfort and condition.
- Be aware of the feelings patients have when they are being carried. It feels awkward when you are lifted and controlled by others. Explain to the patient what you are going to do with each move. Warn him of bumps and loud sounds before they happen.

REVIEW QUESTIONS

SHORT ANSWER

1. What is a Reeves stretcher?

2. Describe the "power grip."

MULTIPLE CHOICE

1. The three classifications of patient moves are emergency, nonurgent, and
   _____.
   A. critical   B. standard
   C. delayed   D. urgent

2. While moving a patient down a flight of stairs, you should use the
   _____ whenever possible.
   A. incline drag   B. stair chair
   C. extremity carry   D. flexible stretcher

3. If there is no suspicion of head or spinal injury, but the patient is still
   unresponsive, how should he be positioned for transport?
   A. In the semi-Fowler's position   B. In the prone position
   C. In the recovery position   D. In the inversion position

4. The use of an orthopedic stretcher is contraindicated if the patient
   _____.
   A. has a suspected spinal injury
   B. is suffering from hypoperfusion
   C. is unresponsive
   D. has a swollen, deformed lower extremity

5. When maneuvering a heavy patient on a wheeled stretcher, you should
   _____.
   A. keep your elbows in the locked position
   B. always try to pull the majority of the weight
   C. adjust the stretcher height to several inches below waist level
   D. keep the weight close to your body

SCENARIO QUESTIONS

You are driving the ambulance back to the station at the end of your shift. It
has been raining steadily, and suddenly the pickup truck ahead of you begins
to slide out of control and rolls over several times. It comes to rest—upside
down—in an open field beside the freeway. You pull over and activate the
ambulance's hazard lights. Your partner radios dispatch and begins setting out
flares as you approach the cab. You find two unresponsive passengers inside
the truck, one on top of the other. Neither individual seems to have been
wearing a seat belt during the crash.

1. Once the vehicle is stabilized, how should you remove the first patient
   from the vehicle?
   A. Taking appropriate cervical-spine precautions, secure the patient to a
      long backboard and pull the patient from the vehicle.
   B. Utilize a vest-type extrication device to secure the patient's spine and
      transfer to a long spine board once out of the vehicle.
   C. Measure and apply a cervical collar and use the "modified extremity
      lift" to relocate the patient to the ambulance.
   D. Grab the patient's shoulders and drag him straight out of the vehicle.

2. After the second patient has been removed from the vehicle and is properly secured to a long spine board, she begins to show signs of shock. How should you position the patient?

   A. Raise the patient's legs 8 to 12 inches by loosening the straps and placing a folded blanket under her feet.

   B. Raise the foot-end of the long spine board 8 to 12 inches.

   C. Remove the long board straps, reposition the patient onto her left side (while maintaining manual spinal immobilization), and reapply the straps.

   D. Prop the head-end of the spine board up to the height that makes the patient most comfortable.

You and your partner are dispatched to a vehicle–bicycle collision. The bicyclist was knocked off of the road and down a sloping 60-foot ravine. You navigate down the rough terrain and find the bicyclist propped in a sitting position against a large rock. He is responsive but confused, covered with abrasions and has deformity to both legs.

1. What device should be used to carry the patient out of the ravine?

   A. A scoop stretcher.   **B.** A portable stretcher.

   C. A Stokes stretcher.   **D.** A stair chair.

2. How should this patient be prepared for transport out of the ravine?

   A. He should be fitted with a cervical collar, secured to a short spine board, and moved to a long spine board.

   B. He should be gently turned from his seated position, while a rescuer maintains manual immobilization of his head, and lowered onto a long spine board.

   C. Due to his critical condition, he should be lifted up by a rescuer using the "firefighter's carry."

   D. A flexible stretcher should be carefully slid underneath the patient, allowing him to be moved while still in the sitting position.

C A S E   S T U D I E S

CASE STUDY 1	**DOWN IN THE BATHROOM**

You are dispatched to a multistory apartment complex for a woman who has fallen down. Upon your arrival, you are directed to a third-floor apartment where an approximately 60-year-old female has fallen in the bathroom while getting out of the shower. She is responsive and alert, lying on her left side and complaining of severe pain in her right hip. She denies hitting her head and has no neck or back pain.

1. What will be your plan of action for getting this patient out of the bathroom?

2. How many people do you think it will take to get her moved?

You now have her safely moved into the middle of the living room and have obtained a baseline set of vitals. Everything appears to be stable and within normal limits. Your next challenge is how to get her down to the ambulance. You estimate her weight to be around 180 pounds.

1. What device do you feel would be the best to move her down to the ambulance if she must remain supine due to pain?

2. The elevator for the building is out of service. What will be your plan for getting her down three flights of stairs?

CASE STUDY 2 HE NEEDS TO GO TO THE HOSPITAL—AND I CAN'T GET HIM OUT OF THE HOUSE!

Your ambulance is dispatched to a call for "general weakness." You arrive to find a private-duty nurse and the patient's wife who meet you at the end of the driveway. There are no signs of obvious danger, and the nurse approaches the ambulance before you exit the passenger door, saying, "You'd better back in. Maybe get some help. He's a big one."

It turns out that she was not kidding. The patient weighs 690 pounds and has not been out of the house in over a year.

1. What does this information mean to you as you size up the call?

2. What is the weight rating of your (or the average) ambulance stretcher?

The nurse began coming in daily to assist the patient in caring for himself. She tells you that the patient normally moves from bed only minimally but now is profoundly weak and is having "a bit" of respiratory distress. You go in the house and find the man in bed and responsive. He tells you that he is having trouble breathing. You note that he cannot speak a full sentence without catching his breath. He is propped up using sofa cushions. The patient is in a raised-ranch-style home in the last bedroom on the left after going up a half staircase.

1. What operational/technical needs do you have for getting this patient to the ambulance?

2. What additional assistance/equipment would you call for?

Active Exploration

Surely the quickest way to put an early end to an otherwise promising career in EMS is to throw one's back out. It is simply not possible to place too much emphasis on the importance of proper body mechanics when lifting and moving patients. Without even realizing it, the majority of us never learn, and more important, never practice, good body mechanics. It is rare that we ever lift anything more than a few pounds and we can generally stay out of harm's way despite poor technique. Poor body mechanics will eventually get you into trouble when moving patients. It may not be the first or second or tenth time you reach to move a patient, but it will eventually get you and when it does, it could be a career-ending injury.

For most of us, practicing good body mechanics feels very awkward and we quickly return to the old way of doing things. The following exercises are designed to help you develop and become accustomed to using proper body mechanics when moving and lifting patients.

Activity 1: $10,000 Video

No one likes to watch themselves on the TV screen, but there are times when it is very beneficial. Working on your golf or baseball swing is a good example where seeing yourself and making small changes can make big improvements in efficiency and performance. Developing good body mechanics is much the same, and the EMT can make improvements in body mechanics by following these suggestions:

1. Obtain a video camera and a fresh tape. You will also need at least two other fellow students to participate in the exercise.
2. Have one student play the role of patient and have the other two students play the role of the EMT-Bs who will be moving the patient.
3. Begin with simple, less complex moves such as moving the patient from the floor to the bed or from a chair to a stretcher.
4. While the two EMT-Bs are demonstrating the move, the fourth person will videotape the entire move.
5. Following each move, immediately play back the tape and critique the move from the standpoint of proper body mechanics.

As suggested above, begin with simple moves and correct and perfect them as you move along, gradually increasing the complexity of the moves.

If you have enough people, giving one additional person the duty of safety officer is a great idea. As you move through the different moves, change roles so that each of you can work on your own skills.

Activity 2: Technique Wins over Strength

One of the biggest challenges for many new EMT-Bs is the operation of the wheeled stretcher, or gurney as it is referred to in some regions of the United States. Like any other skill the new EMT-B must learn, operating the wheeled stretcher takes proper coaching and practice. Most EMT-B students struggle with raising and lowering the stretcher in unison and with a smooth gentle flow. The biggest reason for this is simply technique and *not* the weight, as they often think. Experience has shown that with proper coaching and lots of practice, the art of stretcher operation can be mastered by even the smallest of students. It has been suggested that working with the stretcher is 70 percent technique and 30 percent brute strength. This is why even the smallest of EMT-B students with enough practice can overcome the challenges of the wheeled stretcher.

Use the following activity to improve your skills with this device:

1. Using an empty wheeled stretcher, work with a fellow student who is approximately the same height as you.

2. Go over all the components together and quiz each other on each of the functions.

3. Once you are comfortable, begin with the stretcher in the raised position and practice the following exercises:

- Lower it all the way down in one smooth motion.
- Raise it all the way up in one smooth motion.
- Lower it down one "notch" at a time. Be aware that different stretchers have different increments.
- Raise it up one notch at a time.
- Switch positions and repeat all of the above.

Next, repeat all of the same steps using different-sized partners, taking note of whether it makes it easier or more difficult when they are taller or shorter.

Eventually, you will want to add a patient to the equation. Begin with a small patient and gradually increase the size.

RETRO REVIEW

1. A patient lying on his back is said to be _____.

   A. prone   **B.** supine

   C. pronated   **D.** anterior

2. A communication system that displays the location of a caller on the dispatcher's screen is called_____.

   A. GPS-enabled 911   **B.** 911

   C. enhanced 911   **D.** enabled 911

3. Which of the following is *not* a stage of death and dying?

   A. Enabling   **B.** Denial

   C. Bargaining   **D.** Acceptance

THINKING AND LINKING

CHAPTER TOPIC	HOW IT RELATES TO YOU AND OTHER COURSE AREAS
Emergent, urgent, and nonemergent moves	Almost every call will require a lifting and moving decision. Some will be relatively simple, such as how to move an uninjured patient from the floor to the stretcher. More serious examples include moving a patient with an injured spine who is wedged between a wall and the bed—or a person from a motor vehicle collision.
Lifting and moving devices	You will apply this to almost every call as well. Moving a patient from an ATV crash deep in the woods and moving a cardiac patient down stairs are two examples.
Body mechanics	You must do all lifts and moves very carefully and with respect to your responsibility to the patient as well as your need to prevent injury to yourself.

6

Airway Management

CHAPTER SUMMARY

Assessing and managing a patient's airway will be one of the most important skills you perform as an EMT-B. The human body cannot survive without an adequate level of oxygen being brought in and an adequate level of waste product (carbon dioxide) being expelled. This is the process of respiration. It will be your first priority with any patient to determine whether he has a patent airway and whether he is breathing adequately. Your next priority will be to decide whether you need to assist him, either by providing supplemental oxygen or assisting with ventilations. These decisions will greatly impact the outcome for your patient.

AIRWAY STRUCTURES

The following are the major structures of the respiratory system:

- Nose
- Mouth
- Pharynx
- Oropharynx
- Nasopharynx
- Uvula
- Epiglottis
- Trachea
- Cricoid cartilage
- Larynx
- Bronchi
- Carina
- Bronchioles
- Lungs
- Alveoli
- Diaphragm

INADEQUATE BREATHING

When a patient is breathing at a rate or depth outside of normal ranges, the patient is said to be breathing inadequately. If he is breathing too slowly, the patient is not inhaling enough oxygen. If the patient is breathing too fast, the breaths are shallow, and the patient will not move oxygen into the alveoli. The average person inhales approximately 500 mL of air, with only 350 mL entering the alveoli for oxygen and carbon dioxide exchange. The remaining 150 mL is in airway structures that are not capable of this essential gas exchange.

To assess a patient's breathing, you must look for adequate rise and fall of the chest and ensure that it is equal on both sides. You must also listen carefully for air entering and leaving the nose, mouth, and chest. You should not hear any abnormal sounds in the airway. If the patient is unresponsive, you should feel for air moving out of the airway. You will also want to assess the patient's skin color, as poor skin signs are often a sign of hypoxia.

If you find any of the following signs, your patient may be breathing inadequately:

- Unequal or absent chest movement
- Abdominal movement with no chest movement
- Absent or limited air movement from the nose or mouth
- Diminished or absent breath sounds
- Abnormal breath sounds
- Breathing rate that is outside normal ranges
- Breathing that is too shallow, very deep, or appears labored
- Abnormal skin signs
- Prolonged respirations indicating an obstruction
- Patient has trouble talking because of shortness of breath
- Use of accessory muscles above the clavicles and between/below the ribs
- Nasal flaring

AIRWAY MANAGEMENT

The procedures for managing respiratory emergencies include opening and maintaining the airway and providing artificial ventilations for a patient who is not breathing or not breathing adequately. For a patient who is breathing adequately, you will provide supplemental oxygen. You may need to provide suctioning for both responsive and unresponsive patients.

There are two methods for opening the airway. The head-tilt, chin-lift maneuver is used for a patient with no suspected trauma. For a patient with suspected trauma, the jaw-thrust maneuver should be the first choice. Once the airway is placed in the open position, it is important to clear the airway of any secretions, blood, vomitus, or any other obstruction. Suction should be readily available when maintaining a patient's airway.

If you open the airway and determine that your patient is not breathing, one of the following procedures must be initiated. They are listed in the order of preference.

1. Mouth to mask
2. Two-rescuer bag-valve mask
3. Flow-restricted, oxygen-powered ventilation device (FROPVD)
4. One-rescuer BVM

During artificial ventilations you should:

- Observe chest rise and fall with each ventilation.
- Observe the patient's heart rate return to a normal rate.
- Observe the patients' skin color improve.
- Ventilate at an adequate rate.

If any of these do not occur, you need to adjust your ventilation technique. Remember that you may also assist a patient who is breathing too slowly with artificial ventilations. With patients who are responsive, it is important to explain the procedure and to reassure them.

Mouth-to-mask ventilations are performed with a pocket face mask. This procedure delivers up to approximately 16 percent oxygen with each breath from the rescuer and approximately 50 percent if supplemental oxygen is attached to the inlet. When properly used, the pocket face mask can deliver higher volumes of air to the patient than the BVM.

The bag-valve mask, or BVM, is a handheld device. It comes in different sizes for adults, children, and infants. Use the BVM with supplemental oxygen at the rate of 15 lpm. The most challenging part of using a BVM is maintaining an adequate seal with the face mask. Therefore, the two-rescuer method is preferred. One rescuer maintains the face-mask seal with two hands, while the second rescuer squeezes the bag.

The FROPVD uses oxygen under pressure to deliver ventilations through a mask. The device has a trigger that allows the rescuer to deliver ventilations as necessary. Most FROPVDs have a relief valve that helps minimize the chances of overinflation.

Airway adjuncts help maintain an open airway. You may use the oropharyngeal airway in an unresponsive patient who has no gag reflex. The nasopharyngeal airway (NPA) can be tolerated by some responsive patients who still have a gag reflex. Both devices aid in keeping the airway clear and open. You must still maintain a head-tilt, chin-lift, or jaw-thrust maneuver and monitor the airway. The adjuncts come in different sizes and you must measure them properly if they are to work effectively.

The patient's airway must be kept clear of secretions, blood, vomit, and other obstructions. Suctioning will help maintain a clear airway. Suction units are either portable or wall mounted in the ambulance. Either system must create a vacuum of no less than 300 mmHg. You should check these devices daily. There are different types of suction tips that can be used, depending on the type of fluid that needs to be suctioned. When suctioning, remember to:

- Use appropriate BSI precautions.
- Never suction for longer than 15 seconds.
- Suction only while removing the suction tip or catheter from the patient's airway.

OXYGEN THERAPY

Oxygen therapy is not just for patients with difficulty breathing. Many other conditions require that supplemental oxygen be administered. These include chest pain, blood loss, broken bones, and hypoxia, to name a few.

Oxygen is supplied in cylinders of various sizes. The oxygen is under pressure in these cylinders and therefore safety is of prime importance when handling oxygen cylinders.

A pressure regulator is attached to the cylinder to allow for a safe working pressure. A flowmeter is attached to the regulator and allows you to deliver the oxygen at a selected flow rate. You may also use humidifiers to provide moisture to the oxygen being delivered.

Supplemental oxygen can be administered to patients who are breathing in one of two ways. A nonrebreather mask will deliver 80 to 95 percent oxygen when a flow rate of 12 to 15 lpm of oxygen is used. Inflate the reservoir bag before placing the mask on the patient. A nasal cannula provides a lower concentration of oxygen, between 24 and 44 percent. You should use the nasal cannula with a flow rate of 2 to 6 liters of oxygen. Most patients will benefit from a higher concentration of oxygen.

Excellent airway assessment and management is crucial for getting a positive outcome for the patient. Artificial ventilation is not a skill used every day, so it is important to practice it often. As a new EMT-B, be familiar with the airway management equipment you will be using and its location in the jump bags and ambulance.

MED MINUTE

There are several medications that can cause significant respiratory depression and inadequate breathing. Medications prescribed for pain control, anxiety, seizures, and other conditions, when accidentally or intentionally taken in greater quantities, cause respiratory depression and respiratory arrest, which can lead to death.

MEDICATION CLASS	USES	EXAMPLES
Narcotics	Pain relief	Acetaminophen with codeine (Tylenol #3 or #4 with codeine), propoxyphene (Darvocet), oxycodone (Percocet), OxyContin, methadone, hydrocodone (Vicodin)
Benzodiazepines	Anxiety	alprazolam (Xanax), lorazepam (Ativan), diazepam (Valium)

PATHOPHYSIOLOGY PEARLS

As mentioned previously, good airway management is paramount to a patient's survival. Although aggressively managing an airway is critically important, it is equally important to know when to simply monitor the airway without being overly aggressive.

The airway of a patient with epiglottitis is a good example of one that would benefit from a less aggressive intervention. Epiglottitis is an acute, severe, life-threatening disease of the upper airway. Epiglottitis has traditionally been referred to as a pediatric disease, but this is not necessarily the case anymore. The majority of epiglottitis cases are caused by Hib (*Haemophilus influenzae* type B). As a result of the introduction of the Hib vaccine in the 1980s, epiglottitis is being seen more in young adults than in children.

In epiglottitis, a local infection of the epiglottis occurs followed by an increase of bacteria in the blood. The epiglottis and the structures connected to or immediately surrounding it become inflamed and swollen, leading to a compromised airway at the level of the epiglottis, often causing respiratory difficulty.

The typical presentation for epiglottitis is a rapid onset of a fever that may or may not be accompanied by a sore throat. The patient will likely refuse to eat or drink because of the irritation this may cause and will eventually be unable to tolerate their own secretions, causing the patient to drool. The patient may develop signs of upper airway obstruction with inspiratory stridor and some degree of respiratory difficulty. The patient will sit with his neck extended in the sniffing position. This position is maintained to assist the patient in optimizing the degree to which the airway can remain open. This patient will typically avoid coughing, as this further irritates the inflamed tissue.

Treatment of epiglottitis is focused on preventing airway obstruction. The first treatment step is the administration of high-flow oxygen through blow-by technique, as tolerated by the patient. The goal of all prehospital care providers should be to ensure that the patient remains calm. There is absolutely no need to force an inspection of the patient's airway and you should not attempt it. Attempting oral intubation in a patient with epiglottitis is contraindicated in the field because of the potential irritation caused by laryngoscopy. This irritation will likely cause complete occlusion of the airway by inducing soft-tissue swelling and edema.

If the patient deteriorates and requires assisted ventilation in the prehospital setting, slow, deep ventilations by BVM are best. If BVM ventilation is not effective in ventilating the patient, you should assume that the patient has complete airway obstruction at the level of the epiglottis. Paramedics and other advanced-level providers would then need to perform either a needle or surgical cricothyroidotomy to provide ventilatory support for this patient.

Sources

Crain E, Jeffrey C, Clinical Manual of Emergency Pediatrics, 4th Edition, New York, NY: McGraw-Hill, 2003.
Markenson D, Pediatric Prehospital Care, Upper Saddle River, NJ: Brady, 2002.
Taussig L, Louis L, Pediatric Respiratory Medicine, St. Louis, MO: Mosby, 1999.

REVIEW QUESTIONS

SHORT ANSWER

1. Describe both the primary benefit and the major fault with the Bourden gauge flowmeter.

2. What is the difference between respiratory failure and respiratory arrest?

MULTIPLE CHOICE

1. It is generally recommended to switch to a new oxygen cylinder when the old one reaches _____ psi.

   A. 200   **B.** 50
   C. 500   **D.** 250

2. Which of these suction catheters has the largest diameter?

   A. 4 French   **B.** 8.0 Flextip
   C. 16 French   **D.** 22 Yankauer

3. The majority of airway problems are caused by _____.

   A. vomitus

   B. the patient's tongue

   C. swelling of the airway structures

   D. foreign bodies

4. A nasopharyngeal airway is contraindicated if _____ has been found in the nose.

   A. blood   **B.** vomitus
   C. cerebrospinal fluid   **D.** soft-tissue damage

5. When using a flow-restricted, oxygen-powered ventilation device (FROPVD) on a patient with _____, be very careful not to overinflate.

   A. chronic obstructive pulmonary disease (COPD)

   B. pneumonia

   C. an aortic aneurysm

   D. chest trauma

SCENARIO QUESTIONS

You are dispatched to attend to a case of a possible drug overdose. You find the patient, a 17-year-old male, unresponsive and lying supine on the floor of his bedroom. He has a weak, rapid pulse and is not breathing. There is vomitus on his clothing.

1. The first thing that you should do for this patient is to _____.
   A. open his airway with the head-tilt, chin-lift and suction any vomitus
   B. insert an NPA and begin ventilating with a BVM
   C. check his mouth for vomitus. If present, turn the patient to the side and suction his mouth
   D. place the patient in the prone position so any vomitus can drain as you are artificially ventilating him

2. At what rate would you ventilate this patient?
   A. One breath every 5 seconds.
   B. Two breaths every 15 seconds.
   C. One breath every 3 seconds.
   D. 100 per minute.

3. Make sure that each of your ventilations _____.
   A. contains at least 85 percent oxygen
   B. delivers 1,000 to 12,000 mL of air
   C. causes the patient's chest to rise
   D. provides 200 to 400 mL of oxygen

You and your partner are at the video store looking for a movie—just in case it turns out to be a slow shift. You hear a woman frantically begin calling for help. In the next aisle you discover an unresponsive elderly man lying on the floor. Your partner runs to the ambulance to retrieve the primary-care bag and to notify dispatch. You quickly determine that the man is not breathing and see that he has a stoma. The woman is screaming hysterically and yelling at you to "do something!"

1. To properly open this patient's airway, you should _____.
   A. use the head-tilt, chin-lift maneuver
   B. place the patient's head in the "sniffing" position
   C. utilize the jaw-thrust technique
   D. leave the head and neck in a neutral position

2. If you are unable to artificially ventilate through the stoma, consider _____.
   A. sealing the stoma and attempting ventilation through the mouth
   B. sliding an NPA into the stoma and trying again
   C. using substantially more air pressure
   D. performing abdominal thrusts

Your agency has been hired to provide on-set medical services for a film company that is working in town. As you and your partner are standing near the ambulance, a production assistant runs up to you and says that one of the carpenters has cut himself with a power saw. You grab your equipment and follow the woman, who leads you to the patient. You find him sitting on the ground cradling his left hand. You notice a circular saw, quite a bit of blood, and several fingers on the ground in front of the man. "Let's get some O_2 on him," your partner says.

1. Why is providing supplemental oxygen important in this situation?
   A. Concentrated oxygen causes an endorphin release and will have a calming effect on the man.
   B. The patient's blood will need a higher saturation of oxygen to compensate for the loss of red blood cells.
   C. It will prevent hypoperfusion.
   D. Severe trauma can cause a decrease in respiratory rates.

2. Approximately what percentage of oxygen is in the earth's atmosphere?
   A. 89 percent
   B. 14 percent
   C. 21 percent
   D. 2 percent

3. How would you provide supplemental oxygen to this patient?
   A. Cannula with 15 lpm
   B. Rebreather mask with 15 lpm
   C. Blow-by with 25 lpm
   D. Nonrebreather mask with 15 lpm

CASE STUDIES

CASE STUDY 1	DOWN AND OUT

You are dispatched to a local homeless shelter for an unresponsive person. Upon your arrival, you are met outside by a man who states that one of his employees discovered the man lying unresponsive outside of the shelter, just before calling 911. He states that he does not know the man.

As you approach, you notice an approximately 50-year-old male lying on his left side apparently unresponsive. You notice a puddle of what looks like vomitus next to his face.

1. **What are your initial concerns with this man and how will you begin your assessment?**

2. **What equipment will you want to have ready as you begin your assessment?**

You are unable to accurately assess his breathing with him on his side. You decide to roll him onto his back for a better look. Once he is on his back, you discover that his respirations are 8 per minute and shallow and you hear slight gurgling with each breath.

1. **How will you manage this man's airway at this time?**

2. Is it necessary to ventilate this patient and if so, how will you accomplish this?

CASE STUDY 2   **GO WITH THE FLOW**

For each of the following mini case studies, choose the appropriate oxygen-delivery device and flow rate.

1. A 24-year-old patient who was playing soccer and injured his right lower leg. He is alert and in considerable pain.

2. A 69-year-old man with a long history of chronic respiratory problems who called because of a change in the color of his phlegm. He is alert, resting comfortably, and appears to be in minor respiratory distress.

3. A 21-year-old patient who was found on the side of the road after being ejected from a vehicle in a rollover crash. His respirations are shallow at about 5 or 6 per minute.

4. A 56-year-old woman was at the ATM when she was robbed. She resisted and the perpetrator stabbed her in the chest just below the armpit. She is breathing 24 times per minute. The breaths seem deep.

5. A 78-year-old woman passed out in the mall. You find her sitting on a bench looking pale with a rapid pulse.

6. A 34-year-old man appears to have taken an overdose of medication and consumed alcohol. He has a pulse, but you do not detect any breathing at all.

Active Exploration

It has probably become very clear to you by now that airway management is a very high priority when it comes to patient care. In fact, other than personal safety, airway management *is* the most important priority when treating patients. The following activities will assist you in developing your skills in this area.

Activity 1: While You Were Sleeping

Assessing a patient's respirations involves identifying no fewer than three characteristics: rate, depth, and ease of respirations. It is fairly easy to assess these qualities in the responsive patient having difficulty breathing; however, it becomes a bigger challenge when the patient is unresponsive and whose chief complaint is not related to difficulty in breathing. The following activity will allow you to practice your skill in assessing the characteristics of breathing.

The next time you encounter someone who is sleeping, take a moment to carefully observe his respiratory status. You do not have to touch him, just get close enough to observe his chest and/or abdomen for rise and fall.

1. Observe the rise and fall of the chest/abdomen. Take note as to which of these areas moves more, the chest or the abdomen. Observe the "depth" or tidal volume. Would you classify it as normal, shallow, or deep? Is it easy to tell how much volume he is moving with each breath?

2. Next observe the rate. Count how many times he is breathing in and out. Does that rate fall into the "normal" range for the person's age?

3. Next note the "ease" with which the person is breathing. Is he making noise while breathing? If so, what is this a sign of? Observe the pattern of respirations. Are they regular and evenly spaced, or are there extended gaps between breaths? What medical conditions might cause irregular breathing patterns in ill or injured patients?

It is one thing to learn to assess breathing on fellow students who are healthy and breathing normally and entirely another to attempt the same on an unconscious patient. By practicing your respiratory assessment skills on sleeping volunteers of all shapes and sizes, you will quickly become more confident in your abilities and be better prepared for the real thing.

Activity 2: Take a Deep Breath

Assessing lung sounds is one of the more challenging skills for the novice EMT. Like many of the skills you learn as EMT students, you sometimes get in the habit of "going through the motions" and forget to really pay attention to what you are trying to accomplish. This happens most often with new students who are assessing pupils. You always shine the light into each eye but neglect to carefully pay attention to the actual response of the pupils. This is a common pitfall in the classroom because you know that your "patients" are normal and of course their pupils will be responding accordingly.

Breath sounds often fall into this category as well and you should pay special attention to learning to assess breath sounds. Grab a fellow student and a stethoscope and follow these steps:

1. Find a quiet space where you can listen for breath sounds without distraction. Ensure that the earpieces are properly fitted into your ears and listen for several seconds in each of the lung fields, top, middle, and bases.

2. Have the "patient" breathe normally at first, then have them take deep breaths as you listen. Pay close attention to the sounds you hear in all lung fields. Do they differ in each field or from side to side?

3. Now have your "patient" run for 2 minutes. When he returns, have him sit upright and listen again in all lung fields. Compare what you hear with the resting lung sounds. How are they different?

Learning to assess lung sounds as well as other vital signs in the classroom setting can cause you to become complacent. Students often neglect to pay close attention because they assume that vital signs will be normal. Taking the time and effort to simulate abnormal vital signs by asking your "patients" to run is just one way you can get experience taking vitals that are outside the normal parameters.

RETRO REVIEW

1. An oriented patient with mild to moderate difficulty in breathing, receiving oxygen via nonrebreather mask, would likely be transported downstairs _____ using _____.
   - **A.** walking, manual assistance
   - **B.** sitting, a wheeled stretcher
   - **C.** sitting, a stair chair
   - **D.** lying, a Reeves stretcher

2. The bones of the lower leg are called the_____.
   - **A.** radius and ulna
   - **B.** carpal and metacarpal
   - **C.** femur and patella
   - **D.** tibia and fibula

3. The shoulder is _____ to the elbow.
   - **A.** distal
   - **B.** proximal
   - **C.** medial
   - **D.** lateral

THINKING AND LINKING

CHAPTER TOPIC	HOW IT RELATES TO YOU AND OTHER COURSE AREAS
Adequate vs. inadequate breathing	There are three levels of breathing: adequate, inadequate, and not at all. Adequate and not at all are relatively obvious. Inadequate is not. Be on the alert for inadequate breathing and treat it aggressively in any patient you encounter.
Oxygen and administration devices	Most of your patients will receive oxygen. Oxygen (sometimes referred to as "high-flow Os" or "the wonder drug") has tremendous benefit and very little risk. Give it to your patients who need it. You will also have to use, check, and change oxygen tanks and regulators every time you give oxygen. As you begin to study medical-emergency patients (Module 4) and trauma patients (Module 5), you will notice that most of these patients will be given oxygen. Serious illness in pediatric patients (Module 6) is usually centered around respiratory problems where oxygen is beneficial.
Suction	Medical or trauma patients who have an altered mental status (ranging from lethargic to unresponsive) will likely require suctioning at some point. A small amount of stomach contents entering the lungs can cause pneumonia and death.

Scene Size-up

CHAPTER SUMMARY

A timely and accurate scene size-up will keep you, your fellow emergency workers, and bystanders safe and allow for the delivery of efficient emergency care to the patient. In a matter of minutes, you should identify any hazards, the number of patients, mechanism of injury (MOI) or nature of illness (NOI), and whether you require any additional resources. A good scene size-up can make or break a call.

The scene size-up is the start of your patient assessment. Your scene size-up is an ongoing process because situations can change quickly during an emergency call. Start observing the scene as you approach and again before you leave your vehicle. Be alert for any immediate or potential hazards. Determine whether additional resources such as fire suppression or extrication are needed. Once you have determined that the scene is safe to approach at a vehicle crash, set up a danger zone. The extent of the zone will be dependent on the type of hazards found at the scene.

Violence is a hazard you may encounter. Be observant for loud voices, signs of drug or alcohol use, unusual silence, and weapons. As always, retreat if you observe any signs of danger. Do not return to the scene until it has been secured by police.

As you perform your scene size-up, determine what you will need for appropriate BSI precautions. Are gloves sufficient, or are eye protection and a gown needed as well? Personal protective equipment (PPE) should always be readily available.

The next step is to determine either the MOI for a trauma call or the NOI for a medical call. Determining how a patient fell or how his vehicle was impacted during a collision gives you a hint of what injuries to suspect. Evidence at the scene, such as a bent steering column or a starred windshield, can also raise suspicions about specific injuries. Head-on collisions create the potential for injuries to any part of the body. Head and neck injuries are common in rear-end collisions. Side-impact collisions can cause neck injuries and internal or skeletal injuries from the head to the thighs. Rollover collisions and rotational impacts are potentially the most serious because the patient may have sustained multiple impacts during the incident. It may be helpful to determine where the patient was sitting in the vehicle before the crash and whether he was wearing a seat belt. The type of seat belt is also important. A patient wearing just a lap belt is at a greater risk of internal abdominal injuries.

During the evaluation of the MOI, you also need to consider the type of trauma. Trauma can be penetrating or blunt. Penetrating trauma is an injury that passes through the skin into the underlying tissue. Blunt trauma does not break the skin but has the potential to injure internal organs and vessels.

During a medical emergency, you can gather information regarding the NOI from several sources. If the patient is responsive and reliable, he is usually the best source of information regarding his illness. You may also obtain information from family or bystanders. The scene itself will give you clues about the patient's condition, such as medications or living habits.

The final stage, but not the least important, is determining the number of patients and whether you have the resources to handle the call. The earlier you recognize the need for extra help, the sooner it will arrive and the smoother and more efficiently the call will proceed.

PEARLS FROM THE PODIUM

- Do a thorough scene size-up on each call. It sets the foundation for the call to go well.
- Do not enter dangerous scenes if you do not have appropriate training, equipment, and support.
- Do not begin the initial assessment of any patient until the size-up is complete.
- Experience tells us that once you begin emergency care for your patient, it is easy to "tunnel in" and forget to call for help as you go along.
- If you are unsure whether additional resources will be needed, it is better to call for them and then cancel them than to wait too long to call.

REVIEW QUESTIONS

SHORT ANSWER

1. What is cavitation?

2. Explain the term *index of suspicion*.

MULTIPLE CHOICE

1. The most important consideration regarding body substance isolation precautions is to have BSI equipment _____.
   A. properly labeled
   B. on at all times
   C. readily available
   D. in your personal vehicle

2. Penetrating trauma wounds are classified by the _____ of the item that caused the injury.
   A. velocity
   B. size
   C. composition
   D. shape

3. If you cannot determine the exact nature of a patient's injuries, the _____ will help predict general injury patterns.
   A. US DOT EMS Handbook
   B. patient
   C. receiving medical facility
   D. mechanism of injury

4. You arrive at a call and see two police officers, a fire crew, and another ambulance already on the scene. The first thing that you should do is _____.
   A. perform a scene size-up
   B. check in with the incident commander
   C. contact dispatch to determine whether you are still needed
   D. locate and treat any patients who are not being cared for

5. An important aspect of the scene size-up is determining whether you have sufficient _____ to handle the call.
   A. courage
   B. resources
   C. experience
   D. time

SCENARIO QUESTIONS

You are driving the ambulance through midday traffic en route to a vehicle collision at the intersection of Washington and 122nd Avenue. As you approach 128th Avenue, the traffic comes to an abrupt halt because the traffic lights are out. Using appropriate emergency driving techniques, you are able to navigate around the stopped traffic only to find that the lights at each subsequent intersection are also dead. Your partner notices thick smoke rising over the traffic several blocks ahead and says, "That looks like it's right at 128th Avenue."

1. Based on the conditions as you approach the scene, what should you be anticipating?
   A. Additional vehicle collisions.
   B. Downed power lines.
   C. A vehicle fire.
   D. All of the above.

2. If there is an electrical line down at the scene, you should park the ambulance _____.
   A. several blocks away, until the utility company clears you to enter the area
   B. at least one full span of wire away from the pole to which the broken line is attached
   C. at least 200 feet away
   D. with your tires on top of it, to prevent it from snaking around the scene

3. The danger zone around a vehicle that is on fire should extend at least _____ in all directions.
   A. 100 feet
   B. 50 feet
   C. 250 feet
   D. 500 feet

Your assistance has been requested at a residence for an individual with a scalp laceration from a fall. As you get out of the ambulance, you hear shouting coming from the residence. Moments later, a 40- to 45-year-old male who is bleeding profusely from a deep cut above his left ear comes out to meet you. The patient explains that he had fallen while hanging a picture, but as you begin treating him, he admits that his wife had attempted to stab him with a knife. "Then she ran out of the kitchen and went upstairs," he says. Just then, you hear a door slam somewhere in the house and through the open front door you see a person moving quickly down the stairs.

1. What is the first danger signal in this situation?
   A. The slamming door.
   B. The initial dispatch information.
   C. The patient telling you that his wife had attempted to stab him.
   D. The shouting that you heard upon your arrival.

2. What should your next step be in this situation?
   A. Tell your partner to contact the police while you continue treating the patient.
   B. Try to determine exactly what is going on before overreacting.
   C. Immediately retreat to a safe position and contact dispatch for law-enforcement assistance.
   D. Attempt to defuse the situation by keeping the husband and wife separated.

CASE STUDIES

CASE STUDY 1	CALLING ALL RESOURCES

You are dispatched to the scene of a multiple-vehicle collision (MVC) on a major multilane freeway. You are told by dispatch that there are multiple patients and that you are one of several emergency vehicles responding. They have also dispatched an air ambulance.

1. How many potential hazards might you expect to find en route or once at the scene?

2. What will be your first priority should you be the first resource on the scene?

You arrive at the scene immediately after the first fire engine. They are addressing the issue of traffic and the spilling liquids from one of the vehicles. There are multiple patients and some appear to be trapped in their vehicles.

1. With the major hazards under control, what hazards still pose a threat to you as you begin treating patients?

2. What additional resources will you request for this scene?

Your ambulance is dispatched to a two-vehicle MVC. The dispatcher tells you that there are "minor injuries." What the dispatcher does not tell you is that one of the vehicles involved is a tractor-trailer with a tank back. From a distance, you see that the tanker is upright and that people are standing about 100 feet from the truck on the side of the highway. The police have not arrived at the scene.

1. What should you do before approaching the scene?

2. What additional resources might you need at the scene?

3. What information can you obtain before you approach?

You observe that the placard has the number "1993" with a red background.

1. What does this mean?

2. Where could you look up the information needed?

The fire department is able to determine that the tanker is not leaking and is structurally safe. You approach the scene.

1. What parts of the scene size-up still need to be completed?

Active Exploration

The scene size-up is one of the more complex elements of overall patient assessment and frequently gets overshadowed by the primary task of assessing the patient. You need to understand and reinforce this early in your EMT training so that you can address appropriately all the necessary aspects of scene management. The following activities are designed to get you to think critically and consider all aspects of the scene size-up.

Activity 1: A Picture Is Worth a Thousand Words

Your textbook is rich with photos depicting a wide variety of emergency scenes and injuries. Begin with the photos contained in Chapter 7 and complete the following activity.

1. Select any image of an emergency scene and write down your answers to the following questions:
   a. What type of PPE do you think is needed for the scene depicted?

   b. What obvious hazards can you identify?

   c. What hidden or potential hazards can you identify?

   d. Can you identify the MOI or NOI? What injuries are you likely to find based on the MOI or NOI?

   e. How many patients can you see? Is there evidence of other possible patients?

   f. What additional resources may you need for the emergency? How will you request them?

Once you have written your responses to two or three photos, compare your responses to those of a fellow student. Did he identify something that you did not or vice versa?

As an EMT student, you should begin to look for opportunities to use your skills even outside of the classroom. If you see an emergency scene on television or in a trade publication, take a moment to conduct a scene size-up.

Activity 2: What's in Your EMS System?

One of the most important things you can do as a new EMT-B working in your area is to know exactly what resources are available. You must do some creative research and find out whether the following resources are available and through which specific agency. You can begin by asking fellow students, but eventually you may need to call local EMS, fire, and law-enforcement agencies to find your answers.

- Advanced extrication tools (Jaws of Life)
- HazMat response teams
- Air-ambulance resources (helicopters and airplanes)
- Critical-incident counselors
- Hostage-negotiation teams
- SWAT teams
- Trauma center
- Other specialty centers for the care of burns, pediatric cases, limb reattachment, and so on

Knowing what resources are available in your area and knowing how to request them is an important part of being an EMT-B in the EMS system.

RETRO REVIEW

1. When an EMT does not ensure that care for a patient is continued at the same level or higher, it is called _____.
   A. negligence   **B.** standard of care
   C. abandonment   **D.** scope of practice

2. Which of the following statements about crime scenes is true?
   A. EMTs should ensure evidence is preserved before beginning emergency care.
   B. EMTs are not concerned with evidence preservation.
   C. EMTs can begin emergency care after police have secured all evidence.
   D. EMTs should consider evidence preservation while treating the patient.

3. The organization responsible for administering national examinations for First Responders, EMT-Bs, EMT-Is, and EMT-Ps is the _____.
   A. NREMT   **B.** NAEMT
   C. DOT/NHTSA   **D.** NAEMSE

THINKING AND LINKING

CHAPTER TOPIC	HOW IT RELATES TO YOU AND OTHER COURSE AREAS
Scene safety and BSI	Originally taught in Chapter 2, you now see where this fits in the call/assessment process. *Every* call starts with a thorough scene size-up for safety and in order to be able to take the proper BSI precautions.
Hazardous materials and other dangers	The "Ambulance Operations" chapter (Chapter 33) and "Special Operations" chapter (Chapter 35) deal with dangers from leaking fuel, hazardous materials, and highway incidents.
Mechanism of injury	Chapter 10, "Assessment of the Trauma Patient," continues the assessment process. Your determination of the MOI in the size-up is a key factor in determining how the remainder of the trauma assessment will continue. A significant MOI means the patient could have serious hidden injuries—even if he looks "OK"— and your assessment takes this into account.
Number of patients	The "Special Operations" chapter (Chapter 35) provides additional information on how to triage (sort or prioritize) multiple patients. These calls are relatively rare, which makes it even more important to identify multiple-patient situations early.

8

The Initial Assessment

CHAPTER SUMMARY

The initial assessment, which will be your first step in the actual assessment of a patient, is used to immediately identify any life-threatening problems—which you will also need to remedy as you discover them. When performing an initial assessment, you will first form a general impression and then assess mental status, airway, breathing, and circulation. You will conclude the initial assessment by determining the patient's priority for transport.

Assessing the environment around a patient, coupled with the patient's appearance and chief complaint, will develop your general impression of the patient. Do not underestimate how much a patient's surroundings can tell you about his current condition and even his history (e.g. an overturned chair, prescription medicine bottles, extreme temperatures, and so on).

Why were you called to assist this patient? The answer to that question, in the patient's own words, is the chief complaint. You may find that some chief complaints are very specific, such as "my left elbow hurts," and some are unhelpfully vague, such as "I just don't feel good."

Looking, listening, and smelling are important actions in forming a general impression. Look to see whether the patient seems to be in pain or is having trouble breathing, listen for moaning or noisy respirations, and sniff for any indications of hazardous fumes, urine, feces, or vomitus.

Never ignore "uneasy feelings" or seemingly baseless concerns when you arrive at a scene or begin forming a general impression of the patient. With experience, it is not uncommon to develop a "sixth sense" about potential hazards or the severity of a patient's condition. Do not, however, depend solely on these feelings or senses. They should be used in conjunction with the rest of your assessment skills.

Assessing a patient's level of responsiveness, or mental status, is normally easy. Most patients will be alert and able to talk to you. You will occasionally find patients who are not awake but will respond to talking or shouting and others who will only respond to pain, like a sternal rub or toe pinch.

An easy way of remembering the levels of responsiveness are the letters **AVPU**, which stand for Alert, Verbal, Painful, or Unresponsive.

What if a patient is fully awake but confused? In these cases, you will determine the patient's mental status by finding out what he is "oriented to." Most EMS systems use person, place, and time to determine orientation. Does the patient know *who* he is? Where he is? How about the date or time?

A depressed mental status may indicate a lack of sufficient oxygen to the patient's brain or that the patient is in shock, both of which are serious life-threats. A patient who presents (or deteriorates) below "Alert" on the AVPU scale should be placed on high-concentration oxygen via a nonrebreather mask and transported immediately.

You will next assess the **ABC**s (Airway, Breathing, and Circulation) in your search for life-threats. If the patient is talking or crying loudly, you know that the airway is open. If the airway is not open or is compromised, utilize the head-tilt, chin-lift maneuver, or the jaw-thrust to open the airway and suction if necessary. You should also consider oropharyngeal or nasopharyngeal airways. Use accepted procedures to clear blocked airways.

Once you know that the patient has an open airway, assess for adequacy of breathing. You will need to begin rescue breathing for a patient in respiratory arrest, and if he is unresponsive with a breathing rate of less than 8 times per minute, provide positive-pressure ventilations with 100 percent oxygen. If the patient is alert and breathing adequately but at an elevated rate (24 times per minute or more), you should provide high-concentration oxygen via nonrebreather mask. What if the patient has an elevated rate but is *not* taking adequate breaths? You will use one of the techniques found in Chapter 6 to ventilate the patient with supplemental oxygen.

Once the airway and breathing are secure, turn your attention to the patient's circulation. Check for the presence of a pulse, the quality of skin signs, and for any evidence of bleeding. If there is no pulse, begin CPR—keeping in mind that there may be a life-threatening circulatory condition other than cardiac arrest, such as severe bleeding.

A light-skinned patient with proper perfusion will have warm, pink, and dry skin—which will become cool and moist with a decrease in circulation. Dark-skinned patients with proper circulation will have pink nail beds and lips.

You must find severe bleeding and immediately control it. A patient can bleed to death within 1 to 2 minutes if a large vessel, or several smaller ones, have been ruptured. Always be alert for the onset of shock in patients who have suffered a significant mechanism of injury and make your transport decisions accordingly.

Once the immediate threats to your patient's life have been controlled, you must decide whether to transport right away or remain at the scene for further assessment and emergency care. In general, if the patient has a decreased level of responsiveness or life-threats that either cannot be resolved or have the potential of recurring, you must transport immediately. You would then continue assessments and emergency care en route to the hospital.

Remember, regardless of the patient's age, condition (medical or trauma), and level of responsiveness, the steps of your initial assessment should remain the same. You will always form a general impression, assess mental status, check the ABCs (immediately correcting any life-threats), and determine the priority for transport.

Be systematic about your initial assessments, otherwise there is the possibility that you may overlook something and neglect to notice (and correct) an immediate threat to your patient's life.

PEARLS FROM THE PODIUM

- On serious calls, it is common to have one EMT-B at the patient's head to continuously monitor and maintain the airway. This may include head-tilt or jaw-thrust, suctioning, and in some cases providing ventilations.
- One of the most important determinations you must make is whether a patient who is breathing is doing so adequately.
- The statement "the patient is talking to me so his ABCs are OK" is not always true. Look for work of breathing and an inability to speak full sentences as indicators of potential problems. Patients who are "talking" only a few short words at a time are not really talking and are very sick.
- Operating a BVM, especially for a prolonged time is not easy. Two rescuers do the job best.
- Patients can bleed quite a bit and have it absorbed by clothing. This is why the hands-on bleeding check helps find significant but hidden bleeding.
- The initial assessment is where you identify and treat immediate life-threats. Insert an oropharyngeal airway (OPA), suction, administer oxygen, seal open chest wounds, stabilize flail segments, and control life-threatening bleeding and any other life-threatening problems as part of the initial assessment.
- One of the most common errors—and one that is a critical error on practical examinations—is not completing the initial assessment before moving on to the next steps of the assessment process.

REVIEW QUESTIONS

SHORT ANSWER

1. What is an intervention?

2. What is the danger in not being systematic and consistent in your initial assessment?

MULTIPLE CHOICE

1. If the patient is alert and breathing adequately but his respiratory rate is above _____ breaths per minute, administer high-concentration oxygen via nonrebreather mask.

   A. 18   B. 24
   C. 20   D. 16

2. Which of the following is not a reliable sign when checking circulation in a 20-year-old patient?
   A. Distal pulse
   B. Skin color
   C. Capillary refill
   D. Pedal pulse

3. A general impression is based on an immediate assessment of the environment and the patient's chief complaint and on _____.
   A. appearance
   B. SAMPLE history
   C. vital signs
   D. mental status

4. Judgment based on experience in observing and treating patients is called _____.
   A. categorical judgment
   B. observational judgment
   C. experiential judgment
   D. clinical judgment

5. You form a general impression by looking, listening, and _____.
   A. talking
   B. smelling
   C. touching
   D. documenting

SCENARIO QUESTIONS

You are dispatched to a home after a 6-year-old boy contacted emergency services for his mother. The child indicated that his mother "wasn't acting right" and that she "wouldn't stay awake." Once you are on the scene, the boy leads you to the garage where you find the patient, a 25- to 30-year-old female, unresponsive on the concrete. You notice gold coloration around her mouth and nose and a paper bag near her hand.

1. Which of the following would *not* be part of your "general impression"?
   A. The patient's approximate age.
   B. The patient's position.
   C. The paper bag.
   D. The patient's respiratory rate.

2. What steps would you have taken before determining that the patient was "unresponsive"?
   A. Spoken to her, shouted at her, and pinched her finger or toe.
   B. Observed her, spoke to her, and provided painful stimulus.
   C. Tapped her shoulder and shouted.
   D. Watched to see whether she was alert and provided painful stimulus.

You pull up to the scene of a vehicle-versus-motorcycle crash. You observe a heap of twisted metal with handlebars on one side of the road and a station wagon with minor front-end damage on the other. Your partner checks on the driver of the car while you set out to find the motorcycle rider. You discover him lying supine in a ditch about forty feet from the scene. He is barely responsive to verbal stimulus and breathing noisily and with tremendous difficulty. There is also a large amount of blood on and around the patient.

1. Which intervention would come first for the patient in the ditch?
   A. Manual stabilization of the head and neck.
   B. Controlling the loss of blood.
   C. Providing positive-pressure ventilations with supplemental oxygen.
   D. Performing the jaw-thrust maneuver.

2. The MOI would be used in your decision making in all of the following parts of the initial assessment except for _____.
   A. transport priority
   B. airway
   C. general impression
   D. breathing

CASE STUDIES

You are dispatched to a traffic collision involving a vehicle and a motorcycle. Upon your arrival, you assess the scene and determine that the motorcycle broadsided the vehicle at a high speed. A firefighter on the scene advises you that the driver of the vehicle is not injured and that the driver of the motorcycle is in the ditch and has been unresponsive since they arrived at the scene. You approach the patient and find him to be facedown in the ditch. A firefighter is stabilizing the patient's head and helmet with both hands.

1. Describe in detail how you would conduct your initial assessment of this patient.

2. Under what circumstances would you want to remove the patient's helmet?

After a careful initial assessment, you determine that the patient's respirations are 8 per minute and shallow. His pulse is 88, strong, and regular, and he is bleeding from the nose and mouth.

1. Would you want to roll this patient faceup? If so, why?

2. What equipment will you use to manage his airway and breathing status?

It is 3:00 AM when you are called to a patient experiencing difficulty breathing. You arrive to find a 78-year-old male patient sitting on the edge of his bed with his feet dangling over the side. He is resting his arms on his knees. It appears that he is having considerable difficulty breathing, and you notice he appears a bit sweaty.

1. What have you observed thus far? What does it tell you?

2. Describe your general impression.

You begin to talk to the patient and begin an initial assessment. He is alert and oriented. As he answers your questions, you find that he cannot complete a full sentence without catching his breath. You find his airway open and clear, his breathing somewhat rapid but adequate, and his pulse rapid. As you check the pulse at the wrist, you find that his skin is moist and a bit cool.

1. What interventions would this patient receive as part of the initial assessment?

2. Is this patient going to receive a high or low priority for transport?

3. Would this patient benefit from your calling advanced life support (ALS) to the scene or meeting a paramedic en route?

The patient's history includes prior heart attacks and diabetes. He tells you he awoke with difficulty breathing and cannot seem to catch his breath. You prepare the stair chair and move the patient to the ambulance. As you get the patient settled into the ambulance for the trip to the hospital, you observe that his difficulty in breathing has worsened. He now tries to talk but finds saying anything very difficult. His respirations have become faster and shallower. He appears a bit sleepy.

1. How would you respond to the patient's change in condition?

Active Exploration

Aside from safety, the initial assessment is arguably the most important component of the entire patient assessment. The primary objective of the initial assessment is to identify and treat all life-threatening problems, period. At no time will you proceed on to the SAMPLE history or any physical exam if something within the initial assessment needs attention. There will be many times, in fact, when you will spend the entire time from the moment you arrive at the scene until handing the patient over to the emergency department staff managing problems found in the initial assessment. What does it matter that the patient has a possible fractured extremity if you are unable to keep the airway clear of fluids? Your priority is always the initial assessment and the elements of airway, breathing, circulation, and bleeding. Once these elements have been adequately addressed, then, and only then, will you focus on less critical components of the patient assessment. The following activities will help you learn the components of and develop your skills relating to the initial assessment.

Activity 1: Done in 60 Seconds

This activity is designed to reinforce the elements of the initial assessment and to help the student complete the assessment in under 60 seconds.

Grab two fellow students for this activity. One of you will play the EMT-B and step out of the room for a moment. The other two must develop a scenario that requires emergency care being provided during the initial assessment. Keep it simple but include things that *must* be addressed in the initial assessment.

For instance, tell the EMT-B he is responding to a man down in an alley. The scene is safe. Have the "patient" lying faceup and unresponsive. Have him hold his breath as the EMT-B enters and begins the assessment.

The goal is to have the EMT-B recognize that the "patient" is not breathing and provide the indicated emergency care. You can decide ahead of time that if the EMT-B determines that the "patient" is not breathing and opens the airway, the "patient" will immediately begin breathing.

You can conduct the same scenario with the "patient" facedown to reinforce the skill of conducting an initial assessment in the facedown position.

You can use other elements such as noisy respirations, weak or slow pulse (just have the observer state the pulse is 40 and weak when the EMT-B assesses the pulse), varying levels of responsiveness, simulated bleeding, and so on.

Have the observer time the assessment and provide feedback on the performance. Your goal is to address all the elements of the initial assessment and provide the indicated emergency care in less than 60 seconds.

Activity 2: Who am I?

A common assessment tool used to describe a patient's level of responsiveness is the A&O scale: "A" standing for "Alert" and "O" standing for "Oriented." There are four levels to the A&O scale, and they are as follows:

- X 1 = Oriented to person (who he is)
- X 2 = Oriented to person and place
- X 3 = Oriented to person, place, and time
- X 4 = Oriented to person, place, time, and event

A person who is conscious and alert can be described as A&O x 4. A person who knows who he is and where he is but is unsure of what time it is and what happened would be described as A&O x 2.

For this activity, have one person play patient and decide in advance his A&O status on the basis of this scale. Have the other person play EMT-B and conduct an initial assessment including level of responsiveness. The goal is for the EMT-B to accurately identify the patient's status using the A&O scale.

RETRO REVIEW

1. The oropharyngeal airway is measured from the _____.
   A. tip of the mouth to the Adam's apple
   B. tip of the nose to the angle of the jaw
   C. corner of the mouth to the tip of the earlobe
   D. corner of the mouth to the larynx

2. Which of the following would not be considered a component of negligence?
   A. A duty to act existed.
   B. The patient suffered psychological harm.
   C. The EMT acted outside of his scope of practice.
   D. The EMT acted within protocols.

3. A device that would be used to carry patients a distance over rough terrain is the _____.
   A. Reeves stretcher   B. stair chair
   C. wheeled stretcher   D. Stokes basket

THINKING AND LINKING

CHAPTER TOPIC	HOW IT RELATES TO YOU AND OTHER COURSE AREAS
The initial assessment	Every patient gets one.
The general impression	This may seem vague to you now, but it is very important. Trauma patients with multiple injuries or a significant MOI and medical patients who are very sick will be more obvious if you look for clues when you approach. Experienced providers usually can identify serious patients from a distance. Identifying potentially critical patients early sets the foundation for the remainder of the call. Your book, class work, instructor, and ride time will help you identify critical patients when you see them.
The ABCs	Performed on each patient, in that order. The ABCs actually combine material from many chapters in the book involving protecting the spine, mental status, airway, breathing, oxygen administration, circulation, bleeding control, treating chest wounds, and more. The initial assessment and the ABCs are a critical part of the assessment process.

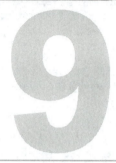

CHAPTER 9

Vital Signs and SAMPLE History

CHAPTER SUMMARY

Vital signs taken after your initial assessment and then periodically through-out the emergency call allow you to better identify subtle changes, good or bad, in your patient. Obtaining a medical history, including the events lead-ing up to the need for EMS response, can help you determine appropriate emergency care for your patient. These two components of your focused his-tory and physical exam (FHPE) should be obtained as soon as you have completed your initial assessment and addressed any immediate life-threats.

Vital signs are indicators of your patient's condition that you can measure. They include pulse, respirations, skin signs, pupils, and blood pressure. The first set of vital signs you obtain is called the baseline vital signs. You will compare all subsequent vital-sign findings to the baseline set during the call to see whether your patient's condition is changing. It is also very important to assess mental status, even though it is not considered a vital sign.

Assess the patient's pulse for rate, rhythm, and quality. A healthy adult pulse rate is between 60 to 100 beats per minute. It should be regular and easy to palpate. You should first attempt to locate a radial pulse, in the wrist above the thumb. In infants (children younger than 1 year old) use the brachial pulse in the upper arm. If neither a radial or brachial pulse can be felt, use the carotid pulse in the neck. Count the pulse for 30 seconds and multiply by 2. If the pulse is irregular, count for a full 60 seconds. You should be con-cerned if an adult's pulse rate stays above 100 or below 60 beats per minute.

Assess the patient's breathing for rate, rhythm, and quality. An adult at rest should breathe between 12 and 20 breaths per minute. Be concerned about a patient whose respiratory rate stays below 8 or above 24 breaths per minute. Breathing rhythm is typically not a concern in a responsive patient. An unresponsive patient who has an irregular breathing pattern can be in immediate danger. Determine whether the patient's breathing is normal, shallow, labored, or noisy. Breathing should be fairly effortless and quiet. If your patient is struggling to breathe and using accessory muscles, or making noises such as wheezing or gurgling, he is in distress. Count the number of breaths in 30 seconds and multiply by 2 to obtain breaths per minute.

Skin color, condition, and temperature can help you to determine the circulatory status of your patient. You should observe a pink color in a patient's nail beds, inside of the lips, or lower eye lids. Cyanosis, jaundice, or flushed colors indicate problems. Children who are in shock may have a blotchy appearance called "mottling." A patient's skin should be dry, not diaphoretic (sweaty). Capillary refill should be evaluated in children under six. If the nail beds are pressed, the normal color should return in no more than 2 seconds.

A patient's pupils should be assessed for size, reactivity to light, and equality. Pupils should dilate slightly in low light and constrict when bright light is shone at the eye. Pupils should react equally and be the same size.

Blood pressure is measured early in your patient assessment and periodically throughout the emergency call. The systolic pressure is the pressure exerted on the vessel walls when the left ventricle is contracting. The diastolic pressure is the pressure that remains in the vessels when the left ventricle is not contracting and is refilling. Blood pressure is measured in millimeters of mercury (mmHg). For adults up to 40 years of age, you can estimate an acceptable systolic blood pressure: For men, add 100 to their age. For women, add 90 to their age. Normal diastolic pressures range from 60 to 90 mmHg. Typically, systolic pressures below 90 mmHg are considered seriously low. Systolic pressures above 150 and diastolic pressures above 90 mmHg are considered high blood pressure.

Blood pressure can be obtained by two methods. Auscultation is when a stethoscope is used to listen for sounds as you deflate the blood-pressure cuff. Palpation is when either the radial or brachial artery is palpated for return of a pulse as you deflate the blood-pressure cuff.

You should take the vital signs of a stable patient every 15 minutes. For an unstable patient, you need to take the vital signs every 5 minutes. You should also obtain vital signs after you perform a medical intervention such as assisting a patient with his inhaler or nitroglycerin.

Each set of vital signs should be documented on your run report including the time they were obtained.

As an EMT-B, you will also be able to measure the level of oxygen circulating through your patient's circulatory system with a pulse oximeter. This device measures the proportion of oxygen in the blood and displays it as a percentage. Oxygen saturation in a healthy person is generally between 96 and 100 percent. Readings of 91 to 95 percent indicate slight hypoxia, 86 to 90 percent relate to significant hypoxia, and severe hypoxia is indicated by readings of 85 percent or below. It is important to remember that you are utilizing a piece of equipment that can give inaccurate readings. Always treat your patient according to how he is presenting, not from readings off a piece of equipment.

A SAMPLE history is an acronym used to help you remember important information you need to collect from the patient, family, or bystanders.

    S—Signs and Symptoms
    A—Allergies
    M—Medications
    P—Pertinent past history
    L—Last oral intake
    E—Events leading up to the injury or illness

PEARLS FROM THE PODIUM

- One set of vital signs will reveal very little about a patient; you must take several sets to reveal a trend in the patient's condition. Be careful not to get too relaxed just because your baseline vitals appear normal.

- If the scene is too noisy to hear blood pressure well with a stethoscope, use the palpation method. You are better off getting something to use as a baseline rather than nothing at all. Be sure to document properly the fact that you obtained the blood pressure by palpation.

- Remember to use the carotid pulse of the unresponsive patient to assess pulse status. A patient with a low blood pressure may not have a palpable radial pulse.

- Do your best to assess respiratory rate when the patient is not talking and without the patient knowing. This will allow you to get the most accurate value possible.

- Another way of thinking of the quality of respirations is to use rate, depth, and ease as your assessment characteristics. Rate speaks for itself; depth is either deep, shallow, or normal (good tidal volume); and ease can be stated as normal or labored.

- If the environment is well lit, it will be useless to use a light source to assess pupil response. Instead, cover the eye with your hand and allow plenty of time for the pupil to adjust. We suggest you ask at least two to three history questions while covering the eye just to ensure that you give it time to adjust.

- The SAMPLE acronym is only a tool to help you remember what to ask in terms of history. It is not essential that you ask these questions in any specific order.

REVIEW QUESTIONS

SHORT ANSWER

1. Why is it important to obtain vital signs and a SAMPLE history?

2. Once applied to the patient, what information does a pulse oximeter provide?

MULTIPLE CHOICE

1. A snoring sound from the patient's airway indicates that _____ is (are) present.

    A. an obstruction from the tongue

    B. an obstruction from infection

    C. vomitus

    D. secretions

2. The "P" in the acronym "SAMPLE" stands for _____.

    A. Pulse

    B. Pertinent past history

    C. Percentage

    D. Patient

3. Anemia, _____, and certain kinds of poisoning (such as carbon monoxide) can produce false high-oxygen-saturation readings.

   A. hypoglycemia   **B.** hypoperfusion
   C. hypovolemia   **D.** hypoxia

4. When taking a patient's pulse, the two factors you should be concerned with are rate and _____.

   A. depth   **B.** regularity
   C. number of beats per minute   **D.** location

5. Yellow-tinted skin is an indication of _____.

   A. liver abnormalities
   B. lack of oxygen in the red blood cells
   C. congestive heart failure
   D. severe blood loss

SCENARIO QUESTIONS

You are obtaining a SAMPLE history on a 95-year-old Chinese woman. The patient's granddaughter tells you that the patient moved from Beijing about six years ago and has been relatively healthy since the move. After completing your SAMPLE history, you know the following: the patient has abdominal pain, she has no allergies, she currently takes no medication, she has no significant medical history, and she was trying to get out of bed when the pain began.

1. Which letter in the memory aid SAMPLE did you forget during the questioning?

   A. M   **B.** L
   C. E   **D.** S

2. What should you try to do when questioning this patient?

   A. Talk slowly and very loudly.
   B. Speak to the granddaughter and avoid addressing the patient directly.
   C. Ask open-ended questions whenever possible.
   D. Only ask "yes" and "no" type questions.

You are called to a home by a husband because his wife is experiencing shortness of breath. The woman is very embarrassed by the attention and keeps saying that she hopes none of the neighbors see the ambulance. Your partner takes the patient's vital signs and tells you, "Her BP is up there: 142 over 90." The woman's husband says, "She's never had high blood pressure." A few minutes later, after the patient has been on supplemental oxygen, your partner tells you that the patient's blood pressure has dropped to 126/84 and that her pulse has decreased slightly. The patient insists that she feels fine, and you find that her skin is pink, warm, and dry.

1. The current trend of this patient's vital signs most likely indicates _____.

   A. hypoperfusion   **B.** myocardial infarction
   C. temporary stress   **D.** hypertension

2. Your partner is obtaining the patient's blood pressure by _____.

   A. auscultation   **B.** brachial gradation
   C. pedal constriction   **D.** palpation

CASE STUDIES

You are dispatched 45 minutes away to a person who has had a fall. Upon your arrival, you find an approximately 30-year-old male who has fallen from a second-story roof. He responds to verbal stimuli and according to witnesses was unresponsive for at least 10 minutes following the fall. A local volunteer firefighter is on the scene and provides you with a set of vital signs taken approximately 20 minutes after the fall. These are blood pressure 110/72; pulse 92, strong, and regular; respirations 16, shallow, and unlabored; skin pink, warm, and dry; and pupils equal and reactive.

1. **What conclusions can you draw based on the patient's baseline vital signs?**

2. **What additional history might you want to obtain? From whom will you try and get it?**

You determine that the man has a good airway and that he is breathing adequately although shallowly. You decide to place him on oxygen by nonrebreather mask at 15 lpm and obtain a second set of vital signs. They are as follows: blood pressure 90/60, pulse 112, respirations 24 and shallow. His skin signs are pale, cool, and clammy and his pupils are responsive but sluggish.

1. **Why do you think this man's second set of vital signs are different from the baseline set?**

2. **How often will you want to take additional sets of vital signs and why?**

You are called to a 78-year-old man in a nursing facility who is complaining of shortness of breath. You arrive to find the patient in a bed by the window. He greets you with a quick joke and a smile. You notice that in between the words of his joke, he stops to catch his breath. He denies having problems today, but this is contradicted by the nurse who enters the room and tells him that he is going to the hospital for shortness of breath. She says, "He has COPD and his stats are down." She hands you a big pile of paperwork and leaves the room.

1. **What have you learned about the patient's history up to this point?**

2. How can you obtain additional information?

3. What does the low oxygen saturation mean?

4. How reliable will the history the patient provides you be?

5. Using the OPQRST mnemonic, what other questions would you ask to gain additional pertinent information?

6. What parts of the SAMPLE history do you still need?

Active Exploration

As a student, you should be getting lots of practice taking vital signs on healthy people, your fellow classmates. While this is important and necessary to help develop your vital-sign skills, it does not provide much of a variety. This exercise will expose you to vital signs that are somewhat out of the norm and help you develop skills associated with trending a patient's vital signs.

Activity 1: Take a Hike

If possible, select someone whom you have not had the experience of taking vitals on before. This way you cannot anticipate what he might be. Now follow these steps:

1. Take a complete set of baseline vitals and record them on a piece of paper along with the time.
2. Send your "patient" for a run. Have them run a reasonable distance or up and down some stairs, long enough to get their pulse above 100 beats per minute.
3. When they have done so, have them quickly lie down and take another set of vital signs. In the interest of time, you may focus on the blood pressure, pulse, and respirations. Record these next to the baseline set.
4. Wait 5 minutes and take another set and record them along with the others.
5. Continue taking sets of vital signs about every 5 minutes until the vitals have returned to normal.
6. Now compare all the vital signs, and see whether you can identify a pattern.

This exercise is terrific for building your vital-sign skills and can be done either in or out of class. You can do this as often as you like and on as many different people as possible. We suggest that you keep a log of people you have completed this exercise with and compare everyone's results. Make note of the person's age and whether there is any pertinent medical history.

Activity 2: A Quart Low

This next exercise is used to develop a skill used commonly in the clinical setting and occasionally in the field setting. Regardless of whether it is commonly used in your area or not, it is an excellent tool for building your vital-sign skills.

Note that this is merely an assessment. Taking "orthostatic" vital signs is an assessment tool used to identify a patient who may be low on fluid volume (hypovolemic). These patients often present with a general feeling of weakness, light-headedness or dizziness, and of just not feeling well. There may be a history of nausea and vomiting that has led to mild dehydration. Follow these steps to complete a set of "orthostatic" vital signs:

1. Obtain and record a complete set of baseline vital signs with the patient in the lying-faceup (supine) position.
2. Assist the patient to a sitting position and allow his body to adjust for a minute or so, then take and record another blood pressure reading and pulse.
3. Assist the patient into the standing position and allow his body to adjust for a minute or so, then take and record another blood pressure reading and pulse.
4. Allow the patient to return to a position of comfort and compare the vitals signs.

A general rule of thumb for orthostatic vitals is when there is a change of at least 20 points in readings of either of the blood pressure readings (systolic or diastolic) or the pulse, the patient is said to be "orthostatic." In a patient who is orthostatic, you should anticipate a drop in blood pressure and an increase in pulse rate when they move from a supine position to a standing position. It is an important tool that can be used when you suspect that a patient might be low on fluid volume. It is NOT a diagnostic tool. This is also a great way to practice your vital-sign skills and your ability to evaluate readings with a critical eye.

RETRO REVIEW

1. The pelvic socket into which the ball at the proximal end of the femur fits to form the hip joint is called the _____.
   A. acromion
   B. calcaneus
   C. dorsalis
   D. acetabulum
2. The EMT-B's primary ethical consideration is to make patient emergency care and well-being a priority, even if this requires some _____.
   A. personal sacrifice
   B. specialized training
   C. advanced planning
   D. financial assistance
3. What is an important rule of airway suctioning?
   A. Suction for no more than 20 seconds.
   B. Always use appropriate infection control practices.
   C. Never use a rigid tip for pediatric patients.
   D. Only activate suction while withdrawing the catheter.

THINKING AND LINKING

CHAPTER TOPIC	HOW IT RELATES TO YOU AND OTHER COURSE AREAS
Blood pressure	Changes in a patient's blood pressure can be very significant, whether caused by vessel dilation—as in the case of anaphylaxis (explained in Chapter 20)—or simply a lack of fluid volume (see severe bleeding in Chapter 26). Just remember that it is usually a *late* indicator of trouble.
Oxygen saturation	Obtaining a patient's oxygen saturation percentage (SpO^2) can provide valuable information regarding the effectiveness of oxygen therapy or artificial ventilations (both covered in Chapter 6). Do not forget that certain types of poisoning (e.g. carbon monoxide—explained in Chapter 21), shock (Chapter 26), and hypothermia (an environmental emergency covered in Chapter 22) can all cause inaccurate SpO^2 readings.
Medications	It is very important to get a *complete* list of patient medications during the SAMPLE history. Even though many of the drug names may mean little to you as an EMT-B (although you will get a basic drug overview when you reach Chapter 15), the information that you gather will greatly assist advanced life support (ALS) or hospital personnel. Many elderly patients will have very extensive lists of prescribed medications. (You will learn more about dealing with older patients in Chapter 32.) It can be a good idea to have the patient's spouse begin compiling a list of the prescription medications (or actually gathering the bottles) while you are completing the patient assessment.

10

Assessment of the Trauma Patient

CHAPTER SUMMARY

Focus. That is the key to performing an effective assessment of the trauma patient. It allows you to balance between spending too much time at the scene and neglecting to provide effective emergency care in your rush to transport. For trauma patients, it is essential that you are able to quickly pinpoint, or assess, their needs.

The word trauma simply means "injury" and injuries can range from cut fingers to massive, fatal wounds. Often, the extent of an injury cannot be determined in the prehospital setting, as in the case of an internal injury. That is why it is imperative that you identify the mechanism of injury (MOI), which is simply the force(s) that caused the injury.

Immediately after completing an initial assessment of the trauma patient, you will move into the focused history and physical exam. The way you proceed from there will be directed by the significance of the MOI.

If you have determined that a particular MOI is not significant, the first thing to do is *reconsider*. Always reconsider the MOI and its potential effects on the patient. Can it be worse than you thought? Is there something that you are not seeing? If you still believe that the MOI is not significant (and there are no immediate life-threats), you can simplify the focused history and physical exam—and spend additional time at the scene. Focus your exam on the patient's chief complaint and areas where you believe, based on the MOI, injuries may have occurred. You should include baseline vitals and a SAMPLE history along with your physical examination.

You will examine patients in two ways—by visual inspection and by touch, called *palpation*. You will be looking for contusions, abrasions, punctures, penetrations, burns, and lacerations and palpating for deformities, tenderness, and swelling. An easy way to remember what to check for is by using the mnemonic DCAP-BTLS (pronounced *Dee-Cap B-T-L-S*).

Deformities are body parts that no longer hold their normal shape, such as with a displaced fracture. Contusions are bruises. Abrasions, a very common injury, are scrapes. Punctures or penetrations are holes in the body that can be caused by sharp objects or projectiles. Burns have many appearances, from slightly red to black and charred. Tenderness means there is pain during pressure such as palpation. Lacerations are cuts. Swelling is caused by injured capillaries bleeding under the skin.

Since you cannot evaluate what you cannot see, it will be necessary to remove or cut away any clothing over the areas that you are assessing. Explain this process to patients, reassure them, and protect their privacy. Also ensure that they are not unnecessarily exposed to the elements.

If you suspect a spinal injury (based on MOI, patient complaint, or your own assessment), immediately apply manual in-line stabilization of the patient's head and neck, apply a cervical collar, and utilize a spinal immobilization device. Sizing the collar correctly will prevent problems such as excessive neck movement and breathing difficulty—this is especially critical with pediatric patients. Complete your initial assessment and take care of any life-threats before applying a cervical collar. You should also palpate the back of the neck, reassure the patient, remove any necklaces or earrings, and maintain manual stabilization until the patient is completely secured to a backboard.

If your assessment findings indicate that the patient is a high priority for transport, or if there is a significant MOI, you should ensure manual stabilization of the head and neck, consider summoning advanced-life-support (ALS) assistance, reassess the patient's mental status, and perform a rapid head-to-toe trauma assessment.

Examples of significant MOIs are ejection from a vehicle or being in the same passenger compartment as a fatally injured person. When vehicle collisions are responsible for injuries, it is important to inspect the entire vehicle to look for clues regarding the severity of the MOI. Was there intrusion into the passenger compartment? Is the windshield deformed and could the deformity have been caused by your patient's head? Make sure you lift any deployed airbags and inspect the steering wheel and dashboard for any deformities that may indicate an impact.

Never underestimate the possibility of "hidden injuries," which can become serious—even fatal—in the hours and days following a crash. Seat belts, for example, are common causes of internal abdominal injuries. Be especially alert with pediatric patients, as it takes much less force to cause severe injuries in children and infants.

As you prepare to complete a rapid trauma assessment on the patient with a significant MOI, remember that you will be using many senses, not just your eyes. You will touch to find swelling and tenderness, listen for airway problems or broken bones (crepitation), and smell for hazardous fumes, urine, feces, or vomitus.

The rapid trauma assessment itself should only take a couple of minutes and can be invaluable in finding life-threats that you missed during your initial assessment or injuries that could quickly become dangerous to your patient's life. You should follow the same systematic approach on *every* rapid trauma assessment to ensure that you do not miss a potentially serious condition.

Check the patient's head, neck, chest, abdomen, pelvis, extremities, and back (in that order) for DCAP-BTLS as well as other signs and symptoms specific to those locations (e.g. paradoxical chest movement, priapism, abdominal rigidity, and so on).

Always tell the patient what you are doing and try to maintain eye contact while asking questions or listening to answers. Assume spinal injury in all trauma cases involving impacts to the upper body or head and when the MOI is a significant fall.

The next step in the emergency care of the trauma patient, after the initial assessment and the rapid trauma assessment, is the *detailed physical exam.* A detailed physical exam can be completed at the scene (for lower-priority patients) or en route to the hospital. Although detailed physical exams are usually limited to trauma patients with significant (or unknown) MOIs, you can complete one on any trauma patient if you have a suspicion that there may be other, hidden injuries. You will be repeating, and expanding upon, the same steps that you followed during the rapid trauma assessment, except that as you examine the patient's head, neck, chest, abdomen, pelvis, extremities, and posterior body, you will be moving slower—assessing more extensively. You will also add examinations of the face, ears, eyes, nose, and mouth. Remember that responsive trauma patients will need comfort and reassurance.

You will conclude your detailed physical exam by reassessing the patient's vital signs and notifying the receiving emergency facility of the patient's condition. At this point, you may also have the opportunity to splint any extremity fractures or deformities that you were not able to take care of at the scene.

Detailed physical exams are generally not used for medical patients because there are very few items of significance that you as an EMT-B will be able to find—and even less that you can do about them. Chief complaints, histories, and vital signs should be your main focus when assessing medical patients.

What if you come across an unresponsive individual that could conceivably be a medical patient or a trauma patient? The safest approach is to assume a trauma and complete your rapid trauma assessment followed by a detailed physical if you have the time. Also, try to obtain a history from any potential witnesses.

PEARLS FROM THE PODIUM

- It is easy to be distracted by the sight of open wounds and deformities. Try not to let these things distract you from your priorities.

- Remember to carefully evaluate the mechanism of injury for all trauma patients as this will help you anticipate internal injuries.

- Trauma patients should be treated on the basis of the MOI and not on the presence or absence of pain.

- When deciding whether a patient has suffered a significant MOI, ask yourself whether the patient has suffered an injury to the head, torso, or pelvis, areas that can easily hide internal bleeding. These patients must receive a rapid trauma assessment. A patient can suffer what might be seen as a significant MOI, but if it only affects an arm or leg, it is not likely to involve injury to internal organs. This is actually considered a nonsignificant MOI because it does not involve multiple body systems.

- When treating unresponsive patients with an unknown MOI, assume they may have a spinal injury and treat them accordingly.

REVIEW QUESTIONS

SHORT ANSWER

1. Which senses should you be using while performing a rapid trauma assessment?

2. Under what circumstances would it be appropriate to apply a cervical collar?

MULTIPLE CHOICE

1. Visible neck veins while the patient is lying supine commonly indicate _____.
   - **A.** jugular vein distention
   - **B.** accessory muscle use
   - **C.** traumatic asphyxiation
   - **D.** normal circulation

2. Which of the following should be your first step when treating a patient with a possible spinal injury?
   - **A.** Sizing and applying a cervical collar.
   - **B.** Assessing for extremity sensation and motor function.
   - **C.** Manually stabilizing the patient's head and neck.
   - **D.** Moving the patient onto a spine board.

3. What causes initial swelling in trauma-related injuries?
   - **A.** Damaged capillaries.
   - **B.** Steady contractions of torn muscle tissue.
   - **C.** The release of histamine and heparin into the tissues.
   - **D.** Severe dilation of the blood vessels.

4. Bruising behind the ear of a trauma patient is called _____ and is a late indication of a skull injury.
   - **A.** a Burdick's mark
   - **B.** Battle's sign
   - **C.** a Murphy bleed
   - **D.** Bowman's sign

5. The *chief complaint* is the primary problem, as determined by _____.
   - **A.** medical direction
   - **B.** the First Responder
   - **C.** EMS guidelines
   - **D.** the patient

SCENARIO QUESTIONS

You arrive at the State College swim center to provide emergency care for a person who has had a fall. You find the patient, a 19-year-old female, responsive but crying and complaining of tremendous back and head pain. Witnesses tell you that the patient had fallen from the top of the 18-foot dive ladder onto the concrete below.

1. You should obtain this patient's baseline vital signs after _____.
   A. the SAMPLE history
   B. initial assessment
   C. the rapid trauma assessment
   D. determining the chief complaint

2. While at the scene of a patient who sustained a significant MOI, you should perform a(n) _____ on this patient.
   A. detailed physical exam   B. rapid trauma assessment
   C. focused trauma physical   D. extended fall evaluation

3. A cervical collar should be applied to this patient _____.
   A. after completing the rapid trauma assessment
   B. as soon as the MOI is identified
   C. as soon as you arrive at the scene
   D. after completing the detailed physical exam

You are treating a patient who was thrown from his motorcycle after striking a car. You have found that the patient has several angulated lower extremity injuries, pelvic and abdominal tenderness, paradoxical chest movement, and diminished right-side breath sounds. En route to the hospital with the patient secured to the backboard, you note flat jugular veins.

1. The assessment findings on this patient indicate _____.
   A. internal bleeding   B. the onset of hyperperfusion
   C. impending respiratory arrest   D. abdominal dissection

2. Paradoxical chest movement is also called "_____ chest."
   A. detached   B. frail
   C. floating   D. flail

3. Diminished breath sounds on one side of the chest are a sign of _____.
   A. pulmonary distention   B. cardiac tamponade
   C. lung collapse   D. intercostal hematoma

CASE STUDIES

CASE STUDY 1   FIRE ON THE SCENE

You are dispatched to a multiple-vehicle crash a few miles outside of town. En route, you have been advised by the law enforcement on the scene that there are multiple patients with one fatality. Once on the scene, you are met by a fire captain who has triaged the patients and directs you to an unresponsive person who was ejected when one of the vehicles rolled over. You approach the patient and find what appears to be a female in her 20s, unresponsive and facedown.

1. What will be your priorities as you begin to assess and provide emergency care for this patient?

2. Will you want to roll this person onto her back? If so, why?

You have rolled the patient faceup and have inserted an OPA and placed her on 15 lpm by nonrebreather mask. She has a weak pulse of around 90 and has not responded to any stimulus so far.

1. Which assessment path do you feel is most appropriate for this patient and why?

2. Will it be necessary to perform a detailed physical on this patient? If so, when will you do it?

CASE STUDY 2   WATCH THAT LAST STEP–IT'S A BIG ONE!

You are called to a shopping mall for a patient who has had a fall. You arrive to find a patient sitting on the ground at the base of the escalators. The scene is safe, and you do not see any BSI hazards. You introduce yourself to the patient. She is alert and oriented. She tells you that she misjudged the last step as she was exiting and "twisted her ankle."

1. Is this a significant or nonsignificant mechanism of injury?

2. Are there injuries you should consider in addition to the ankle?

3. Would this patient receive a rapid trauma exam or a focused exam on the injured area?

4. What signs would indicate that the patient has a more serious problem?

Active Exploration

Patient-assessment skill is the foundation for all prehospital providers beginning with First Responders and moving right up to the Critical Care Nurse. It is safe to say that a poor assessment will almost always lead to poor emergency care and a good assessment will almost always result in good emergency care for the patient. For this reason, it is essential that, as an EMT student, you continually work on developing and improving your patient-assessment skills even once you have completed your training. The following exercises have been developed to do just that.

Activity 1: Hide and Seek

This exercise is best done on someone who is not aware of how it works but can be used as a good exercise even if you have practiced it before. You can use yourself as a patient or, better yet, get a third person to act as a patient.

1. Gather several small to medium-sized items such as an OPA, NPA, hard suction catheter, bite stick, pencil eraser, marker pen, or similar items.

2. Hide two or three items on your body beneath your clothing. It may be helpful to tape them in place so that they do not slip out of place. Place them in the harder-to-reach places such as behind the knee, the small of the back, or on the inside of the upper arm.

3. Now have your partners perform a trauma assessment on you and see whether they detect the hidden items.

It is a real eye-opener when they complete the assessment without finding any of the hidden items. It reinforces just how important it is to use both hands and thoroughly assess all parts of the body for deformity.

Activity 2: The Silent Treatment

This activity is especially good at reinforcing the hands-on aspect of any patient assessment. As EMT students, you often place the majority of emphasis on memorizing the skill sheet and being able to recite it during a skills exam. This often results in EMTs who verbally conduct a patient assessment while standing over the patient and complete the skill without ever touching the patient. This is unacceptable and must be counteracted with an equal emphasis on the physical aspects of the patient assessment.

1. You will act as the observer and carefully watch as your partner performs a trauma assessment on another person.

2. The exam must be performed silently without a word from the student performing the assessment.

3. You will observe the assessment and grade the EMT student on the basis of his ability to perform a thorough physical exam.

The student may want to talk during the exam, but you must remind him to remain silent the entire time. His actions must speak for him, and you should be able to tell what he is doing simply on the basis of what he does and not on what he says.

A variation of this same exercise can be practiced with the student performing the assessment blindfolded.

RETRO REVIEW

1. Bullets cause injuries in two ways: direct projectile damage and _____.
   A. fragmentation   **B.** incineration
   C. cavitation   **D.** blunt trauma

2. When fleeing danger, your best option is to use distance, cover, and _____ to protect yourself.
   A. defensive tactics   **B.** concealment
   C. discarded equipment   **D.** communication

3. A(n) _____ is used to lift a patient with no suspected spine or extremity injuries from a sitting position to a stretcher.
   A. direct carry   **B.** draw-sheet maneuver
   C. short spine board   **D.** extremity lift

THINKING AND LINKING

CHAPTER TOPIC	HOW IT RELATES TO YOU AND OTHER COURSE AREAS
Mechanisms of injury	Mechanisms of injury are either significant or not significant. Trauma patients with a significant MOI (auto rollover, and so on) need to be transported as quickly as possible—as you can never truly stabilize a trauma patient's condition in the field. You will see more about treating and transporting trauma patients once you reach Module 5.
MOI and immobilization	Patients with significant MOIs should always be immobilized under the assumption that a spinal injury has occurred. Let the staff at the receiving hospital rule out spinal injury—you will have neither the equipment nor the expertise to do it in the field.
Rapid assessment	You should complete a rapid trauma assessment on all significant MOI patients prior to leaving the scene. You may discover complications caused by soft-tissue injuries, bleeding, musculoskeletal injuries (Module 5), or even preexisting medical problems (Module 4)—any of which could cause the patient's condition to deteriorate during transport. Having a good overview of the patient's illnesses and/or injuries will assist you in reacting quickly (and effectively) to any complications that arise.

11

Assessment of the Medical Patient

CHAPTER SUMMARY

After you have performed your initial assessment and corrected any life-threats, you will then obtain a focused history and perform a physical exam, when treating a medical patient. The FHPE has four parts: history of the present illness, SAMPLE history, focused physical exam, and baseline vital signs. The order in which these are performed will depend on whether your patient is responsive or unresponsive. Remember that the responsive patient is your best source of information regarding his medical condition.

With a responsive patient, your focused history begins by initiating a conversation with your patient. Ask open-ended questions that will encourage the patient to better describe what he is experiencing. Utilizing the mnemonic **OPQRST** will help you remember many of the most important questions to ask.

- **O**nset
- **P**rovokes
- **Q**uality
- **R**egion/**R**adiation
- **S**everity
- **T**ime

    The next step is to obtain a **SAMPLE** history.

- **S**igns/symptoms
- **A**llergies
- **M**edications
- **P**ertinent past history
- **L**ast oral intake
- **E**vents leading to the illness

A patient may have a prior history related to his present complaint. The following are three common situations that you may encounter where the patient has been prescribed medication by his physician to treat an illness. These are:

- A patient with chest pain who has been prescribed nitroglycerin.
- A patient with difficulty in breathing who has a prescribed inhaler.
- A patient with a specific allergy reaction who has a prescribed epinephrine auto-injector.

As an EMT-B, you may be able to assist these patients with their medications. Once you have determined the chief complaint and obtained the focused history, you can then target your physical exam based on the chief complaint. Obtain baseline vitals, perform any interventions, and prepare to transport your patient.

Your sequence will be slightly different for an unresponsive patient. Since you cannot get history information directly from this patient, you will start with your physical exam and baseline vital signs. Suspect spinal injury with any unwitnessed unresponsive patient and take spinal precautions if necessary. If there are family members or bystanders nearby, you can obtain as much of the patient's history as possible from them. Question them about what happened and whether the patient was complaining of anything prior to the event, and so on. Your physical exam will need to be more detailed because your patient is not able to give you the chief complaint. Your physical exam will be very similar to a rapid trauma assessment. You may discover a medical-identification necklace or bracelet during your physical exam that will provide you with important information. Obtain baseline vital signs, perform any interventions, and prepare your patient for transport.

For all of your patients, you must also consider whether they would benefit from the additional services provided by an ALS provider.

PEARLS FROM THE PODIUM

- Medical patients with vague complaints can be very challenging for new and experienced EMT-Bs alike. Your success with these patients will depend on good history-taking skills.
- Asking questions more than once and in different ways will often reveal important history information. A patient who denies any "medical problems" may reveal more of a history when you ask him whether he is taking any medications and he states that he is taking insulin and a "water pill."
- Your job is to gather the facts, as many as you can find. Resist the temptation to "decide" what the problem is and follow a path that may lead you in a wrong direction.
- It is all right to use the patient's own words when relaying information to the next level of care or when documenting your emergency care. If the patient states that there is a giraffe sitting on his chest, then a giraffe it is.
- The OPQRST mnemonic, similar to the SAMPLE acronym, is a tool to help you remember important history questions. They do not need to be asked in any specific order.

REVIEW QUESTIONS

SHORT ANSWER

1. What are two specific actions that you can take to make gathering a SAMPLE history from a child more productive?

2. Name three examples of medical emergencies where the patients may actually be carrying part of the treatment.

MULTIPLE CHOICE

1. The most commonly used medical-identification devices are necklaces, bracelets, and _____.
   A. wallet cards   B. ankle bracelets
   C. tattoos   D. patches

2. Which one of the following individuals would be considered a *medical* patient?
   A. A man in respiratory distress following an electrical shock
   B. An infant who began vomiting shortly after falling from a chair
   C. A woman suffering an allergic reaction following a bee sting
   D. A boy who has coughed up blood after being struck in the chest by a baseball

3. Which of the following statements with reference to medical patients is false?
   A. Most of the pertinent information you obtain will come from the SAMPLE history.
   B. If the medical patient is unresponsive, you can obtain information from family members or bystanders.
   C. A head-to-toe physical examination is critical for medical patients.
   D. The medications the patient is taking will provide information about the patient's condition.

4. When assessing a responsive medical patient, you will conduct a _____ physical exam.
   A. rapid   B. comprehensive
   C. general   D. focused

5. The question, "Can you describe your pain for me?" would come from which part of the OPQRST mnemonic?
   A. Quality   B. Time
   C. Severity   D. Onset

SCENARIO QUESTIONS

You are dispatched to a local motel where a housekeeping employee found a guest lying unresponsive on the bed in one of the rooms. The patient, a female in her 50s, does not respond to your voice but briefly flutters her eyelids when you rub your knuckles on her sternum. The patient has lost bladder and bowel control, and there is a small amount of vomitus on the pillow.

1. What is your first concern with this patient?
   A. Getting her transported to a medical facility.
   B. Looking for clues to her unresponsiveness.
   C. Ensuring and maintaining an adequate airway.
   D. Looking for signs of drug use or possible overdose.

2. How might you find information about this patient's medical history?
   A. Look in her belongings for an address book and attempt to contact anyone who might know her.
   B. Search for prescription bottles, medical equipment, or medical-identification devices.
   C. Continue trying to obtain a coherent response from the patient.
   D. In this situation, you cannot. Instead, you should focus on transporting her immediately.

You and your partner step off of an elevator in an apartment complex, en route to a call concerning a sick child. A young woman waves you over to her apartment. Once inside, she tells you that her son has been very sick all week and begs you to help. The responsive boy is five years old and you can tell right away that he is not doing well. His mother tells you that he has been very hot and refusing to eat and that he vomits any fluid that he is given.

1. After an initial assessment, which of the following should be quickly performed next to gain information on the patient's condition?
   A. Conduct a rapid physical exam.
   B. Obtain baseline vital signs.
   C. Conduct a focused physical exam.
   D. Gather the history of the present illness.

2. When assessing the child's baseline vital signs, you should check his _____.
   A. respirations, pulse, skin, heart rate, sensations, and pupils
   B. pulse, capillary refill, skin, pupils, motor function, and blood pressure
   C. blood pressure, respirations, capillary refill, pulse, skin, and pupils
   D. capillary refill, skin, respirations, blood pressure, pulse, sensations, and motor function

CASE STUDIES

CASE STUDY 1   THE CHURCH LADY

It is early on a Sunday morning and you are dispatched to a local church for a person who has "difficulty breathing." Upon your arrival, you are directed to the church office where you find an approximately 70-year-old female lying on a couch. One of the people caring for the woman introduces her as Lucille and tells you she started having trouble breathing about 20 minutes ago. As they were walking her into the office, she began to get dizzy and needed to lie down. That was when they called 911.

You introduce yourself to Lucille and ask her how she is feeling. She tells you, with some difficulty, that her chest hurts and that she cannot seem to catch her breath.

1. How will you proceed with your questioning pertaining to her chest pain and difficulty in breathing?

2. What assessment path is most appropriate for Lucille and why?

Lucille states that her difficulty in breathing started first and the pain in her chest began shortly thereafter. She states that she only takes a "water pill" and denies any other prior history.

1. What position do you feel is the best for Lucille and why?

2. What oxygen therapy do you feel is most appropriate for Lucille?

CASE STUDY 2   I'M COUGHING UP A LOT OF BAD STUFF

Your ambulance is dispatched to deal with respiratory distress in a 78-year-old male patient. You arrive at a safe scene and find a male patient sitting up in a chair. His wife tells you that he has difficulty breathing, but he waves her off by saying "She overreacts. I've been coughing up gobs of phlegm. That's all." He proudly displays a tissue with white phlegm and noticeable yellow streaks.

1. What is your initial impression of the patient?

2. What do you think about the conflicting reports between the patient and his wife?

3. What role does the pulse oximeter play in determining the need for oxygen?

4. How much oxygen would you give this patient? By which device?

5. Is this patient a high or low priority for immediate transport?

6. What other questions would you ask as part of the SAMPLE history?

7. During transportation, what position do you think he would likely find most comfortable?

Active Exploration

Medical patients offer a challenge that is quite different from that of the trauma patient. With the trauma patient, the EMT-B can use the mechanism of injury to provide clues to the types of injuries likely to be found. With the medical patient, the clues are much harder to find and can become nearly impossible if the patient is unconscious. As an EMT-B, you must develop good history-taking skills in order to master the assessment of the medical patient. The following activities will help you develop these skills.

Activity 1: What's Wrong With Me?

You will need your book and a fellow student for this activity. To prepare, each of you should quickly write down the signs and symptoms of a particular medical complaint such as stroke, heart attack, insulin shock, appendicitis, and so on. Use your book and any other resources you may have at hand. It is best to use a 3 × 5 card to write the ailment on one side and the signs and symptoms on the other side.

Now sitting back to back, one of you must ask the other "yes" or "no" questions in an attempt to determine the specific medical problem. The goal is to identify the medical complaint using the fewest questions.

Activity 2: Fill in the Blanks

For the most part, the assessment path (head-to-toe sequence) that you are to perform in the field will be very similar regardless of whether the patient has an illness or an injury. What is different will be what you might be looking for during each phase of the assessment. Working with a fellow student, practice the following activity:

1. Decide who will play "coach" and who will play "student."
2. Using the worksheet provided, and beginning at the top of the worksheet moving down, the coach will state the item or area of the assessment.
3. The student must verbally describe what is to be done or assessed in detail for that specific area of the assessment.

4. The coach must write down in the space provided what the student verbalizes.
5. Once you have progressed through the entire assessment, share the sheet with the student and discuss any deficiencies.

An alternative to this method is for the solo student to simply complete the blank worksheet and compare it with the answer sheet provided.

The worksheet and answer sheet do not represent complete and total assessments. These are merely to be used as learning aids and a beginning point for learning this skill. Your instructor may wish to add or delete items of the worksheet as appropriate.

WORKSHEET FOR FILL-IN-THE-BLANKS ACTIVITY

PATIENT ASSESSMENT - MEDICAL

SCENE SIZE-UP	ACTION/VERBAL RESPONSE
* *Assess scene safety* (CRITICAL CRITERIA)	
Determine nature of illness	
Determine number of patients	
Assess need for additional help	
Take cervical spine precautions as necessary	

INITIAL ASSESSMENT	ACTION/VERBAL RESPONSE
Verbalize general impression of patient	
Determine responsiveness/ level of consciousness	
Determine chief complaint	
Identify apparent life threats	
* *Assess airway/initiate appropriate airway management* (CRITICAL CRITERIA)	
* *Assess breathing/initiate appropriate oxygen therapy* (CRITICAL CRITERIA)	
* *Assess circulation* (CRITICAL CRITERIA)	
* *Assess and control severe bleeding* (CRITICAL CRITERIA)	
Assess skin signs	
State priority of patient for transport	

DETERMINE APPROPRIATE ASSESSMENT PATH	FOCUSED HISTORY-PHYSICAL or RAPID MEDICAL ASSESSMENT
Perform focused history and physical examination or if indicated complete rapid medical assessment	

Signs and Symptoms (assess history of present illness)	
"**O**" - Onset	
"**P**" - Provocation	
"**Q**" - Quality	
"**R**" - Region/Radiation	
"**S**" - Severity	
"**T**" - Time	
Allergies	
Medications	
Past pertinent history	
Last oral intake	
Event leading to present illness (rule out trauma)	
Vital Signs	
Interventions	
Transport (reevaluate the transport decision)	

Detailed Physical Exam	
Head	
Face	
Eyes	
Ears	
Nose	
Mouth	
Neck	
Chest	
Abdomen	
Pelvis	
Legs	
Arms	
Back	

ONGOING ASSESSMENT	
Repeat initial assessment	
Obtain secondary vital signs and compare with baseline	
Repeat focused assessment regarding patient complaint or injuries	

RETRO REVIEW

1. Never delay oxygen to a(n) _____ patient in order to obtain an accurate pulse oximeter reading.
   A. elderly
   B. respiratory distress
   C. medical
   D. emotionally disturbed
2. The minimum flow rate for a nonrebreather mask is _____.
   A. 8 lpm
   B. 2 lpm
   C. 6 lpm
   D. 4 lpm
3. Significant changes to the record keeping, storage, access, and discussion of patient-specific medical information were the result of _____.
   A. NAFTA
   B. the Dell-Franklin Act
   C. HIPAA
   D. HR252(a)

THINKING AND LINKING

CHAPTER TOPIC	HOW IT RELATES TO YOU AND OTHER COURSE AREAS
Medical ID devices	In addition to common methods of displaying medical information (necklaces, bracelets, anklets, wallet cards, and so on) some patients will use not-so-common methods—such as tattoos.
	The most common items that you will find on medical ID devices are: allergies (covered more in Chapter 20) and preexisting medical conditions like asthma (Chapter 16), heart problems (Chapter 17), and diabetes (Chapter 19).
Known vs. no known history	If your patient is already aware of what is causing his medical emergency, there is a chance that he may also possess the treatment (e.g., an epinephrine auto-injector for a severe allergic reaction—see Chapters 15 and 20 for more details).
	Remember, you should always consider medical emergencies with no known cause as high priorities for transport.
Unresponsive patients	If you are treating an unresponsive medical patient, keep in mind that there may be trauma injuries present also. There is always the potential for head and spine injuries (Chapter 29) with patients who fall after becoming unconscious.
	You will also need to maintain the airway for any unresponsive patient and always anticipate the need for suctioning (review Chapter 6).

CHAPTER

12

Ongoing Assessment

CHAPTER SUMMARY

So, you effectively assessed the patient at the scene and took the appropriate steps to minimize any life-threatening conditions. Does that mean your job as an EMT-B is done? Far from it! Continual reassessment of the patient is critical because unnoticed changes in condition, whether gradual or rapid, can have disastrous consequences.

The ongoing assessment is a tool used to detect changes in a patient's condition after the detailed physical exam. These changes may be obvious, like sudden unresponsiveness, or very subtle, such as restlessness, anxiety, or sweating.

The cycle of ongoing assessments begins after you have resolved any life-threatening problems and, when possible, completed the physical exam. You should never neglect the ongoing assessment process unless you are focused solely on life-saving interventions—in which case your partner could complete the assessments. As a general rule, ongoing assessments should be completed every 5 minutes for unstable patients (altered mental status, difficulty with respirations, airway concerns, severe blood loss, and so on) and every 15 minutes for stable patients. If you suspect that a patient's condition has changed, repeat the initial assessment as soon as possible to evaluate for any new or recurring life-threats.

If your patient is responsive, be aware that he may be feeling anxious or embarrassed en route to the hospital. You should clearly explain all procedures and speak in a reassuring tone. Try to stay at a pediatric patient's level and maintain eye contact.

During the ongoing assessment, you will be repeating the initial and focused assessments while obtaining new vital signs for comparison (pulse, respirations, blood pressure, skin, and pupils). Always write down the patient's vital signs and the time you take them. You will also take the opportunity to evaluate the effectiveness of any interventions that you have performed. When evaluating interventions, do it objectively—as if you had never seen the patient before—and make adjustments as necessary. Just because an intervention was effective initially does not mean that it will continue to be so and equipment may malfunction or be displaced. Continually check oxygen levels, masks, tubing, bandages, splints, backboard straps, and so on.

Remember, the initial assessment is the step where you look for life-threatening problems by checking the patient's mental status, airway, breathing, pulse, and skin signs. Life-threats may develop or recur before the patient reaches the hospital.

You should consider several specific differences when treating infants and children. The mental status of unresponsive pediatric patients can be checked by shouting or flicking their feet—with crying being an acceptable response. When assessing circulation, remember to check for a two-second capillary refill time. For infants with very small nail beds, you can check for capillary refill on the back of a hand or on the top of a foot.

As you repeat the focused assessment, you may find injuries or conditions that you did not notice the first time. Initiate interventions as needed.

By completing ongoing assessments and documenting the patient's changes over time (a process called "trending"), you will be able to see the general progress of a patient—whether improving, deteriorating, or staying the same. Always relay the patient's trend (including accurate vital signs) to receiving medical personnel.

PEARLS FROM THE PODIUM

- The ongoing assessment is performed every 5 minutes for an unstable patient and every 15 minutes for a stable patient.
- Ongoing assessments are how repeated vital signs are obtained. This provides trends.
- Trends in vital signs give more accurate information than any individual set of vital signs.
- The ongoing assessment rechecks the ABCs, checks the effectiveness of interventions you have performed, and reevaluates the patient's chief complaint.
- During transportation, you may find that a splint has loosened or an oxygen tank is near empty and must be switched. This is why assessments are ongoing throughout the call.

REVIEW QUESTIONS

SHORT ANSWER

1. What does "trending" mean?

2. What are the four components of an ongoing assessment?

MULTIPLE CHOICE

1. When may you skip the ongoing assessment?
   A. When you are performing life-saving interventions.
   B. When the patient is alert and very stable.
   C. When the receiving facility is less than 10 minutes away.
   D. All of the above.

2. Repeat the ongoing assessment every _____ minutes for an unstable patient.
   A. 15   B. 7
   C. 5   D. 10

3. You can check the mental status of an infant by shouting or _____.
   A. rubbing the sternum
   B. poking the palms with a hard object
   C. making eye contact
   D. flicking the feet

SCENARIO QUESTIONS

There are no ALS units available, so your Basic Life Support (BLS) ambulance is dispatched to a cardiac-arrest call. You arrive to find a pulseless and apneic 62-year-old female. You initiate CPR and attach the AED. After two sets of stacked shocks, the patient regains a pulse but does not begin breathing on her own. As you transport the patient to the hospital 25 minutes away, you continue providing positive-pressure ventilations with high-concentration oxygen and checking her pulse.

1. Which of the statements in regard to the ongoing assessment of this patient is false?
   A. Nothing would be assessed in an ongoing fashion.
   B. The ongoing assessment would assess the adequacy of positive-pressure ventilations.
   C. The pulse would be checked to ensure that CPR is not required.
   D. The oxygen tubing and cylinder would be checked to ensure that the patient was receiving oxygen.

2. How many full sets of vital signs should you be able to complete before reaching the hospital?
   A. one   B. three
   C. none   D. five

You are en route to the hospital with an unresponsive 3-month-old male. Respirations and pulse are currently present and adequate. Prior to your arrival, a neighbor had provided chest thrusts and removed an object from the child's airway, at which time the child had spontaneously resumed breathing. He has yet to regain consciousness.

1. When checking capillary refill, if the infant's nail beds are too small, you should _____.
   A. press on the back of his hand
   B. use the skin color alone to assess circulation
   C. press on the sole of his foot
   D. gently pinch the earlobe

2. At what point during the ongoing assessment would you discover that the infant's airway is no longer patent?
   A. When repeating the focused assessment.
   B. When repeating the initial assessment.
   C. While reassessing vital signs.
   D. While performing the detailed physical exam.

C A S E   S T U D I E S

CASE STUDY 1   LIGHTS ARE ON BUT NOBODY'S HOME

You are treating a possible stroke patient and have completed your focused medical and detailed physical exam. Your patient is a 69-year-old male who was sitting at home when his wife noticed that he was staring off into space and was unable to respond verbally.

Upon your arrival, the patient was sitting semi-Fowler's in a recliner, awake and unable to respond verbally. His blood pressure is 190 over 98; pulse 88, weak, and regular; respirations 10 and shallow, skin pale, warm, and dry; and pupils equal and sluggish.

1. **What concerns you most about this patient based on his presentation so far, and what will you be concerned with as you begin to transport?**

2. **What interventions will you initiate for this patient and what is the best position for transport?**

You have placed him on oxygen, moved him to the stretcher, and placed him in the recovery position. You wheel him out to the ambulance for a 25-minute ride to the hospital.

1. **What will your ongoing assessment consist of for this patient?**

2. **What will you do if after 5 minutes on oxygen his skin signs remain poor and he is getting less responsive?**

Look at the following sets of vital signs. For each set, look for trends and changes. Match the vital-sign changes with the situations below that cause them. In this exercise, consider all patients to be healthy adults before this event.

This exercise will require some research throughout your Emergency Care textbook.

A. Normal vital signs (no illness or injury)
B. Developing shock (patient bleeding internally)
C. Head injury (increasing pressure on the brain)
D. Uninjured patient in a car crash who was very nervous, then calmed down

1. _____
   P: 104 R: 24 BP: 138/86 Pupils: equal/react Skin: warm/dry
   P: 88 R: 16 BP: 120/76 Pupils: equal/react Skin: warm/dry
   P: 86 R: 16 BP: 122/78 Pupils: equal/react Skin: warm/dry

2. _____
   P: 76 R: 12 BP: 116/68 Pupils: equal/react Skin: warm/dry
   P: 80 R: 12 BP: 120/72 Pupils: equal/react Skin: warm/dry
   P: 80 R: 14 BP: 120/70 Pupils: equal/react Skin: warm/dry

3. _____
   P: 84 R: 16 BP: 124/64 Pupils: equal/react Skin: warm/dry
   P: 92 R: 22 BP: 126/68 Pupils: equal/react Skin: cool/dry
   P: 108 R: 24 BP: 120/60 Pupils: equal/react Skin: cool/moist

4. _____
   P: 72 R: 14 BP: 140/86 Pupils: equal/react Skin: warm/dry
   P: 68 R: 18 BP: 152/88 Pupils: equal/react Skin: warm/dry
   P: 56 R: 10 BP: 192/92 Pupils: react/sluggish Skin: cool/dry

Active Exploration

The work of an EMT-B is never done. From the moment you first make patient contact to the moment care of the patient is handed over to the next level of provider, you should be continuously monitoring and evaluating your patient. Sometimes it means that you are in the face of an unresponsive patient listening for breathing and watching for adequacy of chest rise. At other times, it may be a casual conversation as you gather history information on the way to the hospital. No matter what the situation, you must realize and remain conscious of the fact that every time you look at or speak to a patient you are treating, you are assessing his condition.

The last component of both the medical and trauma patient assessments is called the ongoing assessment. This is where the EMT-B reassesses the ABCs, vital signs, and the effectiveness of any interventions that have been initiated. The following activities are designed to help reinforce the importance of the ongoing assessment as part of your overall patient assessment.

Activity 1: Ongoing Street Scenes

Using your Emergency Care textbook, turn to any one of the "Street Scenes" sections at the end of one of the chapters. Read the scenario presented and answer the following questions relating to the ongoing assessment of the patient described in the scenario.

- Describe how you will reassess the ABCs of the patient.

- When you reassess vital signs, will you expect them to be the same or different? Why?

- If you think they are going to be different, what are they likely to be?

- What are you likely to find on the repeat of the focused assessment? What changes will you be looking for?

- How will you know whether the interventions that you have initiated are helping the patient?

- What will you change if the patient appears to be getting worse?

It is also important to practice these "virtual" ongoing assessments on both trauma and medical patients as they may differ slightly. One of the most important things you will begin to do as you gain experience is anticipate changes in the patient's condition based on his chief complaint. This ability will allow you to provide the most appropriate emergency care sooner and advise others of critical changes.

Activity 2: What to Expect

Anticipating how a patient might appear or change as his condition improves or worsens is an important skill every EMT-B must work to develop.

Using the "Street Scenes" that you worked with in the previous exercise, work with a fellow student to answer the following questions:

1. On the basis of the injury or illness, how will the patient present if nothing is done to treat the problem?

2. What signs and or symptoms will you look for that might indicate the condition is getting worse?

3. What changes will you make to the emergency care you are providing?

4. On the basis of the injury or illness, how will the patient present if his condition begins to improve?

5. What signs and or symptoms will you look for that might indicate the condition is getting better?

You should begin to play the "what-if" game in every scenario and on every patient you encounter. Think to yourself, "What would he look like if he begins to get worse? How will I know? What would I do for him?" When you ask yourself these questions, you will begin to formulate appropriate responses and become better prepared to manage the patient who does not respond to your treatment.

RETRO REVIEW

1. The mental status of an unresponsive infant should be checked by
   _____.
   - **A.** rubbing his sternum
   - **B.** gently pinching his legs
   - **C.** flicking his feet
   - **D.** rubbing his head

2. The _____ stretcher does not offer any support directly under the
   patient's spine.
   - **A.** Stokes
   - **B.** orthopedic
   - **C.** wheeled
   - **D.** basket

3. While checking the medical patient's neck during a rapid physical exam,
   you should assess for DCAP-BTLS, jugular vein distention, and _____.
   - **A.** rigidity
   - **B.** incontinence
   - **C.** sensation
   - **D.** medical ID devices

THINKING AND LINKING

CHAPTER TOPIC	HOW IT RELATES TO YOU AND OTHER COURSE AREAS
Trending	You will need to continually assess your patient in order to determine whether his condition is deteriorating or improving. How else would you know whether your interventions are effective? Watch for changes in blood pressure, pulse, breathing rates, skin signs (Chapter 9, and mental status (Module 4).
	Also, write everything down (Chapter 14)—and *not* on the back of your glove! Effective (and potentially life-saving) trending is impossible with jumbled details and forgotten vitals.
Stable vs. unstable patients	Ongoing assessments will be a little more relaxed with stable patients—but when you have an unstable patient, you may find yourself completing one assessment just in time to start the next.
	It is easy to get distracted and lose track of time in the back of an ambulance, but it is very important to stay focused. Neglecting to assess an unstable patient as often as required can endanger the patient's life and leave you open to lawsuits (Chapter 3).
Checking interventions	Just because you have implemented an intervention does not mean that it will be (or remain) effective. Conditions change and sometimes equipment can even stop working. A good example of that is a patient whose oxygen saturation (SpO_2) is dropping even though the nonrebreather mask is fitted properly and the tubing is not kinked—but the O_2 tank has run out. If you do not thoroughly check interventions, you may never notice.

CHAPTER 13

Communications

CHAPTER SUMMARY

In the course of your job as an EMT-B, you will need to be proficient in three areas of communication: radio/cellular, verbal (when reporting to hospital staff), and interpersonal (when dealing with patients, the patients' families, and other EMS personnel). Keep in mind, also, that you will be interacting with people of all ages, races, nationalities, and languages—and many times in highly stressful situations.

The widespread use of radio communication between dispatchers, ambulances, and hospitals has contributed to significant improvements in the EMS system. There was a time when ambulance crews had to phone the dispatch center to find out whether they had any calls, and hospitals were never warned about incoming patients.

The hardware for radio communication consists of a base station (a two-way radio at a fixed site), mobile radios (two-way radios usually mounted in vehicles), portable radios (handheld two-way radios), and repeaters (devices that boost radio-signal strength so that mobile and portable radios can send and receive clearly over extended distances).

Technological advancements are now supporting EMS communications via cellular systems, microwave systems, and push-button digital systems. These advancements are relegating traditional two-way radios to a "back-up" role in EMS communications.

Since EMS is just one of the many public-service agencies utilizing the airwaves, the Federal Communications Commission (FCC) issues licenses to prevent more than one agency from using the same frequency. The FCC also has very strict rules regarding the use or interruption of emergency frequencies and what type of language may be used.

The EMS communication process begins when an emergency dispatcher receives a telephone or radio call requesting medical assistance. Once the proper information is obtained (situation, location, number of patients, potential dangers, and so on), the dispatcher will send the appropriate unit(s) to the scene. The dispatcher will document all information pertinent to each call, including the time the ambulance was dispatched, when it arrived and departed the scene, when it arrived at the hospital, and, finally, when the crew was through with the call and ready to receive a new one.

As an EMT-B, you will also be required to give patient reports to other medical personnel. This may be by radio, cellular phone, verbally (in person), or in writing. You will want to avoid tying up radio frequencies or phone lines with unnecessary information. Some EMS protocols forbid the transmission of a patient's personal information over the radio, so make sure to check your local regulations. If your patient is critical, make that information known, but always keep your radio transmissions clear and concise.

An effective radio/cellular report has 12 parts: identification of unit and level of provider, estimated time of arrival (ETA), the patient's age and sex, the chief complaint, a brief (but pertinent) history of the present illness, any major past illnesses, mental status, baseline vital signs, pertinent findings of the physical exam, the emergency care given, and the patient's response to that care.

After you complete the radio/cellular report to the hospital, continue ongoing assessments as needed. Additional information or changes in the patient's condition (particularly deterioration) can be forwarded to the receiving facility in follow-up radio/cellular reports.

If you must contact on-line medical direction for a particular situation, always make sure to speak very clearly and give accurate information. Once a physician has given you an order, repeat it word for word and obtain confirmation of your accuracy. If the physician's order seems inappropriate, do not be afraid to question it—there may have been a miscommunication.

Once at the hospital, you will be expected to provide the receiving staff with a written report of the patient's condition. Since there will most likely be some urgency, however, and written reports can take time, your first report to them will be verbal. You should introduce the patient by name and repeat the same information that you gave during the radio/cellular report, adding any new developments or concerns.

Effective communication between two or more people (called "interpersonal communication") is a skill that takes years to develop. Unfortunately, some people's ability to communicate is not as developed as it could be, which can be made even more difficult during crisis situations.

In order to develop better rapport and have more effective communication with patients, families, friends, and bystanders, you should make frequent eye contact, be aware of what your body language might be saying (and make the appropriate changes), use a language that can be understood by the person you are talking to, be honest, use the patient's proper name, and, perhaps most important, *listen*.

When speaking to a mentally disabled patient or one who is hard of hearing, speak slowly and clearly—remembering not to turn away from a deaf patient, as he may be reading your lips. Blind patients will most likely be able to hear normally, so it is inappropriate to speak loudly or unnaturally to them. It is also a good idea to explain procedures in a step-by-step manner to a blind person, as he cannot see what you are preparing to do.

If you find yourself treating a patient who speaks a different language than you, try to find an interpreter at the scene or use a reference book. If neither option is available, your dispatch center or the receiving facility may have a person available via radio or phone who can translate.

Very commonly, you will be called to assist elderly patients who (primarily due to age) tend to get injured or become ill more often than younger people. You will also encounter more hearing, sight, and cognitive difficulties among this rapidly growing segment of the population.

PEARLS FROM THE PODIUM

- Communication exists in many forms, both verbal and nonverbal.
- You will need to communicate with patients, their families and coworkers, and other medical professionals.
- Effective and accurate communication is essential when transferring patient information to other medical professionals.
- You will use a radio for communication. This includes portable, mobile, and base-station radios. Cell phones may also be used in your system.
- Of all the things patients will remember about you and the emergency care you perform, the thing most remembered will be the way you communicate.

REVIEW QUESTIONS

SHORT ANSWER

1. Why is eye contact with your patient important?

2. What does "staging" the ambulance mean?

MULTIPLE CHOICE

1. A(n) _____ is used to increase the range of two-way radio signals.
   A. repeater
   B. booster node
   C. RF modulator
   D. converter

2. If on-line medical direction gives you an order that seems inappropriate, you should _____.
   A. comply but document your concerns
   B. attempt to contact the physician's supervisor
   C. refuse to comply
   D. question the physician

3. While explaining a medical procedure to your patient, do not _____.
   A. let him know that it may be painful
   B. use medical terms
   C. explain each individual step
   D. position yourself below his eye level

4. Two-way radios and _____ are common communication devices used on modern ambulances.
   A. satellite phones
   B. GPS intercoms
   C. cellular phones
   D. analog touch screens

5. Since communicating effectively with children can often be very challenging, it is a good idea to _____.
   A. speak only to the parents
   B. just spend your time providing emergency care
   C. carry a puppet on the ambulance
   D. involve the parents as much as possible

SCENARIO QUESTIONS

A man slipped and fell in a supermarket and your ambulance got the call. You arrive to find a 30- to 35-year-old Hispanic male seated in a chair and holding a wad of blood-soaked paper towels on his left elbow. It is immediately apparent that the man is unable to see, and when you introduce yourself, you discover that he cannot speak English.

1. When dealing with visually impaired patients, avoid _____
   A. asking about the cause of their blindness.
   B. overexplaining what is happening or what you are doing.
   C. speaking unnaturally.
   D. asking such questions as, "Do you know what happened?"

2. If there are no bystanders who can speak Spanish, you should _____.
   A. contact on-line medical direction
   B. speak loudly and use simple sentences
   C. begin assessing the patient
   D. leave the scene, since you are unable to obtain consent

You are called to a farm on the edge of town for a man down. Upon your arrival, you find a 17-year-old male who had been working on a hay baler when his right arm was caught and amputated above the elbow. He is responsive, alert, and the bleeding has been controlled. The patient's severed arm is mangled, entangled in the machine, and cannot be recovered.

1. The patient tells you that he has just gotten a college football scholarship and wants to know whether you think that the doctors can save his arm. What do you tell him?
   A. That it is not possible to answer that question until he is evaluated at the hospital.
   B. That you think there might be a chance that his arm can be reattached.
   C. That you just do not know.
   D. That his arm was badly damaged in the machine and could not be recovered. This makes reattachment very unlikely.

2. Which of the following is the most complete and accurate radio report to the receiving medical facility?

   A. "Main County, BLS Rig 9 here. We're about 22 miles out with a 17-year-old young man who lost his right arm in a farming accident. His pulse is 97, respirations 24 and a BP of 112 over 74. No pertinent history and we're currently treating him for shock, although so far he's stable. We'll be in touch if anything changes."

   B. "Community General, this is BLS4 en route to your location with a 20-minute ETA. We've got a 17-year-old male patient with a right arm amputation, proximal to the elbow. The arm was caught in a hay baler and couldn't be recovered. The patient has no pertinent medical history and is alert, oriented, and never lost consciousness. His vital signs are: pulse 97; respirations 24 and unlabored; skin is pale, cool, and moist; and blood pressure is 112 over 74. The exam indicates that the right arm trauma is the sole injury and bleeding is controlled. We've placed the patient in the Trendelenburg position with a nonrebreather and 15 liters of O_2 and are keeping him warm. The patient's level of pain has increased from seven to nine but mental status is unchanged and there's been only a slight increase in pulse and respiration. Do you have any orders for us?"

   C. "Delta Regional, we're inbound with a right arm amputation on Joey Hitsman from Noble City. He's 17 years old and the arm was severed at the elbow and not recovered. Be advised that this young man was going to play football for State College so you may want to have a counselor available. His vitals are stable, BP a little depressed, but he's doing pretty good. We'll be there about 1635."

   D. "Metro ED, this is ABC Unit 7 with a 15-minute ETA. We're bringing a 17-year-old male with a right arm amputation, distal to the elbow, caused by the intakes on a hay baler. We unfortunately couldn't get the arm. The patient is alert, oriented times three, and says that he never lost consciousness. Vitals are steady with a pulse of 97, respirations 24 and unlabored, skin is pale and clammy. BP is 112 over 74. There's no other trauma and the bleeding is under control. The patient's feet are currently elevated and he's on 15 liters of O_2. He's gone from seven to nine on the pain scale, but he's still awake and alert. His pulse and respirations have increased a little also, but so far negligibly. Is there anything medical direction needs?"

CASE STUDIES

CASE STUDY 1   COPY THAT

You are dispatched to a man down at a construction site at the corner of Baker and 1st Street in the downtown area. You have been advised that Engine 8 and law enforcement are also responding to the scene.

1. How will you acknowledge to dispatch that you have received the call and will respond as dispatched?

2. What information will be important to have regarding the other responding units?

You are first on the scene and your scene size-up reveals a large hoist truck on its side with what appear to be power lines down. Several people are waving you over to where a person is lying on the ground.

1. How will you advise dispatch that you are on the scene?

2. What additional information will you want to advise dispatch of regarding this scene?

CASE STUDY 2   THE CALL-IN

While providing emergency care to a patient can be challenging, few things cause more anxiety for new EMT-Bs than the radio report to the hospital. Read the following radio report and decide what is good— and what can be improved. We will use the same patient from Chapter 9 who was in respiratory distress.

YOU: "Memorial Hospital, how do you read this unit?"

MEMORIAL HOSPITAL: "Loud and clear. Go ahead."

YOU: "Memorial Hospital, we are en route to your location with a 78-year-old male patient whose chief complaint is respiratory difficulty. He is a resident of the Hope Eternal Nursing Home. He has a history of COPD and is on oxygen while in his room. His vital signs are pulse 96, strong, and regular; respirations 24 and slightly labored, BP 144/94, skin warm and dry, pupils equal and reactive to light. Our ETA is 10 minutes."

1. What is missing from the report?

2. What is good about the report?

Active Exploration

Imagine what a job it would be if we could not speak with our patients, what a challenge it would be to figure out what is wrong. As you may already know, just because we *can* speak, it does not mean we are able to communicate.

Trying to explain something to someone who just does not get it can be very frustrating, and when it involves an ill or injured patient, it can be life threatening. Developing excellent communication skills is important for all medical professionals.

The following activities will help reinforce the importance of good communications and provide some insight into your own ability to communicate well.

Activity 1: Monkey Say, Monkey Do

This is a popular communication game used to develop verbal skills. You will need a partner for this exercise, preferably a fellow student. Begin by gathering a blank piece of paper and a pencil or pen for each of you. You will also need something like a clipboard or magazine to write on.

1. Sit back to back and place the paper and pencil on the floor in front of you.
2. One of you should pick up the paper and, using the pencil, draw four geometric shapes at random locations and of random sizes on the paper. For instance, you might draw a triangle, a circle, a rectangle, and a straight line in random locations on the paper.
3. When you are done, direct your partner to pick up his paper and pencil.
4. Using your picture as a guide, and using only verbal commands, direct your partner to duplicate what you have drawn on his blank piece of paper.

Neither of you may look at the other's paper until all four elements have been completed. Once you have finished, take a look and compare both pictures. Are they similar? If not, why do you suppose they are not? What went wrong?

A variation of this activity can require that no clarifying questions be asked by either person. Only one-way communications can be used.

Activity 2: Loud and Clear

This activity will help you become more familiar with conducting a patient handoff to the next level of care. You will need to have your Emergency Care textbook handy and a fellow student to lend a hand.

Using the documentation samples at the ends of many of the chapters, formulate a hospital radio report as if calling the hospital from the ambulance. It may help to write down exactly what it is you want to say before you give your report.

This activity works best if you can use a pair of two-way radios or walkie-talkies for the report. With radios in hand, each of you should find separate locations and take a few minutes to formulate a report. When you are ready, give your report to your partner, using the radio. Have your partner write down exactly what you say over the radio.

Once you both have given your reports, compare notes and critique each other's verbal report.

A variation on this activity is to use a small tape or digital recorder to record the report and play it back for the reporting EMT-B.

RETRO REVIEW

1. An EMT-B's obligation to provide emergency care to a patient is known as a _____.
   - **A.** duty to act
   - **B.** care initiative
   - **C.** duty to serve
   - **D.** scope of practice
2. A(n) _____ is objective, whereas a _____ is subjective.
   - **A.** symptom, sign
   - **B.** opinion, symptom
   - **C.** sign, symptom
   - **D.** indication, sign
3. Leukocytes are more commonly known as _____.
   - **A.** red blood cells
   - **B.** platelets
   - **C.** cancer cells
   - **D.** white blood cells

THINKING AND LINKING

CHAPTER TOPIC	HOW IT RELATES TO YOU AND OTHER COURSE AREAS
Cellular phones	You may find yourself working for an ambulance service that uses cellular phones with a "two-way radio" feature as its primary method of communication. These devices give the ease of immediate communication associated with traditional radios but without the cross talk of the other units on the same frequency. They also allow the transmission of private patient information that would not be appropriate over an open radio frequency (Chapter 3).
Why a portable radio?	You may find yourself 50 feet (or more) from your vehicle before discovering that a scene is unsafe. There could be downed power lines, fire, hazardous materials (Module 7), violence (Chapter 2), and so on. It may not be safe (or possible) to return to the ambulance—in which case you will need a way to summon help without being able to access the mobile radio.
	Remember to use freshly charged batteries in your portable at the start of each shift (you will learn more about preparing equipment for service in Chapter 33) and double-check that you are on the correct channel before trying to contact dispatch.
Honest communication	Patients may not have your training or experience, but they can tell when you are lying about their situations. One of your responsibilities as an EMT-B will be to answer patient questions honestly—even if it means telling a patient that he may not survive.

14

Documentation

CHAPTER SUMMARY

As an EMT-B, your written documentation is permanent. It becomes part of the patient's hospital record and enters your EMS system's Quality Improvement program and may even be subpoenaed and become part of a legal case. Not only will your documentation assist with proper care of the patient in the present but it can also reach far into the future. Document each of your calls with that in mind.

The prehospital-care report (PCR) is the EMT-B's written record of each call. The most important function of the PCR is to be an accurate representation of the patient's condition throughout the call and to present the patient's history and vital signs, the emergency care provided, and changes or lack of changes in the patient's condition following emergency care.

The information gathered is very similar from state to state, but each region has its own method of recording the information. There are written reports (with narrative areas and check boxes for standard information) and computerized reports where the EMT-B shades in boxes or bubbles regarding the call and that are then scanned into a computer.

Advances in technology have also greatly influenced the efficiency of data entry in the EMS system. There are clipboard computers (which can convert and store handwritten notes into computer text), vehicle-based laptop systems, secure Internet data-entry sites and personal digital assistants (PDAs). The methods of documenting calls and transferring that information to hospital staff or EMS administration are being evaluated and streamlined constantly.

The PCR is a legal document that not only provides a record of the emergency care given to the patient but also assists in administrative functions, education, research, and Quality Improvement.

The hospital needs a properly completed PCR in order to effectively treat the patient. The PCR will indicate how the patient was found, any mechanisms of injury, what emergency care was provided, and how the patient's condition progressed during transport to the hospital.

As a legal document, the PCR may be examined in court for a variety of reasons. If the patient was the victim or perpetrator of a crime (criminal court) or if there is a lawsuit claiming negligence (civil court), your PCR will be a very important component of the case.

Your agency administration may require that you collect insurance and/or billing information on the PCR.

PCRs may also be used for education and research purposes. Data and statistics gathered from PCRs in both regional and national categories are compiled to detect patterns and trends in EMS management and emergency care. These trends can then be utilized to improve overall EMS operations or to assess needs for specific regions. An EMS agency will also use PCRs to evaluate the performance of specific EMT-Bs, enabling the supervisory staff to implement additional training programs, and so on.

Finally, PCRs are used by an agency's QI program to evaluate operations and assure compliance with current medical and organizational standards.

Obviously, a PCR has many uses and is of far-reaching importance, but what exactly is contained in one of these forms? Regardless of the technological format, a PCR will usually contain boxes where information is entered or selected. These boxes are called "data elements," and when completed and evaluated in total, can provide an important overall picture of the call. Although the US DOT has developed a *minimum data set*, which is a guideline for the minimum information to be documented, there is no actual regulation.

A PCR is normally broken down into several parts: run data, patient data, check boxes, and a narrative. Run data is information about the agency, ambulance crew, and pertinent dispatch times. The patient data includes such items as the patient's personal information, condition, and the emergency care provided. The check boxes make data collection more efficient by allowing an EMT-B to simply select and mark a box for certain elements. The narrative section allows for information that does not necessarily fit into one of the more structured sections of the PCR. Try to "paint a picture" with your narratives, giving the reader a clear presentation of the important aspects of the call, from your arrival through to your completing the call, in a logical order.

When completing your narrative, make sure you include objective (and pertinent subjective) information as well as pertinent negatives. Objective statements are those that are observable, verifiable, and measurable (e.g., "patient has swollen, deformed extremity"). Pertinent subjective information is important information from an individual's point of view (e.g., "I feel dizzy" or "patient appeared agitated"). A pertinent negative is a finding that has importance because it is not true or is absent. For example, a patient is experiencing chest pain but denies difficulty breathing—in this case, the lack of respiratory difficulty is a pertinent negative.

As you complete your narrative, avoid using radio codes, nonstandard abbreviations, poor spelling/grammar, illegible writing, and improper use of medical terminology.

A simple rule to remember regarding PCRs is "if you didn't write it, you didn't do it." Make sure you include all findings, interventions, and information important to the call and the patient. *Do not* be tempted to include emergency care that you did not perform just because you should have. It can be extremely detrimental to patient care, QI, and EMS research if PCRs are inaccurate.

You should pay close attention to all of the legal issues pertaining to PCRs and other related EMS documentation, such as patient confidentiality, patient refusals, and falsification or misrepresentation.

If you make an error on a PCR, simply draw a single line through the incorrect item or statement and write in the correction. If you scribble over an entry or use a liquid correction fluid, it may appear to others that you are attempting to cover a mistake in the emergency care you provided the patient. Follow your agency's procedure for correcting errors in PCRs that have already been turned in.

There are certain situations (such as multiple-casualty incidents) in which the full completion of a PCR is just not possible. Make sure that you are familiar with your agency's documentation requirements in these situations. During large-scale MCIs (e.g., plane crashes, train derailments, and so on), it is possible that a triage tag will be the only prehospital documentation completed for each patient.

Your agency may require additional documentation for advanced-life-support calls, calls that are particularly complex, or calls that fall into predetermined categories. Some additional types of reporting situations include infectious exposure, injury to EMS personnel, social-service referrals, and child or elder abuse. Check your local protocols, as there are differing requirements nationwide.

PEARLS FROM THE PODIUM

- Your documentation is a legal document. It should be accurate, honest, and complete.
- Your documentation is the only written representation of your call after it is done.
- There are many types of documentation on a run report. Patient data, run data, check boxes (objective), and narrative (subjective) are some examples.
- Documenting should be done objectively. This means you report direct observations and knowledge without opinions or speculation.
- Performing quality emergency care compassionately and documenting the care you give will help you in the event of a lawsuit. It may actually help prevent lawsuits.

REVIEW QUESTIONS

SHORT ANSWER

1. What is a *pertinent negative*? Give an example of one.

2. What are some of the uses of a prehospital-care report?

MULTIPLE CHOICE

1. During an MCI, a patient's chief complaint, injuries, vital signs, and the emergency care received are often recorded on a(n) _____.

   A. PCR

   B. 3 × 5 card

   C. Incident Command Log (ICL)

   D. triage tag

2. Which of the following is the best example of *pertinent subjective* information?

   A. Patient presented with a transient ischemic attack.

   B. Patient was severely depressed at the possibility of his football career being over.

   C. Patient seemed confused when trying to recall events leading to the injury.

   D. Patient complained of "broken right leg" although I suspect a sprain due to a lack of deformity or crepitation.

3. There are two types of errors that can be made during a call: commission and _____.

   A. negligence   **B.** omission

   C. retraction   **D.** falsification

SCENARIO QUESTIONS

It is the first call of your first shift after passing your agency's new-hire training program, and you are transporting a 93-year-old female to the emergency department from a care home. She has been diagnosed with pneumonia and requires 15 lpm of oxygen via nonrebreather mask. Once in the ambulance, you attach her nonrebreather mask to the onboard oxygen and set the flowmeter at 15. During your ongoing assessment, you find that the patient is having increased difficulty breathing and that her oxygen saturation has dropped from 93 to 82 percent. The patient has a DNR, so you try to keep her comfortable as she slowly sinks into unresponsiveness. You then notice that the onboard oxygen flowmeter is at 0. You had neglected to turn on the main valve at the start of the shift, and there was only enough residual oxygen in the system for the flowmeter to reach 15 for a few seconds.

1. If you correct the problem and the patient is responsive again when you reach the hospital, would you be required to detail the incident on the PCR?

   A. No. To do so would open you and your agency to a potential lawsuit.

   B. Yes. The receiving staff needs to know because the patient may experience complications due to your error.

   C. No. You do not want to begin your EMS career with this on your record.

   D. Yes. But you do not need to document the error, just the patient's unresponsiveness and subsequent recovery.

2. How might documenting this error benefit your agency?

   A. Your employment may be terminated, preventing you from making future errors.

   B. The operations department might replace the old oxygen tanks with newer models.

   C. The administration may identify areas where the hiring procedures can be improved.

   D. The QI team may be able to improve the new-hire training program.

You are dispatched to a call for a "severe headache." Upon your arrival, you find a 49-year-old patient sitting in a recliner in the living room of his home. He has pronounced right-side weakness and is having trouble giving appropriate responses to your questions. His wife tells you that he has a history of high blood pressure and is currently taking Lisinopril to control it.

1. You would document all of the following, except _____.

   A. the patient's billing address

   B. the nature of the call

   C. that the patient suffered a stroke

   D. the exact location where the patient was found

2. Which of the following narrative segments is most appropriate?

   A. Patient's spouse states that patient complained of a severe headache before becoming less responsive. The patient has weakness on his right side and answers questions with inappropriate words.

   B. Patient presented with right-side weakness and inability to speak clearly. Respirations 18 regular, pulse 88, BP 174/110.

   C. Arrived at pt's 10:20. Pt presented w/R side wknss and dysphagia. Hx of HTN. Poss. TIA.

   D. Found patient seated in recliner. Patient presented with stroke (right-side weakness and inability to use appropriate words) and per wife, patient has a history of high blood pressure but has never experienced current problem.

CASE STUDIES

CASE STUDY 1	DOWN BUT NOT OUT

You are responding to a call concerning a 71-year-old retired mechanic who was up on a 6-foot ladder changing a light bulb in his garage when he fell and injured himself. He is responsive when you arrive but according to his wife who heard the fall, he was unconscious on the floor bleeding from the head when she found him. She called 911 immediately and placed a washcloth over the cut on his head and waited for the ambulance to arrive.

1. Using the paragraph above, underline those elements that you feel are most important to report in a radio report to the receiving hospital.
2. On the basis of what you know so far, what additional information will the hospital want to know about the incident?

You decide to secure the man to a backboard and treat him with oxygen. While being packaged, he repeatedly asks where he is. His wife provides a history of hypertension and diabetes for which he takes medication. Just before you are about to load him into the ambulance, the man insists that he is all right and demands to be untied.

1. What must be included in your documentation if you end up leaving this man behind and not transporting him?

2. On the basis of the above call, write a narrative describing the patient and the emergency care provided.

CASE STUDY 2   HE'S BANGED UP PRETTY BAD

You are called to a motor vehicle crash where a patient has been thrown from a vehicle. He appears to have been injured quite badly. You arrive to find the patient facedown in the ditch. You see the bone of the upper right leg protruding through the skin just above the knee on the outside of his leg.

1. How would you document the patient's position?

2. How would you document your observation of the patient's leg?

3. How would you document the spine and airway emergency care performed?

4. How would you document the observed injuries listed here?

Long after the patient has recovered from his injury and many emergency calls later for you, the only thing that still remains is the documentation you created following the call. Even on a single busy shift, it can be easy to start mixing up information from one call to another. Good documentation is an essential part of good patient care and a necessary part of all EMS systems.

Like any other skill an EMT-B learns and performs, proper documentation should be studied and practiced as often as possible. In addition to good patient care, a thorough and accurate PCR can keep you out of the courtroom long after the incident.

The following activities are designed to improve your documentation skills.

Activity 1: Fill in the Blanks

You will need your Emergency Care textbook and several blank PCR forms. Turn to any one of the "Street Scene" sections at the end of one of the chapters in your textbook. Using the information in the scenario, complete the PCR as accurately as you can. Whenever there is information missing, just fill it in with information you feel would be relevant to the scenario. Pay particular attention to the "narrative" section of the PCR as this is often the most difficult to complete for new EMT-Bs.

When you have completed several of these PCRs, exchange them with those of a fellow classmate and offer a critique of the accuracy and thoroughness of their documentation.

Discuss any differences in the way the two of you chose to document the findings. Is one way better than another? If so, why?

Activity 2: Please Correct Me

You will need a fellow student and some more blank PCRs for this next activity.

Using a blank PCR, fill it in by trying to make as many intentional mistakes as possible. Leave some areas blank, put wrong information in other areas, and generally do a less-than-thorough job of completing the form using an imaginary scenario and patient. Have a fellow student do the same using another blank PCR.

Once you are both done, exchange PCRs and attempt to identify as many mistakes and inaccuracies as possible. Rewrite the narrative he has provided in a way that would be acceptable.

At first, it is good to make several obvious mistakes that should be easy to spot and correct. As you get better, make your mistakes less obvious and therefore more difficult to find.

You will find that it is not as easy as you might think to intentionally make errors on the PCR. Looking at someone else's documentation with a critical eye will help you become more critical of your own work and therefore make you better at documenting the emergency care you provide.

RETRO REVIEW

1. The U.S. Pharmacopoeia has assigned the colors green and white to identify oxygen cylinders. What gas would be found in unpainted stainless steel or aluminum cylinders?

    A. carbon dioxide   **B.** oxygen

    C. helium   **D.** hydrogen

2. You should never skip the ongoing assessment unless _____.

    A. the hospital is less than 10 minutes away

    B. the patient is stable and responsive

    C. life-saving interventions prevent you from doing it

    D. you are treating multiple patients

3. _____ is the first part of the patient assessment process.

    A. Scene size-up   **B.** Obtaining a history

    C. Checking the patient's airway   **D.** Evaluating the MOI

THINKING AND LINKING

CHAPTER TOPIC	HOW IT RELATES TO YOU AND OTHER COURSE AREAS
Narrative	The narrative section of your PCR should give the reader a clear and simple picture of the events surrounding the call. Your agency's QI team will appreciate it and, if you end up in court, *you* will appreciate it, as your memory about a particular call will fade with time.
	Remember to stay objective in your narrative or you may find yourself in the uncomfortable position of having an attorney accuse you of bias (or worse) or ask you to explain to the jury the source of your "omniscience." Review Chapter 3 for more on the legal aspects of EMS.
Falsification	Falsifying information on your PCR can sometimes be tempting—especially when you realize that you forgot to do something important or when you are having trouble obtaining vitals (Chapter 9). Do not do it. Your patient's initial care at the receiving facility is going to be based on your actions and observations—there could be serious consequences if you falsified your information.
Special reports	Your local EMS and/or law enforcement agency will have forms available for reporting special situations or incidents. You should be familiar with these forms and reporting procedures (Chapter 3) *prior* to running across a case of suspected child or elder abuse (Chapters 31 and 32) or getting exposed to an infectious disease (Chapter 2).

General Pharmacology

CHAPTER SUMMARY

As an EMT-B, it is important that you be familiar with the medications carried on the ambulance as well as the prescribed medications you might need to assist your patients with after obtaining permission from medical direction.

There are six medications an EMT-B can assist with or administer. They are:

- Oxygen—administered to any patient who is hypoxic or has the potential of becoming hypoxic.
- Activated charcoal—A powder usually premixed with water to treat ingested poisons or an overdose. The patient must be able to swallow, and you must obtain permission from medical direction.
- Oral glucose—A form of sugar used to treat known diabetic patients with altered mental status. It is usually supplied in a single dose tube. The patient must be able to swallow.

The following medications must be prescribed to the patient by his physician. An EMT-B may assist the patient with them after getting permission from medical direction.

- Prescribed inhalers—An aerosol form of medication that a patient can spray directly into his airway to treat an episode of difficult breathing. These episodes are often caused by asthma, emphysema, or chronic bronchitis.
- Nitroglycerin—A medication used when a patient experiences suspected cardiac chest pain. It dilates the blood vessels of the heart. It comes in several forms. The two forms that the EMT-B can assist with are tablets and spray. Both are administered sublingually (under the tongue).

- Epinephrine auto-injectors—Epinephrine will constrict blood vessels and relax the airways in a patient having a severe allergic reaction. It is supplied in a single-dose syringe with a spring-loaded needle that, when pressed against the arm or leg, will automatically deliver the medication.

Medications have three names: the chemical name, the generic name, and the trade name. A medication has one chemical and generic name but may have several trade names. As an EMT-B, you are not expected to know every generic or trade name. It is very useful to carry a medication-reference guidebook in the ambulance.

Every medication has indications for use as well as contraindications, or reasons not to use it. An indication is a sign, symptom, or circumstance that makes it appropriate to administer that medication to the patient. A contraindication is just the opposite. It would be a sign, symptom, or situation that would make it inappropriate or even harmful to administer a particular medication to a patient. Side effects are any action of a medication other than the desired actions.

Before administering any medication to a patient, confirm the order from medical direction and write it down. Check the expiration date of the selected medication and verify for yourself the following four "Rights":

- Right patient?
- Right medication?
- Right dose?
- Right route?

Remember to reassess your patient after administration of any medication. Obtain another set of vital signs and compare them to the previous set to see whether the medication had any effect. Document your patient's response to any medication given.

MED MINUTE

Patients can take a wide range of prescription medications for different medical conditions. The following table lists some of the different actions that medications may have on various body systems. Individual classifications and specific medications will be discussed in the chapters where they may be encountered.

BODY SYSTEM AFFECTED	ACTIONS OF MEDICATIONS
Respiratory	Open constricted airways
	Prevent inflammation and mucous buildup in the airways
Circulatory	Regulate the heart rate
	Prevent dangerous heart rhythms
	Relieve pain and improve blood flow to the heart muscle
	Lower blood pressure
	Lower cholesterol and prevent heart disease
	Prevent clot formation and "thin" the blood as a preventative measure against heart attack, embolus, and stroke

(Continued)

BODY SYSTEM AFFECTED	ACTIONS OF MEDICATIONS
Endocrine	Treat hormone deficiencies (e.g., thyroid)
	Treat diabetic conditions
Nervous	Treat depression, anxiety, schizophrenia, obsessive–compulsive disorders, and bipolar disorder
	Prevent seizures
Musculoskeletal	Prevent pain and disability from arthritis and other diseases
	Supplement calcium for bone strength and density

Many medications affect more than one part of the body. Pain relievers, fever reducers, and antibiotics are examples of drugs that are used for many different conditions and body systems.

Medications are powerful and must be used as directed. Accidental or intentional misuse of medications can result in an altered mental status, unresponsiveness, and death.

PATHOPHYSIOLOGY PEARLS

Epinephrine is a drug that will constrict blood vessels and relax the airways in a patient having a severe allergic reaction. To the EMT-B, epinephrine is most commonly supplied in an auto-injector, or a syringe with a spring-loaded needle, that when pressed against the arm or leg, will automatically deliver the medication.

Epinephrine will do wonders for the management of a patient suffering from an anaphylactic reaction. The administration of epinephrine through an auto-injector is highly beneficial and should be considered superior to the standard paramedic administration route. Paramedics are taught to administer epinephrine to anaphylactic patients through a standard needle and syringe via the subcutaneous (sub-Q) tissue.

Think for a second about the progression of a patient in anaphylactic shock: The patient will initially have a histamine release and begin to vasodilate and lose the structure of the capillaries, leading to leakage of water from the blood vessels. When this water is lost, the patient becomes hypovolemic and goes into shock. A patient in shock will immediately begin to compensate by shunting blood from the skin and extremities to the core organs (heart, lungs, brain, kidneys, and others). It is for this reason that an anaphylactic patient should not be given sub-Q medications. It will take a long time for the medication to be picked up by the blood stream if it is sitting in the sub-Q tissue as opposed to a muscle. Muscles are much more vascular (have more blood vessels) and will absorb and use the medication quicker.

Sources

Mulvihill ML, Zelman M, et al., Human Diseases: A Systemic Approach, 5th Edition, Prentice Hall, 2001.

REVIEW QUESTIONS

SHORT ANSWER

1. What is the best method for administering oral glucose? Why?

2. What medications can the EMT-B administer or assist with in the field?

MULTIPLE CHOICE

1. EMT-Bs should have access to a Physician's Desk Reference in order to obtain more information about a patient's _____.
   - **A.** condition
   - **B.** chief complaint
   - **C.** medications
   - **D.** medical history

2. Before administering nitroglycerin to a patient, you should ask whether he has taken _____ recently.
   - **A.** Viagra
   - **B.** aspirin
   - **C.** Valium
   - **D.** Proventil

3. Sublingual medications must be administered _____.
   - **A.** into an endotracheal tube
   - **B.** under the patient's skin
   - **C.** into the patient's muscle
   - **D.** under the patient's tongue

4. The two most common side effects of bronchodilators are _____ and patient jitteriness.
   - **A.** increased respiratory rates
   - **B.** decreased urinary outputs
   - **C.** increased heart rates
   - **D.** decreased blood pressure

5. Oral glucose is contraindicated if the patient _____.
   - **A.** is unresponsive
   - **B.** might be hypoglycemic
   - **C.** recently used a prescribed inhaler
   - **D.** is potentially hyperglycemic

SCENARIO QUESTIONS

You respond to a call from the home of a 57-year-old male who complains of chest pain and difficulty in breathing. He tells you that he has a prescription for nitroglycerin and took one about 15 minutes ago—with no effect. His baseline vitals show that his systolic pressure is at 98 and his pulse at 92.

1. What drug should you immediately administer to this patient?
   - **A.** nitroglycerin
   - **B.** aspirin
   - **C.** oxygen
   - **D.** Albuterol

2. Should this patient try another dose of nitroglycerin?
   - **A.** Yes, because patients can normally take up to three doses.
   - **B.** No, because his systolic pressure is too low.
   - **C.** Yes, because his systolic pressure is 18 points above ideal and the nitro may bring it down.
   - **D.** No, because he has already taken one pill within the last hour.

You and your partner are accommodating a ride-along who has applied for a job with your agency. About two hours into the shift, and while you are proceeding to the scene of a vehicle collision, you notice that the ride-along is having trouble talking coherently. As your partner pulls over, you climb into the back and quickly determine that your passenger has an altered mental status. As you are assessing him, you notice that he is sweating profusely, and you find a Medic-Alert necklace that indicates the person is a diabetic.

1. This patient is still responsive; what should you do?
   A. Perform a detailed physical exam.
   B. Administer glucose subcutaneously.
   C. Apply a nonrebreather mask with 15 lpm of oxygen.
   D. Administer glucose sublingually.

2. If this patient responds positively to your treatment, what was most likely the cause of his altered mental status?
   A. Insufficient insulin production.
   B. Low sugar levels in his bloodstream.
   C. Insufficient oxygen in his red blood cells.
   D. Excessive sugar exposure in his brain.

CASE STUDIES

CASE STUDY 1	AN ATTACK OF ASTHMA

You are responding to a call concerning a child with difficulty breathing, at a local park. Upon your arrival, a parent directs you over to the sidelines of one of the soccer fields where several people have gathered around a child in distress. As you approach the child, you find an approximately 10-year-old girl down on her knees in obvious respiratory distress. A woman who states that she is her mother informs you that her daughter has asthma and has been having trouble breathing for about 10 minutes. When you ask the girl how she is feeling, she is only able to speak in very short sentences. You notice an inhaler lying on the ground between the girl's knees.

1. Is oxygen indicated for this patient and if so, how will you administer it?

2. What will you do with the inhaler on the ground? What questions will you ask the mother regarding it?

The mother states that she gave the inhaler to her daughter as soon as she began having trouble breathing. She has given herself about 5 or 6 doses without any relief before the inhaler ran out. That is why they decided to call 911.

1. What information will you need about the inhaler?

2. Can you use an inhaler from one of the other children on the team who also has a history of asthma?

CASE STUDY 2   MY CHEST HURTS

You are called to a complaint of chest pain in a 60-year-old male patient. You arrive and complete an initial assessment that reveals adequate breathing. Oxygen is applied via nonrebreather mask.

You find that the patient's vital signs are pulse 92 and slightly irregular, respirations 20, blood pressure 122 over 78, pupils equal and reactive to light, and skin warm and dry. The patient was at rest when the pain came on, and he describes it as 8 on a scale of 1 to 10. He describes the pain as crushing and substernal, holding his fist to his chest as he tells you about it. You ask the patient whether he has nitroglycerin. He says he does, and you take it to the hospital with him. He has not taken his nitroglycerin today.

You arrive in the ambulance and continue to assess the patient. His chest pain is still present even after administering oxygen. You consider giving nitroglycerin. You find out that the patient had a heart attack about five years ago. He also has a history of high blood pressure.

1. What specific questions must you ask about the nitroglycerin?

2. What do these vital signs tell you about assisting the patient with his nitroglycerin?

3. What do you need to know about the patient's medical history before giving the nitroglycerin?

4. Use the information above to write down what you would say to medical direction if you were to request nitroglycerin.

5. What is the ideal format for reports to medical direction?

Active Exploration

As technology advances, so does medicine. One of the most visible ways advances in medicine can be seen is in the growing list of prescribed medications that patients are taking. As an EMT-B, you are likely to come across hundreds if not thousands of different kinds of medications over the span of your career. While it is not possible to learn the effects of all of these, learning some of the most common medications will greatly improve your history-taking skills. At the very least, you must learn all that you can about the few medications carried on the typical ambulance and those that the EMT-B is allowed to assist a patient with in the field.

The following activities will help you become more familiar with pharmacology and the various medications that you might encounter in the field.

Activity 1: Who's Ill in My House?

For this activity, you will want to get a notebook and pen handy.

You are about to conduct an anthropological study on the health of your family. Go to the medicine cabinet in your home and gather up all the medications in it. Next, bring them in to the kitchen and set them all out on the table in front of you. Begin by making a list of all the medications, taking special note of those medications that are expired.

Next, you are to gather as much information as possible about the individuals in your home based on the medications and the information contained on each of the containers. What information is contained on the labels? Is it consistent with each of the labels or does one medication contain more information than another? Do the labels indicate what the medication is to be taken for? Who the prescribing doctor is? How often the medication should be taken and for how long?

Note how much medication is left in each of the containers. If you were called to a possible poisoning involving a small child who got into the medication, could you estimate how much the child may have taken?

Activity 2: More About Meds

Using the list you created in the first activity, identify the five most recently prescribed medications and conduct a little research to discover the following information. You may use any resources you wish such as a friend who is a nurse or the Internet.

1. What is the "generic" name of the medication?

2. What is the "trade" name?

3. What is the medication prescribed for?

4. How many different forms does the medication come in (pill, powder, liquid, patch, and so on)?

5. Are there any contraindications for the medication?

6. What are the side effects?

1. Why does AIDS/HIV pose less of a danger to the EMT-B than hepatitis or TB?

   A. A vaccine for AIDS/HIV is available.

   B. The virus does not survive well outside the body.

   C. Only 6 to 8 percent of the population is susceptible to AIDS/HIV.

   D. Seven out of ten people in the United States have either hepatitis or TB.

2. The law of _____ states that a body in motion will remain in motion unless slowed or stopped by an outside force.

   A. gravity   **B.** minutiae

   C. acceleration   **D.** inertia

3. _____ can project radio transmissions over long distances by receiving at low power and rebroadcasting at a higher power.

   A. Boosters   **B.** Modulators

   C. Repeaters   **D.** Transistors

THINKING AND LINKING

CHAPTER TOPIC	HOW IT RELATES TO YOU AND OTHER COURSE AREAS
Assisting with medications	You will come across situations in which you may be required to help your patient take a prescribed medication. Your scope of practice (Chapter 3) will most likely include only prescribed inhalers for respiratory emergencies (Chapter 16), nitroglycerin for cardiac emergencies (Chapter 17), and epinephrine auto-injectors for severe allergic reactions (Chapter 20). Make sure to check local protocols to see exactly what "assist" means in your area—it can range from talking the patient through self-administration to actually doing everything for the patient.
Epinephrine auto-injectors	If you find that your patient has a medical ID device (Chapter 3) indicating a nonpharmacological allergy (peanuts, bee stings, and so on), make sure that you ask about (or look for) a prescribed epinephrine auto-injector. It is not uncommon for anaphylactic patients (Chapter 20) to panic and forget that they already possess a treatment.
Reassessment	Just because you administered (or assisted with) a medication, it does not mean that the patient's medical emergency will be reversed or resolved. It is imperative that you continue to assess the patient (Chapter 12) to determine whether further action will be necessary.

16

Respiratory Emergencies

CHAPTER SUMMARY

Respiratory emergencies are very common. You will encounter patients who are in distress but breathing adequately. Others may not be breathing adequately, and your interventions will need to be much more aggressive. Your ability to distinguish between the two is crucial.

The structures of the airway include mouth, oropharynx, nasopharynx, epiglottis, trachea, cricoid cartilage, larynx, bronchi, lungs, alveoli, and diaphragm. The intercostal muscles and diaphragm contract during the active process of inspiration (inhalation). These same muscles relax during the passive process of expiration (exhalation). The necessary exchange of oxygen and carbon dioxide happens in the capillaries of the alveoli, as well as in the capillaries of the cells throughout the body.

Adequate breathing, that is, breathing capable of sustaining life, falls within specific ranges. Determine your patient's breathing rate, rhythm, and quality when assessing for adequate versus inadequate breathing.

- Rate—Normal ranges: Adults 12–20 breaths per minute.
  Children 15–30 breaths per minute.
  Infants 25–50 breaths per minute.

- Rhythm—Usually regular.
- Quality—Breath sounds should be present and should be equal in each lung. Both sides of the chest should expand equally and adequately. Breathing should not be noisy or require a lot of effort.

Inadequate breathing will present with the following characteristics:

- Rate—A breathing rate outside the normal ranges, either too fast or too slow. A patient who is breathing too slowly is not bringing in enough oxygen per minute and a patient who is breathing too fast cannot move oxygen far enough into the lungs to adequately exchange oxygen and carbon dioxide.

- Rhythm—The rhythm may or may not be irregular.
- Quality—Breath sounds may be noisy, diminished, or absent. The patient's breathing effort may be too shallow. The chest may not rise and fall equally. The patient may be using the accessory muscles to breathe. The patient may look cyanotic and feel cool and clammy.

Respiratory emergencies in children and infants are potentially very serious. A child's airway structures are much smaller than an adult's and, therefore, are more easily obstructed by disease or foreign bodies. The tongue is proportionately larger in a child. The trachea is smaller and less rigid. The cricoid cartilage is less developed. Children and infants depend on their diaphragms more during respiration than do adults. The following are additional signs of inadequate breathing that are common in children:

- Nasal flaring
- Grunting
- Seesaw breathing
- Retractions of the intercostal muscles, as well as of the supraclavicular and suprasternal areas

When you determine that your patient is breathing inadequately, you will provide assisted ventilations by one of the following procedures. They are listed in the order of preference.

1. Pocket face mask with supplemental oxygen
2. Two-rescuer bag-valve mask with supplemental oxygen
3. Flow-restricted, oxygen-powered ventilation device (FROPVD)
4. One-rescuer bag-valve mask with supplemental oxygen

Just as breathing can be adequate or inadequate, so can assisted ventilations. Be sure that the chest rises and falls with each ventilation. If the chest does not rise, make sure that you are maintaining an open airway with a head-tilt, chin-lift maneuver or a jaw-thrust maneuver. Utilize an oropharyngeal or nasopharyngeal airway and suction, if necessary. You may observe an adult patient's pulse decrease to a normal heart rate once adequate ventilations are restored. A pediatric patient's pulse will drop significantly without enough oxygen. Adequate ventilations may raise a child's or infant's pulse to a normal rate. You need to ventilate an adult at least 12 times per minute and infants and children at least 20 times per minute.

Children and infants are susceptible to lower airway problems that may result in swelling of the airway structures. Occasionally, placing anything in the patient's mouth or pharynx may trigger a spasm along the airway, causing further obstruction. Be alert to the following signs indicating a lower airway problem:

- Wheezing
- Increased breathing effort on exhalation
- Rapid breathing without stridor

Symptoms of difficulty in breathing are shortness of breath or tightness in the chest, restlessness, and anxiety. The following are signs of difficulty in breathing:

- Changes in the breathing rate
- Increased heart rate
- Decreased pulse rate (infants and children)
- Changes in breathing rhythm
- Cyanotic, pale, flushed skin
- Noisy breathing such as wheezing, gurgling, snoring, crowing, or stridor
- Inability to speak in full sentences
- Use of accessory muscles for breathing

- Retractions
- Altered mental status
- Coughing
- Flared nostrils, pursed lips
- Patient in tripod position, or leaning forward with feet dangling
- Oxygen saturation of less than 95 percent on the pulse oximeter

The pulse oximeter is a useful tool to determine whether your oxygen interventions are improving your patient's condition. Never delay oxygen administration to obtain a room air reading. Oxygen should be administered to every patient who presents with difficulty in breathing, regardless of his oxygen saturation level.

Your focused history and physical exam will incorporate a patient interview using the OPQRST questions and the SAMPLE history. You will also inspect the chest and auscultate for lung sounds. If the patient is breathing adequately but is still in some distress, you will administer supplemental oxygen with a nonrebreather mask at 15 lpm. Most patients will want to sit up straight if they are having difficulty breathing. If the patient has a prescribed inhaler, you may be able to assist him with it after obtaining permission from medical direction. Be sure to ask the patient whether he attempted to use his inhaler prior to your arrival.

A metered-dose inhaler is a device that delivers a measured amount of fine powder medication each time it is used. Inhalers are for patients whose airway passages constrict or are obstructed owing to their medical condition. The medication in the inhaler will relax the airway and make it easier for the patient to breath. The inhaler must be administered while the patient is inhaling so that the medication enters the lower airway passages. It is beneficial if the patient can hold his breath for as long as possible after inhaling the medication so that it can be absorbed. As with all medications you assist with or administer, check the four rights: right patient, right medication, right dose, and right route.

MED MINUTE

Drugs that affect the respiratory system are vitally important. Some medications widen constricted bronchioles, whereas others work to prevent inflammation. Diuretics (water pills) cause the body to excrete water through urination so it does not build up in body tissues and the lungs. This table gives examples of common drugs in each category. Many other medications may be available with similar effects

CLASS OF MEDICATION	MEDICATION NAME(S)	MECHANISM OF ACTION
Bronchodilators	Albuterol sulfate (Proventil)	Produce bronchodilation by relaxing the smooth muscle of the bronchial tree.
	Xopenex (levalbuterol HCl)	
	Atrovent (ipratropium bromide)	
	Combivent (combines albuterol sulfate and ipratropium bromide)	
Inhaled corticosteroids	Budesonide (Pulmicort)	Reduce inflammation and mucus secretion in the lung patients with asthma and chronic lung diseases.
	Flunisolide (Aerobid)	
	Fluticasone (Flovent, Flovent Rotadisk)	
	Triamcinolone (Azmacort)	

(Continued)

CLASS OF MEDICATION	MEDICATION NAME(S)	MECHANISM OF ACTION
Diuretics	Furosemide (Lasix)	Diuretics, also known as "water pills," through their effect on the kidneys promote excretion of water through urination. Prevent fluid buildup in tissues and can reduce blood pressure.

PATHOPHYSIOLOGY PEARLS

Emphysema, chronic bronchitis, and asthma are diseases that affect millions of Americans and that cause a tremendous amount of suffering and debilitation. They also represent a true challenge to the EMT-B in terms of assessment and proper emergency care. While the EMT-B may find the presentation in each of these conditions to be similar, the root causes of these complaints are quite different.

The U.S. statistics for asthma alone are staggering:

- Americans with asthma: 14.6 million[1]
- Children with asthma: 4.8 million children under age 8[1]
- Asthma prevalence: 5.4 percent of Americans reported having asthma in 1994, a 75 percent increase since 1980[2]
- Asthma prevalence in preschool children: 5.8 percent of children under age 5 had asthma in 1994 (as reported by a family member), a 160 percent increase since 1980[2]
- Asthma deaths: more than 5,000 each year[3]
- Asthma-related hospitalizations: 466,000 in 1994[2]
- Emergency room visits for asthma: 1.9 million in 1995[2]
- Healthcare costs for asthma care: estimated at more than $6 billion a year[4]
- Missed school days: more than 10 million a year[5]
- Loss in productivity by working parents caring for children who miss school due to asthma: an estimated $1 billion a year[5]

But what is at the heart of this disease?

The bronchioles that bring air to the alveoli of the asthma sufferer are chronically (ongoing) thickened, and the specialized mucus-producing cells therein increase their production and number, which causes the airways to become narrowed and clogged with mucus. These changes are thought to occur because of an ongoing physiologic condition, which is very much like what happens during an allergic reaction.

There are two phases to the asthma attack. When the asthma patients are exposed to the trigger(s) to which they are sensitive (dust, pollen, heat, cold, stress, etc.), a substance called histamine is released from histamine-containing cells (mast cells) that reside in the lung and bronchiolar tissue. This substance causes the blood vessels surrounding the bronchioles and alveoli to dilate, the smooth muscle of the bronchioles to constrict, and the specialized mucus-producing cells to secrete more mucus. This phase of the asthma reaction, therefore, causes the already narrowed bronchioles to be

1 *Vital and Health Statistics, December 1995; 10(193): Table 62.*
2 *"Surveillance for asthma - United States 1960-1995," Morbidity and Mortality Weekly Report, April 24, 1998; 47(SS-1).*
3 *Monthly Vital Statistics Report, August 14, 1997; 46(1): Table 6.*
4 *"HHS Targets Efforts on Asthma," Department of Health and Human Services, May 21, 1998.*
5 *"Asthma: A Concern for Minority Populations," National Institute of Allergy and Infectious Diseases, January, 1997.*

further constricted, thus limiting air passage and trapping air in the lungs. Histamine also causes a host of white blood cells (immune-system cells) to move into the bronchiolar walls, causing swelling and further constriction. This second part is referred to as phase 2 of the asthma reaction.

As it turns out, the first phase of the asthma attack usually responds well to drugs that work to relax the bronchiolar smooth muscle and therefore dilate the bronchioles. Drugs such as albuterol (Proventil, Ventolin), metaproterenol (Metaprel, Alupent), and epinephrine (Primatene mist, adrenalin) work directly on the bronchiolar smooth muscle to cause it to relax.

The second phase of the attack responds poorly to these drugs but does tend to respond to drugs that limit or reduce the inflammatory effects of phase 2. Drugs such as flunisolide (Aerobid), beclomethasone (Beclovent, Vanceril), and triamcinolone (Asthmacort) are used to quell this part of the reaction and to help prevent this phase of the reaction from occurring.

REVIEW QUESTIONS

SHORT ANSWER

1. What are the three signs of a lower-respiratory problem in a pediatric patient?

2. Define inadequate breathing.

MULTIPLE CHOICE

1. A pulse oximeter reading of 86–90 percent indicates _____ hypoxia.
   - **A.** moderate
   - **B.** mild
   - **C.** severe
   - **D.** possible

2. _____ is a sign of inadequate respiration that is normally only seen in pediatric patients.
   - **A.** Accessory muscle use
   - **B.** Decreased chest expansion
   - **C.** Seesaw breathing
   - **D.** Cyanosis

3. An infant with a respiratory rate of 45 breaths per minute is _____.
   - **A.** tachycardic
   - **B.** breathing normally
   - **C.** in need of artificial ventilation
   - **D.** breathing too rapidly

4. Low-pitched lung sounds that resemble rattling are called _____.
   - **A.** stridor
   - **B.** rancor
   - **C.** crackles
   - **D.** rhonchi

5. In very rare instances, providing supplemental oxygen to individuals with lung diseases such as emphysema or chronic bronchitis can cause decreased respiratory effort. This is caused by a condition known as _____.
   - **A.** hypoxic drive
   - **B.** bronchoperfusion
   - **C.** instigated hypoxia
   - **D.** respiratory dysrhythmia

SCENARIO QUESTIONS

You and your partner are dispatched to an assisted-living facility for an elderly person who has had a fall. You arrive to find the patient, a 91-year-old male, in substantial pain with obvious pelvic instability and cool, clammy skin. The nurse at the rest home informs you that the patient has chronic obstructive pulmonary disease (COPD) and orders you not to raise his oxygen level above 3 lpm during transport.

1. What reason would this nurse have to demand that you limit the supplemental oxygen?
   A. The patient is relatively stable and would not benefit from additional oxygen.
   B. The patient may have developed a hypoxic drive.
   C. Due to the injuries sustained, there is a chance that this patient could quickly develop oxygen toxicity.
   D. The patient may be further traumatized by a nonrebreather mask, especially if he is accustomed to a nasal cannula.

2. How would you handle this supplemental oxygen situation?
   A. Follow the nurse's order but document it thoroughly.
   B. Simply ignore the nurse's order and place the patient on 15 lpm oxygen with a nonrebreather mask.
   C. Contact on-line medical direction and request instructions.
   D. Increase the oxygen to 15 lpm during transport but set it back to 3 lpm upon arrival at the receiving facility.

3. What is the main respiratory difference between a COPD and a non-COPD patient?
   A. A COPD patient breathes because oxygen levels are low, whereas a non-COPD patient breathes because carbon dioxide levels are high.
   B. A non-COPD patient breathes when oxygen levels are too high, but a COPD patient breathes because carbon dioxide levels get too low.
   C. A COPD patient must maintain a higher level of carbon dioxide than a non-COPD patient.
   D. Unlike the COPD patient, the non-COPD patient would feel the urge to breathe solely on the basis of the amount of oxygen in his system.

You are waiting in the check-in line at a hotel lobby while on vacation. You notice a young boy sitting on a chair not far from you and he appears to be having difficulty breathing. You approach the boy (who is approximately 4 years old) and immediately notice supraclavicular retractions, nasal flaring, and grunting. He is in the tripod position, appears mildly cyanotic, and very tired. You ask whether his parents are in the hotel and he shakes his head slowly and points to the concierge. The concierge tells you that he is watching the boy while his mother runs an errand. You check the boy's pulse and find that it is a little slow.

1. This child is _____.
   A. in danger of respiratory distress
   B. not breathing adequately and needs immediate CPR
   C. having an asthma attack and in need of his inhaler
   D. in very critical condition

2. Is this patient's slow pulse a positive finding?

  A. Yes. Just like an adult patient with respiratory difficulty, a normal or slow pulse indicates adequate oxygen levels.

  B. No. Unlike an adult patient, this child's decreasing pulse during respiratory difficulty means trouble.

  C. Yes. It means that he is maintaining his calm during this respiratory crises.

  D. No. His decreased pulse rate indicates severe hypoxia of the Purkinje system.

3. If you were to help this patient, what would you do first?

  A. Provide a rescue breath every 5 seconds.

  B. Find a phone and call for emergency services.

  C. Ensure that the child's airway is not obstructed.

  D. Begin positive pressure ventilations.

You have just completed the new-hire training program at your agency and are on your first shift with a new partner. You are dispatched to a two-vehicle collision and, upon arrival, you discover that one of the drivers is having difficulty breathing. She is pinned between the dashboard and the seat and is trying to reach an inhaler on the floor next to her. You try to calm the patient as you quickly retrieve her Advair inhaler.

1. Regarding this patient's respiratory difficulty, you should _____

  A. ask, "How many times did you use this inhaler before we arrived?"

  B. administer high-concentration oxygen and continue to calm her.

  C. hand her the inhaler.

  D. utilize an airway adjunct.

2. At what point should you assist the patient to use the inhaler?

  A. Once she has been extricated from the wreckage.

  B. Once you have determined that she has not used the inhaler yet.

  C. While your partner is checking with medical direction.

  D. Not until you have determined the nature and extent of her injuries.

3. If this patient's respiratory difficulty deteriorates to the point where she requires assisted ventilations, how would you ensure that your ventilations are effective?

  A. By providing 20–22 ventilations per minute.

  B. By attaching a pulse oximeter to the patient.

  C. By making sure that the patient's chest rises and falls.

  D. By making sure that the patient's pulse is increasing as you ventilate.

CASE STUDIES

CASE STUDY 1   DON'T LEAVE HOME WITHOUT IT

You are dispatched to a health club to help someone having difficulty in breathing. Upon your arrival, you find an approximately 35-year-old male bent over with his hands on his knees in obvious distress. He advises you that he has a history of asthma and normally carries an inhaler but has left it at home today. You consider this man to be in moderate distress and initiate oxygen as your partner obtains a set of vital signs: blood pressure 144/88; pulse 96, strong, and regular; respirations 32 and shallow; skin is pink, warm, and moist.

1. What signs other than his vitals are you likely to see in this patient that would indicate moderate to severe distress?

2. What oxygen therapy do you feel is most appropriate for this patient?

You now have your patient seated on the stretcher and on oxygen. He seems to be responding to the oxygen as his respiratory rate has decreased to 28. Just then, a friend of the patient runs up and hands you an inhaler and says that you may use it. The friend advises you that he too has asthma and will allow his friend to use his inhaler.

1. Can you use the friend's inhaler since they both have asthma?

2. Will you change (lower) your transport priority for this patient since he seems to be responding to the oxygen?

CASE STUDY 2   HE IS REALLY, REALLY SICK...

Your ambulance is dispatched for a "sick person" at 14347 Cedar Drive. During your approach, you take appropriate precautions and find the scene safe. As you walk toward the residence, you are approached by a young man who tells you his father is inside and says, "He doesn't look good. Hurry!"

As you approach the patient, you notice that he is ashen and appears unresponsive. You observe some labored respiratory effort.

1. What do you know from this information alone?

2. What body substance isolation precautions would you take?

You approach the patient and call his name. No response. He groans to painful stimulus. His respirations are 8 breaths per minute, shallow and extremely labored, his pulse is rapid, slightly irregular, and present at the radial artery. His airway is clear.

1. Would you perform any further evaluations of his breathing?

2. Is his breathing adequate or inadequate? Why?

As you work, you notice a home-oxygen device and a table full of medications. The patient's son tells you that his father has emphysema and some type of heart problem.

1. Is there a problem giving this patient high-concentration (90 percent) oxygen? Will this impact any of your decisions?

2. Would this patient be a candidate for advanced life support? If they were available, would you request medics? Why or why not?

En route to the hospital the patient goes into cardiac arrest. Shortly thereafter, he vomits copious amounts of thick stomach contents.

1. What is the maximum amount of time you would suction this patient for (each time)?

2. What type of catheter would you use to suction this patient?

Active Exploration

Emergencies involving respiratory distress make up a large percentage of the "medical" calls that you are likely to encounter. Understanding how someone presents when he is in respiratory distress and how the distress can eventually lead to failure and ultimately arrest is vitally important.

The following activities will help develop your knowledge of these emergencies and your ability to assess and treat patients in respiratory distress.

Activity 1: Tell Me What It's Like

This activity will help you gain a better understanding of what it feels like to not be able to breathe adequately.

Identify at least two or three people in your world who have a history of respiratory problems of any kind. These can be asthma, emphysema, bronchitis, or congestive heart failure (CHF). You might have to dig pretty hard to find someone with the more serious problems, but you should not have any difficulty finding someone with asthma or bronchitis. Once you do, conduct an interview in which your objective is to find out as much about their problem as possible. The following are some suggestions for questions you might ask:

- When did you first find out you had _____?
- How did you know something was wrong?

- What does it feel like when it gets bad?

- What makes the problem come on?

- Is there anything you cannot do due to your problem?

- What medications, if any, do you take?

- What do the medications do for the problem?

The objective of this exercise is to develop your history-taking skills relative to patients with respiratory problems. In addition, you are trying to find out from them how it feels to have such a problem and what it is like to live with such an illness.

Activity 2: While You Were Sleeping

One of the most difficult vital signs to take in the stable patient is respirations. This is because normal respirations are typically shallow and there is no accessory muscle use to aid the EMT-B in "seeing" the inspiration phase. To help develop the skill of assessing respirations on patients with normal respirations, you must practice on a variety of patients both responsive and unresponsive.

For this activity, your job is to assess the respirations on a sleeping person. You might have to stay up extra late for this one in order to allow other family members or roommates to fall asleep first. Once they have fallen asleep, pay close attention to their respiratory status and identify the following characteristics:

- Rate: Count the rate for 15 seconds and multiply accordingly, then count again for 30 seconds, and for 1 minute. Compare the rates for each sample and notice whether they are consistent or different. What do the results tell you about using small samples when determining rate?

- Depth: pay close attention to the depth of each respiration. How would you describe it to another EMT-B or doctor? Is it normal, shallow, or deep? What moves the most during breathing, the chest or abdomen?

- Ease: Is the breathing easy, or do respirations seem slightly labored?

- Noise: Are the respirations noisy? If so, how would you describe the sound? Is it only on inspiration, expiration, or both? You should have learned by now that noisy respirations indicate some form of partial airway obstruction. Does position affect the noise if the patient moves? What do you suppose is causing the obstruction?

    If possible, try to compare the breathing patterns of infants, children, and adults; it is good experience. How do they differ and why?

RETRO REVIEW

1. Oxygen used for emergency care should always be medical grade and not more than _____ year(s) old.

   A. two   **B.** one

   C. five   **D.** three

2. The final step of the detailed physical exam for a trauma patient is to _____.

   A. assess the extremities   **B.** reassess the vital signs

   C. immobilize any remaining deformities   **D.** assess the spine

3. _____ frequently cause the ejection of any passengers not wearing seat belts.

   A. Head-on crashes   **B.** "T-bone" collisions

   C. Rotational-impact collisions   **D.** Rollover crashes

THINKING AND LINKING

CHAPTER TOPIC	HOW IT RELATES TO YOU AND OTHER COURSE AREAS
Adequate vs. inadequate breathing	As you learned in Chapter 6, there are three levels of breathing: adequate, inadequate, and not at all. A patient's breathing can rapidly deteriorate, so it is important to continually assess the patient (Chapter 12) and treat inadequate breathing aggressively.

Ventilating pediatric patients	Unlike an adult, a pediatric patient's pulse will actually slow down if your artificial ventilations are inadequate (Chapter 6). Since you will most likely be ventilating adults much more often than children, you may find yourself forgetting how critically different adult and pediatric patients are. It is a good idea to periodically review these differences—you will learn more about them in Chapter 31.
Prescribed inhalers	A frightened patient who has accidentally misused his prescribed inhaler (Chapter 15)—and thereby received no benefit—may panic. This can seriously complicate the situation. Take steps to calm the patient and then assist him in using the inhaler again.

Always ask patients who are having trouble breathing whether there is a history of respiratory problems (Chapters 9 and 11) and, if so, determine if an inhaler is prescribed for the condition. |

17

Cardiac Emergencies

CHAPTER SUMMARY

Responding to calls concerning chest discomfort or chest pain is a frequent occurrence for the EMT-B. Chest discomfort can be caused by many things, including pain related to the heart. For these patients, you will provide oxygen and possibly assist the patient with his nitroglycerin. The extreme circumstance in cardiac problems is cardiac arrest. For these patients, you will perform CPR and possibly defibrillate them with an AED.

There are many different ways that a patient can experience cardiac compromise. A coronary artery can become narrowed or blocked so that the heart muscle cannot receive enough oxygenated blood. A valve between the heart's chambers (atria and ventricles) may stop working effectively. It is possible that the heart may begin to beat in an irregular rhythm or at a very fast or slow rate. There are many different signs and symptoms that patients in cardiac compromise may present with. They may have several of the following or only one. Remember that cardiac patients will not always have chest pain or discomfort.

- Difficulty breathing
- Chest discomfort
- Nausea
- Vomiting
- Sweating
- Left- or right-arm pain
- Jaw pain
- Upper-abdomen pain
- Abnormal pulse (bradycardia, tachycardia, or irregularity) or blood pressure (hypotensive or hypertensive)
- Anxiety
- Denial of any problem

Emergency care for a patient with suspected cardiac compromise will include the administration of oxygen and placing the patient in a position of comfort. You should transport a patient immediately if he has no prior cardiac history, has a cardiac history but no prescribed nitroglycerin, or if his systolic blood pressure is less than 100. While making your transport decision, keep in mind what type of treatment facilities are available in your area.

You may assist your patient with his prescribed nitroglycerin if all the following conditions are met:

- Patient has chest pain.
- Patient has a history of cardiac problems.
- Patient has been prescribed nitroglycerin.
- Patient has his own nitroglycerin with him.
- Patient's systolic blood pressure is above 100.
- Patient has not taken Viagra within the past 24 hours (taken in combination with Viagra, nitro can dangerously lower blood pressure).
- You have permission from on-line medical direction for a maximum of three doses.

Ask your patient whether he has taken any nitro prior to your arrival and report this to the hospital when you call medical direction for permission. In most instances, you may assist the patient in administering a maximum of three doses of nitroglycerin. You must evaluate vital signs as well as other signs and symptoms after each dose. The systolic blood pressure must remain above 100 before you can administer the second or third dose.

Some EMS systems and local protocols allow EMT-Bs to administer aspirin to cardiac patients. The following conditions must be met:

- Patient has chest pain.
- Patient is not allergic to aspirin.
- Patient has no history of asthma.
- Patient is not currently on medications to prevent clotting.
- Patient is able to swallow.
- Patient has no other contraindications for aspirin administration.
- You have permission from on-line medical direction.

Patients who experience cardiac arrest have the best chance of survival if all four links in the chain of survival are very strong. The four links are early access to the EMS, early CPR, early defibrillation, and early advanced care. The faster a patient receives emergency care, the greater his chance of survival. As an EMT-B, you are involved in two of these links: early CPR and early defibrillation.

Once you have determined that your patient is breathless and pulseless (in cardiac arrest), the next step is to apply the AED. Defibrillation is appropriate for any nontrauma patient over the age of one, with a shockable cardiac rhythm. If you are part of a two-person team, one of you will set up the AED, while the other initiates CPR. CPR is temporarily stopped while the AED analyzes the cardiac rhythm of a patient in cardiac arrest and determines whether a shock is indicated. If a shock is indicated, the AED will advise the EMT-B to press the shock button on the device to deliver a shock to the patient. No one should touch the patient during the analysis or shock phases. Coordinating CPR with the use of the AED takes some practice. Be familiar with the AED unit you will be using and review your skills at least every 90 days. Consider the following while using an AED:

- State, "I'm clear, you're clear, everybody clear," and look to be sure everyone is clear of the patient before delivering each shock.
- Check the batteries before each shift and carry a spare in the ambulance.

- Most AEDs are programmed to deliver a maximum of nine shocks (three sets of three stacked shocks).
- Due to excessive movement, the AED may not be able to accurately analyze a rhythm while the ambulance is moving.

Patients who regain a pulse following an episode of cardiac arrest will likely go back into cardiac arrest. Be sure you monitor their carotid pulse, maintain their airways and assist with ventilations if necessary. Keep the AED on a patient who has been resuscitated and recheck the pulse at least every 30 seconds.

Practice the following safety considerations while using an AED:

- Do not defibrillate a patient who is lying in standing water.
- Remove medication patches from the patient's chest with gloved hands if they interfere with the placement of the electrode pad.
- Make sure everyone is clear of the patient before delivering a shock.

In addition to the four links in the chain of survival, there are other factors that help determine a cardiac-arrest patient's outcome. Some of these factors include how quickly the EMS is notified, dispatch time, ambulance response time, and the time it takes to assess the patient and deliver the first defibrillatory shock.

MED MINUTE

There are numerous medications used to treat a wide variety of problems of the cardiovascular system. These medications are frequently used to alter the rate or strength of cardiac contraction or to lower blood pressure. This table gives examples of common drugs in each category. Many medications may be available with similar effects.

CLASS OF MEDICATION	MEDICATION NAMES(S)	MECHANISM OF ACTION
Nitrates	Nitroglycerin	Relax smooth muscle, resulting in arterial and venous dilation. Cause pooling of blood peripherally and reduce myocardial oxygen demand.
Beta blockers	Atenolol (Tenormin) Labetalol (Normodyne)	Used in hypertension. Block the actions of the sympathetic nervous system. Lower blood pressure but also can lower pulse.
Calcium channel blockers	Diltiazem (Cardizem) Amlodipine (Norvasc)	Used to slow the heart rate and reduce blood pressure. Act on the heart and blood vessels at the cellular level by blocking movement of calcium ions.
ACE inhibitors	Enalapril (Vasotec) Captopril (Capoten) Lisinopril (Zestril)	Used to reduce blood pressure by inhibiting an enzyme that elevates blood pressure through hormonal controls.
Diuretics	Furosemide (lasix) Hydrochlorothiazide (HCTZ)	Used to eliminate fluid or edema and to lower blood pressure by preventing reabsorption of water in the kidneys.
Digitalis preparations	Digoxin (lanoxin)	Increase force and velocity of cardiac contractions and reduce conduction in the atrioventricular (AV) node of the heart, slowing the heart rate.

PATHOPHYSIOLOGY PEARLS

Cardiovascular disease affects millions of Americans each year. According to the American Heart Association:

- 340,000 Americans die each year of coronary heart disease—more than 930 Americans each day.
- A cardiac-arrest patient's chances of survival are reduced by 7 to 10 percent with every minute he must wait for defibrillation.
- In 2003, 1.1 million Americans will have a first or recurrent heart attack.
- Coronary heart disease remains the nation's single leading cause of death.
- About 7.6 million Americans age 20 and older have survived a heart attack.
- About 6.6 million Americans live with angina pectoris.

Cardiac events are ultimately defined by the degree of cardiac compromise and extent of cardiac cell hypoxia that the heart suffers. A critical physiologic factor that you as an EMT-B must understand is how the heart is oxygenated. It is extremely important to realize that the heart's supply of oxygenated blood is delivered by way of the coronary blood vessels during diastole. As the left ventricle contracts and ejects blood through the aorta, blood is then circulated systemically. The residual blood that remains in the aorta as the left ventricle relaxes is drawn backward into the coronary vessels, which are located at the base of the aorta.

An understanding of this physiology becomes important when the patient experiences any degree of cardiac compromise. Take for example the patient who has poor cardiac contractility secondary to a heart attack. The patient may have an adequate supply of oxygenated blood but because of a weak pump, he cannot effectively eject enough volume to create residual blood flow. In other words, all the blood that the heart pumps will be pushed through the aorta and the coronary vessels, which are the last vessels to be perfused, and the heart will not receive enough oxygenated blood. A thorough understanding of the principle of coronary perfusion will allow you to better appreciate and treat the patient with cardiac compromise. Regardless of the cause of cardiac compromise, the principle of coronary perfusion remains unchanged.

Take, for example, the congestive-heart-failure (CHF) patient. In CHF, it is widely known that the problem is that the heart is no longer effective as a forward pump. This is problematic because the CHF patient experiences a drastic increase in preload, or the pressure, created by blood, within the ventricle when the heart is at rest. When preload is increased, pulmonary capillary pressures (constant pressure created by fluid inside of the small blood vessels of the lungs) are increased and the fluid from inside of the blood vessel is pushed into the lungs. This increase in preload causes the fluid to shift into the lungs and eventually leads to the development of pulmonary edema, which causes the patient to experience dyspnea.

When the fluid leaves the blood vessels, the patient will also experience a rapid decrease in the amount of oxygenated blood that the heart pumps, for two primary reasons. The first reason that the heart is unable to pump enough blood is that it cannot contract fast enough or with enough strength to force all of the blood it receives into the aorta and into the systemic circulation. The second reason the heart lacks oxygen flow is because there is not typically enough blood pumped out of the heart to perfuse or fill the coronary vessels. If the coronary vessels are not filled, the heart does not get oxygenated.

Remember that the more work the heart has to do, the more oxygen it will need. In this case, the heart will be working very hard and is in dire need of high concentrations of oxygen. The EMT-B must understand that getting enough oxygen to the patient and supporting his blood pressure are critically important steps in the management of an ischemic heart.

Sources

"Our quick guide to heart disease, strokes, and risks," December, 2003, AHA Website http://www.americanheart.org/downloadable/heart/1046380555112KTFGTS.pdf.

Rosen P, Barkin RM, et al., Emergency Medicine Concepts and Clinical Practice. 5th Edition, Mosby, St. Louis, MO, 2002.

Tintinalli JE, Kelen GD, et al., Emergency Medicine, A Comprehensive Study Guide, 5th Edition, McGraw-Hill, New York, NY, 2000.

Hurst JW, The Heart, 4th Edition, McGraw-Hill, New York, NY, 1978.

McPhee SJ, Vishwanath RL, et al., Pathophysiology of Disease, An introduction to Clinical Medicine, 3rd Edition, Lange-McGraw-Hill, New York, NY, 2000.

REVIEW QUESTIONS

SHORT ANSWER

1. What are the contraindications to using an AED on a cardiac-arrest patient?

2. What are the links in the cardiac chain of survival?

MULTIPLE CHOICE

1. Which type of AED is able to use less power and, perhaps, cause less heart damage?
   A. Monophasic
   B. Automatic
   C. Biphasic
   D. Hemiphasic

2. A trauma patient with a systolic blood pressure of _____ is commonly seen as hypotensive.
   A. greater than 120
   B. less than 100
   C. less than 150
   D. greater than 100

3. At the EMT-B level, the most important drug in the treatment of cardiac compromise is _____.
   A. nitroglycerin
   B. atropine
   C. oxygen
   D. adrenalin

4. If more than _____ minutes pass between cardiac arrest and defibrillation, there is virtually no chance of survival.
   A. 8
   B. 10
   C. 4
   D. 15

5. Up to half of all cardiac-arrest patients will initially have a(n) _____ rhythm.
   A. V-tach
   B. AF
   C. PEA
   D. VF

You are on standby at the county arena during a monster-truck show when a man in the bleachers begins yelling for help. You approach the stands and see an unresponsive man collapsed over one of the benches. You quickly confirm that he is unresponsive, apneic, and pulseless.

1. The best way to initiate emergency care for this patient is to _____.
   A. open his airway using the head-tilt, chin-lift technique
   B. insert a properly sized oropharyngeal airway
   C. move him out of the stands
   D. provide two rescue breaths

2. At what point should you apply the AED to this patient?
   A. After four full cycles of compressions and ventilations.
   B. As soon as it is available.
   C. At the completion of the current compression cycle following the arrival of the unit.
   D. When ordered by on-line medical direction.

3. After utilizing the AED, the patient has regained a pulse but is still not breathing. How often should you check this patient's pulse while providing rescue breaths?
   A. Approximately every 60 seconds.
   B. As long as your ventilations are adequate, you will not need to.
   C. Once each minute.
   D. Constantly, by keeping two fingers on the patient's carotid artery as you provide ventilations.

You are transporting a hypotensive patient who is experiencing dizziness, crushing chest pain, and dyspnea. You notice that the patient is becoming restless and beginning to sweat. As you are asking him how he is feeling, he becomes unresponsive and loses his pulse.

1. You should immediately _____.
   A. begin CPR
   B. analyze the patient with the AED
   C. check for adequate breathing
   D. deliver three stacked shocks

2. What initial position should this patient have been transported in?
   A. The prone position.
   B. The recovery position.
   C. Lying down.
   D. A position of comfort.

3. How are AEDs programmed to respond to pulseless electrical activity?
   A. The AED will indicate "shock advised."
   B. The AED will remain in the "analyze" mode.
   C. The AED will indicate "no shock advised."
   D. The AED will instruct the operator to "check the pads."

CASE STUDIES

You are responding to a call from an office building for a complaint of "chest pain." Upon your arrival, you find an approximately 50-year-old male seated in a chair, in mild distress. You introduce yourself and inform the man that you are there to help. He informs you that he is experiencing "tightness" in his chest that started about 20 minutes ago while he was walking up some stairs. He states that he has a recent history of angina and takes nitro for the pain. You notice that he is a little pale and that his skin is moist to the touch.

1. **How might you go about differentiating this man's pain from that of musculoskeletal pain? What questions will you ask to help determine this?**

2. **Is oxygen therapy indicated for this patient and, if so, what device and flow will you suggest?**

Your partner obtains vital signs as you place him on oxygen. The patient's blood pressure is 110/86; pulse 88, strong, and regular; and respirations 16 and unlabored. He informs you that he took two of his nitro pills before calling 911 and is concerned that the pills are not taking the pain away.

1. **Can you suggest he take another of his nitro pills? What do you want to know before he does take another?**

2. **What is the best position for this patient during transport and why?**

You are called to the home of a 78-year-old woman for "general weakness." You arrive to a safe scene and a well-kept home. The woman meets you at the door. She walks slowly back to her chair to rest. The woman is responsive, alert, oriented, and is having a bit of trouble breathing. She is able to speak full sentences and appears to be breathing adequately. You finish your initial assessment by applying oxygen by nonrebreather mask and checking her pulse. It is strong and regular but feels a bit fast.

1. **What priority is this patient?**

2. **What is the significance of the information you have obtained thus far?**

You begin to talk with the patient and ask some SAMPLE history questions. She says she has felt weak for the past "day or so." She feels like she cannot catch her breath sometimes when she cleans and she did not sleep well last night. She takes a medication for her high blood pressure and a pill for her diabetes. Her only other medication is a calcium supplement. She had a light lunch, denies any allergies, and cannot be very specific about when the weakness came on. "I just don't feel well," she says. Her vital signs are pulse 96, strong, and regular; respirations 22; skin cool and dry; pupils equal and reactive to light; and a blood pressure of 170/96.

1. **What do the vital signs and SAMPLE history tell you?**

2. **Would you do any elements of a physical examination for this patient?**

You move the stretcher over to the patient and tell her you will lift her onto it. She says, "Oh, that is silly, I'll walk over." She gets up, takes a few steps and begins to feel weak and dizzy. Suddenly, she becomes unresponsive. You were guiding her to the stretcher and were able to lower her safely to the floor. She has no pulse.

1. **When you were reading this scenario, did you think you would be using your AED?**

2. **Did letting her walk cause her to go into cardiac arrest?**

The patient is defibrillated promptly, has return of pulse and breathing, and is transported to the hospital, where she makes a complete recovery. It is a call you will never forget.

Active Exploration

Calls concerning "chest pain" are common in many EMS systems today. Unfortunately, there are many aspects of our culture that seem to increase the likelihood of heart disease and, ultimately, cardiac emergencies. The good news is that advances in medicine seem to move almost as fast and offer many new options for the treatment of both chronic and acute cardiac problems.

As an EMT-B, often the most you can do for patients experiencing chest pain is to offer them reassurance and oxygen and expedite their transport to an appropriate receiving hospital.

The following activities will assist you in becoming more aware of the resources available in your system to deal with these emergencies as well as of your own ability to assess and treat cardiac chest pain.

Activity 1: In Your Backyard

Not all areas of the United States are adequately served by advanced medical resources. As an EMT-B, you should be aware of the resources available in your system to deal with cardiac emergencies. Some hospitals can only stabilize a patient before they must arrange transport to a larger facility. Other hospitals are well known for treating these types of patients, including performing bypass and transplant surgery.

Start by contacting someone whom you know in the medical profession in your area. This could be a nurse, doctor, paramedic, or respiratory therapist. Find out what the capabilities of the local hospital(s) are. Are they equipped and staffed to deal with cardiac emergencies on a 24/7 basis? Are they only capable of conducting diagnostic tests and therefore must transfer the patient to another facility for surgery? Are they capable of performing cardiac surgeries and, if so, to what extent? Can they perform bypass surgery or angioplasty? Are they capable of performing transplant surgery?

If the local resources are not able to provide some or all of these resources, where is the closest facility that can? How are patients transported to these other facilities, by ground or by air?

In your system, are EMTs allowed to bypass a smaller hospital in order to take patients to a specialty facility that can better manage their problem?

As an EMT-B, you have a professional obligation to know as much as you can about the resources available in your local system. Knowing the capabilities and limitations of the various hospitals and knowing the protocols for taking patients to these hospitals can sometimes mean the difference between life and death.

Activity 2: What's the Problem?

For this next activity, you will need your Emergency Care textbook, some 3 × 5 cards, and a fellow student to assist you. You will select one of three "chest pain"-related problems, that is, angina, myocardial infarction, or musculoskeletal pain. Using your textbook, select one problem and create a set of signs and symptoms that are specific to the problem you choose. Be as detailed as possible, including at least two sets of vital signs. The vitals can reflect a stable or unstable patient; the choice is yours.

Once you have created a detailed set of signs and symptoms, devise a scenario for your partner to respond to. You can do this while seated across from the table with one another. Provide your partner with a dispatch and allow him to talk his way through the scene, stating aloud what he would be looking for and eventually conducting a verbal patient assessment of you. You will then provide the signs and symptoms as appropriate.

This is a lot like the old game "20 questions" in that your partner must ask as few questions as possible to figure out what the problem is. Once he thinks he knows, he can guess but must back up his guess with actual findings from the scenario.

This is an excellent way to begin associating signs and symptoms with various medical problems.

RETRO REVIEW

1. Which of the following best defines the term "contraindication" as it pertains to a patient's medication?
   A. A reason to take the prescribed mediation.
   B. A reason not to take the prescribed medication.
   C. The presence of a serious side effect.
   D. None of the above.

2. An immediate assessment of the patient's environment, appearance, and chief complaint is called the _____.

    A. general impression
    B. initial observation
    C. ABCs
    D. overall impression

3. All commonly used medications have at least _____ different names.

    A. six
    B. four
    C. seven
    D. three

THINKING AND LINKING

CHAPTER TOPIC	HOW IT RELATES TO YOU AND OTHER COURSE AREAS
Cardiac compromise	Many elderly patients will experience no pain during a heart attack. If you are responding to an elderly patient who is complaining of general weakness, nausea, "heartburn," or shortness of breath, always bring an AED and an airway kit (you will learn more about the specifics of treating older patients in Chapter 32).
Automated External Defibrillators	With the growing popularity of programs that introduce AEDs into public and business locations, chances are good (and increasing) that you may arrive at the scene and find an AED already in use. You should always evaluate the abilities and procedures of the first responder(s) treating the patient. As an EMT-B, you will probably be the highest trained person on the scene—making you responsible for providing emergency care to the patient from the time of your arrival until the patient is turned over to more advanced care (Chapter 3). Check your local protocols to see whether you need to replace the first AED with your unit's AED.
Documentation	As you complete the PCR following a cardiac emergency (Chapter 14), do not forget to accurately document any AED use (including number of shocks) and the effectiveness of the CPR performed (Appendix C of the Emergency Care textbook). Never falsify your PCR. If you did not check for chest rise during ventilations, do not write that you did. Fictitious PCRs will not give your agency's quality improvement program (Chapter 1) an accurate picture of training and procedural effectiveness.

CHAPTER 18

Acute Abdominal Emergencies

CHAPTER SUMMARY

Acute abdominal emergencies can be challenging because they involve internal organs that cannot be seen. This is one type of an emergency where you must rely very heavily on the patient and/or his family members to gain information. Treatment for all abdominal emergencies is basically the same; therefore, there is no need for you to determine what the specific problem is.

The abdomen contains many organs that perform a variety of functions. To help you remember the location of the organs of the abdomen, imagine that it is divided into four quadrants by two perpendicular lines through the navel. The peritoneum houses the organs. There are two layers of the peritoneum: the visceral (covering organs) and the parietal (attached to the abdominal wall). The kidneys, abdominal aorta, and pancreas are in the retroperitoneal space. This space is outside the peritoneum, between the abdomen and the back. The female reproductive organs also are located in the abdomen.

There are several types of abdominal pain. They are listed below.

- Visceral pain—originates from the organs; will possibly be described as dull, achy, intermittent, and difficult to localize
- Parietal pain—originates from the parietal peritoneum and is caused by localized irritation to the peritoneum; it may be sharp, constant, and located in a specific area
- Tearing pain—not the most common type of pain, usually associated with damage to the abdominal aorta
- Referred pain—pain caused by an injured organ that is often felt somewhere other than where the organ is located

There are many possible causes for abdominal pain. Your goal will be to perform a thorough assessment and obtain important information during your SAMPLE history. Determining the exact cause of the pain is not critical; however, identifying a patient who could potentially go into shock is a priority. You should have a high index of suspicion for internal bleeding when treating any patient with abdominal pain.

During your initial assessment, early observations can clue you into the potential for shock long before you are able to take a blood pressure. An altered mental status; cool, pale, or moist skin; and increased pulse and respirations are signs of shock you can observe very quickly in a patient. Be alert for any blood that may be present in the patient's vomit or feces. As always, make sure you are utilizing appropriate BSI precautions. All patients with abdominal pain should receive 15 lpm of supplemental oxygen by a nonrebreather mask.

After completing your initial assessment, obtain your SAMPLE history. Have the patient describe the pain in his own words. Ask open-ended questions. The OPQRST mnemonic will assist you in what questions to ask while gathering information regarding the signs and symptoms.

Because a woman's reproductive organs are located in the abdomen, you will need to ask additional questions of any female of childbearing age who presents with acute abdominal pain. Any potential for an ectopic pregnancy is a true emergency and requires immediate transport.

When you are treating geriatric patients with abdominal pain, you will be faced with some challenges. Their ability to perceive pain may have decreased, making it difficult for them to describe their pain or discomfort. They may be taking certain medications that prevent their heart rate from increasing, which would mask one of the early signs of shock, an increased heart rate.

Assessing the abdomen involves inspection and palpation. During inspection, observe the abdomen for distension, discoloration, or any abnormal findings. During palpation of the abdomen, note any rigidity, tenderness, or palpating masses. Remember to always palpate the quadrant where the discomfort is located *last*.

Vital signs should be taken every 5 minutes. The patient may appear stable on your first assessment, but any patient experiencing an acute abdominal emergency has the potential of becoming unstable.

Perform the following during your patient assessment:

- Scene size-up—utilize proper BSI precautions.
- Initial assessment—be aware that vomiting may cause airway problems; administer high-flow oxygen.
- Place the patient in a position of comfort. Unresponsive patients with no suspicion of trauma should be placed in the recovery position to help drain any fluid from the mouth.
- Obtain a SAMPLE history, focused physical exam, vital signs.
- Ongoing assessment and vital signs every 5 minutes en route.

Keep in mind that a patient with abdominal pain is likely to vomit or have diarrhea. Pay close attention to adequate BSI precautions and disinfect your ambulance after your call.

MED MINUTE

Patients who take medications for conditions related to their abdomen usually take something for prevention of nausea and vomiting (e.g., patients on chemotherapy) or to prevent diarrhea or constipation. This table gives examples of common drugs in each category. Many other medications may be available with similar effects.

CLASS OF MEDICATION	MEDICATION NAME(S)	MECHANISM OF ACTION
Antiemetics	Promethazine (Phenergan)	Reduce vomiting and the feeling of nausea. Most of these medications have other uses including treating motion sickness and psychiatric conditions.
	Prochlorperazine (Compazine)	
	Chlorpromazine (Thorazine)	
Antidiarrheals	Loperamide (Immodium)	Inhibit peristalsis and prolongs time material is retained in the GI tract.
	Calcium polycarbophil (FiberCon)	Bulk-producing laxative that absorbs fecal fluid and promotes formed stool.
Laxatives	Calcium polycarbophil (FiberCon)	Add bulk and restores moisture levels.
	Docusate sodium (Colace)	Emulsifying and wetting agent allowing moisture to penetrate stool.

PATHOPHYSIOLOGY PEARLS

Pain can arise from many different areas within the abdomen and may feel different depending on the organs that are affected. Two of the more well-known causes of abdominal pain are addressed in this section.

Acute appendicitis is something that has frequently and consistently been discussed as a cause of abdominal pain in prehospital patients. It is important to understand that inflammation of the appendix presents in the same way as inflammation of almost any other organ contained within the abdomen. This is a prime example of why the EMT-B does not need to identify the specific origin of abdominal pain.

The primary cause of appendicitis is an obstruction of the appendix by either fecal matter or mechanical kinking of the appendix upon itself. The obstruction of the appendix by either mechanism leads to acute inflammation of the tissues of the appendix. As the appendix becomes more and more inflamed, mucus production within the organ is increased as a normal immune response to the foreign matter within the appendix. Mucus production is increased in an attempt by the organ to isolate the infectious agent. As the mucus production increases, the appendix begins to swell and become painful.

Early into the infection, a superficial ulceration of the mucosa may develop. After the inflammation progresses without effective blood flow, which is necessary to combat the ensuing infection, the infection spreads from the mucosa to the muscle layers and the appendix becomes filled with pus. As the infection begins to accelerate, the mucosa may actually break down enough to create a hole through the appendix into the peritoneum and the pus will leak out, causing acute peritonitis. If the wall of the appendix is not worn away, pressure will continue to build until the appendix ruptures, again, leading to acute peritonitis and possibly death, if not surgically corrected.

Another cause of abdominal pain is an abdominal aortic aneurysm. The aorta is the main artery of the body and in most cases is capable of handling the high pressures that are created by the left ventricle. An aneurysm is typically preceded by atherosclerosis, which eventually leads to weakening of the vessel wall, and high blood pressure, which applies significant stress to the wall of the aorta. Aortic aneurysms may be worsened by inflammation, genetic predisposition, smoking, or age.

As the wall of the aorta breaks down, it will either balloon out (true aneurysms) or create a tunnel (dissecting aneurysm) on the inside wall of the aorta. True aneurysms, by nature, tend to develop over a period of time and often have no symptoms until late in their development.

Dissecting aneurysms, on the other hand, will develop quickly because of the degree of damage that ensues from the separation of the blood vessel. A patient who has a dissecting aortic aneurysm will complain of "tearing" or "ripping" pain because the aorta, like many other arteries, has nerves within its walls. When these nerves are stimulated, a tearing sensation is felt.

Small aneurysms are generally managed by the administration of drugs to keep the patient's blood pressure under control and to prevent overexertion of the heart. Large aneurysms and dissecting aneurysms of any size are typically treated by surgical intervention.

Sources

Rosen P, Barkin RM, et al., Emergency Medicine Concepts and Clinical Practice, 5th Edition, Mosby, 2002.
Tintinalli JE, Kelen GD, et al., Emergency Medicine, A Comprehensive Study Guide, 5th Edition, McGraw-Hill, 2000.
Hurst JW, The Heart, 4th Edition, McGraw-Hill, 1978.
McPhee SJ, Vishwanath RL, et al., Pathophysiology of Disease, An introduction to Clinical Medicine, 3rd Edition, Lange-McGraw-Hill, 2000.
Saladin KS, Anatomy and Physiology The Unity of Form and Function, 3rd Edition, McGraw-Hill, 2004.

REVIEW QUESTIONS

SHORT ANSWER

1. Explain *referred* pain.

2. What is an ectopic pregnancy?

MULTIPLE CHOICE

1. If a patient tenses his muscles as you are reaching to palpate his abdomen, he is said to be _____.

   A. distending   **B.** guarding

   C. inflecting   **D.** regulating

2. An abdominal aortic aneurysm (AAA) is often accompanied by a _____ pain in the patient's back.
   A. dull
   B. cramplike
   C. tearing
   D. diffuse

3. Coffee-ground-like substances in vomitus or feces may be an indication of _____.
   A. appendicitis
   B. cellulitis
   C. bowel distention
   D. internal bleeding

4. Abdominal pain that is dull and persistent often originates from _____ organs.
   A. lacerated
   B. solid
   C. reproductive
   D. hollow

5. The two layers of the peritoneum are called the _____ peritoneum and the parietal peritoneum.
   A. visceral
   B. retroparietal
   C. umbilical
   D. Langerhans

SCENARIO QUESTIONS

You are dispatched to a residence for an individual with abdominal pain. You find the patient, a 28-year-old female, curled up in a fetal position on her bed. When you ask the patient to describe her discomfort, she explains that it is an intermittent pain and that it feels "crampy." She denies any nausea, vomiting, or diarrhea.

1. Which of the following questions best addresses the *provocation* of this patient's pain?
   A. "How did the pain begin?"
   B. "Can you point to where the pain is?"
   C. "What makes the pain better or worse?"
   D. "Has the pain changed since this morning?"

2. You would suspect that the patient's abdominal pain is most likely originating in a _____ organ.
   A. solid
   B. digestive
   C. hollow
   D. referred

3. Which of the following would *not* be an appropriate question to ask?
   A. "Have you had sexual intercourse since your last period?"
   B. "Do you currently have any vaginal bleeding that is not menstrual bleeding?"
   C. "Are you sexually active?"
   D. "Have you had sexual intercourse in the past 12 to 24 hours?"

You arrive at a care home for an 82-year-old man with severe abdominal pain. You find him sitting in a wheelchair in the facility's activity room. He appears pale, his skin is cool and sweaty, and his pulse is 74 and regular. "I was just sitting here," he tells you. "And I started getting indigestion real bad right here." He points to the center of his abdomen, just inferior to the sternum. As you begin palpating the subject's abdomen, you notice a bulge that is pulsating. The patient has no allergies and regularly takes metoprolol, multivitamins, and aspirin.

1. "Indigestion," or pain just below the sternum, is a common complaint from patients experiencing _____.

   A. a myocardial infarction **B.** an ileocecal perforation

   C. dyspnea **D.** a bowel obstruction

2. As an EMT-B, you should immediately treat this patient for _____.

   A. a suspected aortic aneurysm **B.** angina

   C. acute indigestion **D.** cardiac asystole

3. After initially feeling the pulsating bulge, you should _____.

   A. palpate more to determine whether it is an abdominal aortic aneurysm

   B. place the patient in the Fowler's position and closely monitor his blood pressure

   C. ask the patient whether he has ever had an abdominal aneurysm

   D. immediately administer oxygen via nasal cannula, and transport

CASE STUDIES

CASE STUDY 1	ACUTE ABDOMEN

You are dispatched to a motorcycle crash involving one person. Upon your arrival, you find an approximately 20-year-old male lying supine in the second lane of the highway. Fire personnel are holding c-spine and attempting to get vitals when you reach the patient.

He is alert and complaining of severe pain in his right thigh and right shoulder. You perform a rapid trauma assessment and identify abrasions to the shoulder and considerable swelling and an open wound to the right femur. In addition to the extremity injuries, he complains of extreme pain in his upper right quadrant when you palpate his abdomen. You note that his abdomen feels firm during palpation. The firefighter advises you that the patient's blood pressure is 100 by palpation and that his pulse is 108 and weak.

1. Which of this man's injuries that you have identified is likely to be the most serious and why?

2. What is most likely causing this man's abdomen to appear firm during palpation?

You now have the patient on oxygen and have controlled the bleeding from his right leg. As you prepare him for transport, he becomes less responsive and responds only to painful stimuli. Another set of vitals reveals that the blood pressure is 90 by palpation and the pulse is 130 and weak.

1. How will you prepare this man for transport to the hospital? How will you manage the femur injury?

2. What is most likely the cause for the worsening of this man's condition? What can you as an EMT-B do for this?

You are dispatched for a complaint of abdominal pain at an office complex. You arrive at a safe scene and approach a young woman who is lying on the floor of her office with a cold towel on her forehead. She complains of severe abdominal pain in her "lower abdomen."

The patient is breathing adequately, has no external bleeding, and is placed on oxygen by nonre-breather mask. Her pulse is a bit rapid and her skin is warm and moist.

1. What priority would this patient be?

2. Would you do a SAMPLE history or a physical assessment first?

The patient tells you that she is 19 years old. She is a bit embarrassed that this might just be very bad menstrual cramps. She tells you that she thought she got her period the night before and awoke with unusually serious cramps. She noticed a little bit of blood that stopped in the morning. She tried to do her work but the cramps became more severe during the morning. She got up from her desk and found that it hurt so badly that she had to lower herself to the floor.

1. Can you ask the patient about her menstrual cycle and whether she could be pregnant?

2. If so, what other questions should you ask?

The patient tells you that her period was late this month. While she does not keep close track of the dates, she thought it might be about two or three weeks late. It normally runs pretty regularly. She has been sexually active during the cycle and volunteers that her partner had used condoms. She does not think she could be pregnant.

Palpation reveals tenderness across both lower quadrants that is slightly more severe on the right. Vital signs are pulse 104, respirations 20, skin cool and moist, pupils equal and reactive to light, and blood pressure 104 over 64.

1. Is this complaint pregnancy-related?

2. Is the patient in shock? Are the patient's vital signs as you see them caused by the pain?

Active Exploration

Most injuries to the abdomen can be difficult to detect especially if they were caused by blunt trauma. In many cases involving major trauma, the patient has suffered additional more obvious injuries that can easily distract you and the patient from more serious internal injuries. You might spend several minutes trying to bandage an open fracture of the lower leg and neglect your assessment of the abdomen because by all indications it appears normal.

A thorough and focused assessment of the abdomen is essential when the mechanism of injury suggests possible trauma to the chest or abdomen.

The following activities are designed to help you learn the anatomy of the abdomen and improve your abdominal-assessment skills.

Activity 1: Four Corners

For this activity you will need your Emergency Care textbook, a blank piece of paper to write on, and a fellow student to act as patient.

Begin by drawing two lines on the paper, one vertical and one horizontal, dividing the page into quarters. Now, without looking at your book, pretend these four corners are the four quadrants of a patient's abdomen. Make a list of the specific anatomy that is contained in each of the four quadrants.

Once you think your list is complete, open your book to Chapter 18 and check your list against the illustrations in the book. How did you do?

Activity 2: Practice Perfect Palpation

This next activity will expand on the first by having you apply your knowledge of this anatomy to the hands-on assessment of an actual abdomen.

You will need a fellow student to play the role of patient as you assess the abdomen. Have the "patient" lie supine on the floor. He is to secretly choose a quadrant for which he will complain of pain and the characteristics of the pain. When he is ready, you are to begin a thorough assessment of the abdomen.

Using both hands, press firmly into each quadrant. Watch the "patient's" face for signs of grimacing or pain. Talk the "patient" through the exam with you telling him ahead of time where you will be pressing.

When you come to an area of pain, pause to investigate the pain in more detail. Use the OPQRST mnemonic to assess the pain.

Take turns with your partner and change the location and characteristics of the pain each time you practice. When you are playing patient, provide feedback to your partner as to whether he is pressing too softly or too hard. This will help him develop his assessment skills as an EMT.

RETRO REVIEW

1. How could you quickly assess perfusion on an unresponsive adult patient with painted nails and a bleeding soft-tissue injury in the mouth?
   - **A.** Blanch the back of the hand.
   - **B.** Examine the soles of the feet.
   - **C.** Check the lower eyelids.
   - **D.** Look into the nares.
2. The trending of a patient's condition requires an initial assessment, baseline vitals, and _____.
   - **A.** medical direction
   - **B.** a SAMPLE history
   - **C.** industry statistics
   - **D.** ongoing assessments
3. _____ binds with certain poisons, preventing the body from absorbing them.
   - **A.** Activated charcoal
   - **B.** Vinegar
   - **C.** Syrup of ipecac
   - **D.** Lactated Ringer's

THINKING AND LINKING

CHAPTER TOPIC	HOW IT RELATES TO YOU AND OTHER COURSE AREAS
Abdominal pain/discomfort	There are numerous causes for abdominal pain or discomfort. Luckily, you will not be required to diagnose anything. The goal of your patient assessment is to be able to adequately describe the patient's condition to the receiving facility and to recognize (and treat) immediate life-threats, like shock (Chapter 26).
Physical examination	Many patients will be uncomfortable with a stranger looking at and touching their abdomen—especially once the examination nears the pelvic area. You should be sensitive to this and remember that, as with any physical examination, your professional demeanor (Chapter 1) and ability to explain what you are doing will ease the patient considerably.
BSI and disinfection	You will undoubtedly be called to treat and transport patients with uncontrollable vomiting and/or diarrhea. Protect yourself with appropriate PPE (Chapter 2), and protect your future patients by thoroughly cleaning and disinfecting the patient compartment of the ambulance (Chapter 33). Consider everywhere that projected fluids may end up—from the underside of the gurney mattress to the slots that the cabinet doors run in.

19

Diabetic Emergencies and Altered Mental Status

CHAPTER SUMMARY

As you learned in Chapter 19 of your Emergency Care textbook, altered mental status can be caused by a variety of conditions. Some of these conditions are quite obvious, such as diabetes, and others are more challenging to decipher. The most important issue to remember with any patient is your initial assessment. Regardless of the patients' level of responsiveness or their mental status, you must determine whether they have a patent (open) airway and adequate breathing and circulation. These basic necessities of life must be maintained before further emergency care can be provided.

DIABETES OVERVIEW

Glucose (a form of sugar) is the main fuel for the body. Cells in the body need adequate glucose to function properly. Glucose cannot enter the cells on its own; it needs a transport vehicle. Insulin, a hormone produced by the pancreas, acts as that vehicle. There must be an adequate amount of insulin and glucose in the bloodstream for this transfer to take place.

Diabetic patients do not produce enough insulin, or their bodies are not able to utilize insulin properly. They might administer insulin to themselves by injection, or they may have an insulin pump. The insulin pump delivers metered doses of insulin through a small catheter that is inserted beneath the skin, usually in the abdominal region.

Hypoglycemia (low blood sugar) is the most common medical emergency that a diabetic patient may develop. It may be caused by any one of the following:

- Reduced blood glucose levels due to not eating, or skipping a meal
- An increase in normal activity (uses more glucose than normal)
- Vomiting after a meal
- Taking too much insulin without eating adequate sugar (glucose)

The brain is very sensitive to lowered amounts of sugar in the bloodstream. A drop in blood sugar will quickly result in altered mental status and possibly unresponsiveness if not treated quickly. Patients with hypoglycemia often present with abnormal behavior and sweaty skin (diaphoresis). Once you have confirmed that the patient is a known diabetic and that he is responsive enough to swallow, you must administer oral glucose as quickly as possible; this is critical for maintaining the brain's ability to function. If he is not able to swallow, then maintain the patient's airway and transport promptly.

Excessive blood sugar, or hyperglycemia, occurs when a patient has a decrease in the amount of insulin. This may be caused by the body not producing enough or by missed insulin injections. This condition has a much slower onset, usually days. The patient may feel nauseous and complain of polyuria (frequent urination) and being thirsty.

The following signs and symptoms are characteristic of a diabetic emergency:

- Rapid onset of altered mental status
- Intoxicated appearance or behavior
- Combativeness
- Unusual behavior
- Seizures

OTHER CAUSES OF ALTERED MENTAL STATUS

Seizures can also be the cause of an altered mental status in a patient. Seizures are a sign of an underlying problem such as infection, tumors, alcohol or drug abuse, and trauma, to name a few. Children commonly have seizures following a sudden spike or increase in temperature. Other common causes of seizure are:

- Stroke
- Hypoglycemia
- Hypoxia
- Heat stroke
- Epilepsy

Your emergency care for a patient who is having a seizure is to protect him from harm. This may mean placing him on the floor and moving away objects that could potentially harm him. Do not attempt to restrain the patient. Once the seizure has stopped, protect the airway and transport promptly.

A stroke is another common cause of an altered mental status. A stroke is either a blockage of a blood vessel in the brain or a blood vessel that is bleeding into the brain tissue. Either one of these conditions deprives the brain of oxygenated blood in the affected area. Stroke patients can present with varied signs and symptoms. Paralysis to one side of the body is very common. It may also be difficult to gather information from them due to their inability to communicate because of the region of the brain that is affected.

PATIENT ASSESSMENT AND EMERGENCY CARE FOR PATIENTS WITH AN ALTERED MENTAL STATUS

1. Initial assessment
   a. Airway (patent?)
   b. Breathing (adequate?)
   c. Circulation (adequate?)
   d. Level of responsiveness
2. Apply high-flow oxygen by nonrebreather mask (the brain needs oxygen)
3. Perform a focused history and physical exam
   a. What you discover during the history and physical exam will determine your next course of action
   b. History of diabetes? Is the patient able to swallow? Can you administer oral glucose?

On all patients, determine baseline vitals, request ALS, or transport promptly.

MED MINUTE

Alterations in mental status may be caused by numerous diseases and complications, including diabetes, seizure disorders, and abnormalities within the nervous system. This table gives examples of common drugs in each category. Dozens of medications may be available with similar effects.

CLASS OF MEDICATION	MEDICATION NAME(S)	MECHANISM OF ACTION
Oral glucose	Instaglucose	Increases blood-sugar levels when applied to the oral mucosa and absorbed into the blood stream.
	Glutose	
Oral antidiabetic agents	Glipizide (Glucotrol)	Used for diabetic (type II) patients who produce limited amounts of insulin, to stimulate the pancreas to release insulin when blood-sugar levels are high.
	Glimepiride (Amaryl)	
	Glyburide (Diabeta)	
	Metformin (Glucophage)	
Injectable antidiabetic agents	Insulin (Humulin R, Novolin R, Regular Insulin, Velosulin)	Lower blood-sugar levels by preventing the liver from changing glucose (blood sugar) into glycogen (blood-sugar storage units) and making glucose available for use by the body.

(Continued)

CLASS OF MEDICATION	MEDICATION NAME(S)	MECHANISM OF ACTION
Anticonvulsants	Carbamazepine (Tegretol)	Control seizures by regulating electrical impulses in the brain.
	Clonazepam (Klonopin)	
	Phenobarbital (Barbital)	
	Phenytoin (Dilantin)	
	Valproic Acid (Depakote)	

PATHOPHYSIOLOGY PEARLS

Diabetes is an enormous problem in the United States and contributes to a significant number of deaths and/or disabilities each year. The American Diabetes Association released the following statistics in 2002:

- 18.2 million Americans—6.3 percent of the population—have diabetes.
- 5.2 million Americans do not know they have diabetes.
- 18 million or 8.7 percent of Americans 20 years or older have diabetes.
- 8.6 million or 18.3 percent of Americans 60 years or older have diabetes.
- From 2000 to 2001, about 82,000 nontraumatic lower-limb amputations were performed as a result of diabetes.
- In 2002, the cost of diabetes in the United States was approximately $132 billion.
- The death rate from heart disease is two to four times higher among people with diabetes than among those without diabetes.
- The risk for stroke is two to four times higher among people with diabetes.

Do you know anyone who was on the Atkins diet for a while, and did you notice that his breath had a somewhat sweet or fruity odor to it? Did you wonder why? The answer to this question is very simple; the person was not taking in enough carbohydrates, which insulin stores and helps to break down, and therefore, the body was burning fat as energy for the body.

The diabetic patient who has excessively high levels of glucose in the blood may go into Diabetic Ketoacidosis or DKA. Patients with DKA will present with the fruity odor on their breaths just like a person on the Atkins diet and for similar reasons: they do not have enough insulin available to carry the glucose into the cells where it can be used and they will eventually begin to break down their own fat cells to produce energy. Remember insulin is what makes it possible for the cells of the body to use and break down glucose. If glucose cannot get into the cells, the cells cannot function and eventually the patient will have to rely on another source for energy.

When the body needs energy and cannot get it from the normal route (glucose), it will begin to burn fat. The by-product of broken-down fat is ketoacid or ketones. This is why people who go for long periods of time without eating will have ketones on their breath too: the cells of their bodies are essentially being starved. The problem with DKA is multifaceted: First, because there are so many ketoacids formed, the patient will become acidotic and may die from an abnormally high acid level in the blood. Additionally, the patient will begin to lose a large amount of the water as his body attempts to neutralize the acids and he may go into cardiac arrest because of poor circulating blood volume.

Treatment for the patient with DKA generally includes the administration of IV fluids to correct for the water loss and IV insulin to help get glucose into the cells and stop the destruction of fat, thus reducing the production of acids.

Sources

"National Diabetes Fact Sheet," 2003, ADA Website http://www.diabetes.org/ info/facts/facts_natl.jsp.
Rosen P, Barkin RM, et al., Emergency Medicine Concepts and Clinical Practice, 5th Edition, Mosby, 2002.
Tintinalli JE, Kelen GD, et al., Emergency Medicine, A Comprehensive Study Guide, 5th Edition, McGraw-Hill, 2000.
Mulvihill ML, Zelman M, et al., Human Diseases: A Systemic Approach, 5th Edition, Prentice Hall, 2001.

REVIEW QUESTIONS

SHORT ANSWER

1. What is "status epilepticus"?

2. Why is excessive thirst an indicator of diabetes mellitus?

MULTIPLE CHOICE

1. Increased hunger, accompanied by nausea and an acetone-like breath odor is indicative of _____.

    A. hypoglycemia   **B.** alcoholism

    C. hyperglycemia   **D.** glucositis

2. The most common cause of seizures in adults is _____.

    A. failure to take seizure-control medication

    B. alcohol abuse

    C. high fever or dehydration

    D. head trauma

3. "Vasovagal syncope" is also called _____.

    A. a TIA (transient ischemic attack)   **B.** hypovolemia

    C. epilepsy   **D.** simple fainting

4. Insulin is a hormone produced in the _____.

    A. thyroid   **B.** pancreas

    C. liver   **D.** small intestines

5. _____ seizures occur spontaneously and for unknown reasons.

    A. Metabolic   **B.** Psychogenic

    C. Toxic   **D.** Idiopathic

SCENARIO QUESTIONS

You respond to a call from a public park for an individual who might have lost responsiveness while jogging. Upon your arrival, you find the patient (a 47-year-old female) who is responsive but very confused and complaining of generalized weakness. She has rapid respirations and a pulse. Her blood pressure is 136/92, and you notice that she has a Medic-Alert necklace indicating hypertension and diabetes. She cannot recall what medications she takes.

1. This patient most likely has _____.
   A. suffered an ischemic stroke
   B. become hypoglycemic
   C. suffered an aneurysm
   D. developed a high blood-sugar level

2. How should you provide emergency care for this patient?
   A. Administer high-concentration oxygen and transport in the Fowler's position.
   B. Administer aspirin and transport in the recovery position with oxygen at 15 lpm.
   C. Administer oral glucose, high-concentration oxygen, and transport in the semi-Fowler's position.
   D. Secure the patient to a long spine board, administer oxygen via nonrebreather mask, and transport with the foot-end of the board raised 8 to 12 inches.

You are refueling your ambulance at a service station when the man at the pump just ahead of you suddenly collapses onto the back of his car. You approach and see that the 50- to 55-year-old man is struggling to stand and is slowly sliding to the ground. You identify yourself and help him onto the pavement. "Are you okay?" you ask. His reply is garbled and you are unable to understand what he is trying to say. You notice that the right half of his face is drooping slightly. As you and your partner are transporting the patient to the hospital, his strength and coherence return and his facial droop disappears.

1. This patient has most likely suffered a(n) _____.
   A. stroke (or cerebral-vascular accident (CVA))
   B. transient ischemic attack (TIA)
   C. absence seizure (petit-mal seizure)
   D. hemorrhagic stroke

2. The _____ is used by EMT-Bs to quickly assess the severity of an apparent stroke.
   A. Claremont Ischemia Index
   B. Cleveland Prehospital Stroke Scale
   C. Cerebral Accident Intensity Indicator
   D. Cincinnati Prehospital Stroke Scale

3. You would notify the receiving facility that this patient is showing signs of _____ aphasia.
   A. respiratory   B. expressive
   C. receptive   D. cerebral

You are dispatched to an elementary school for a seizing child. You arrive and find the patient, a 9-year-old boy, convulsing on the floor of his classroom. The teacher, who has already moved all of the desks away from the boy, tells you that he has been convulsing almost constantly since the EMS was called. According to school records, the boy has no history of seizures and neither of his parents can be reached.

1. What are the best emergency-care steps for this patient?

   A. Loosen restrictive clothing, restrain the child to keep him from injuring himself, and provide supplemental oxygen.

   B. Administer high-concentration oxygen, transport immediately, and request an ALS intercept.

   C. Insert an airway adjunct and, once the child's convulsing subsides, prepare for rapid transport.

   D. Administer high-concentration oxygen and wait for the seizure to subside.

2. This patient is experiencing _____.

   A. vasovagal distress
   B. absence-seizure convulsions
   C. status epilepticus
   D. febrile hypoxia

3. Seizures are typically the result of _____.

   A. elevated body temperatures
   B. peripheral nerve pathology
   C. toxins in the brain
   D. irregular electrical activity in the brain

CASE STUDIES

CASE STUDY 1   THE TELLER WHO CAN'T

You are dispatched to an unresponsive person at a local bank. Upon your arrival, you are met outside in the street by one of the bank employees. She tells you the patient is on the third floor and that the elevator is down for maintenance and that you will have to take the stairs. As you approach the patient, you see an approximately 60-year-old female who appears responsive sitting upright in a chair with two others kneeling in front of her trying to ask her questions. A woman identifies herself as the patient's supervisor and states that when she came to meet with her she was staring off into space and not making any sense.

1. **Detail specifically how you will conduct your initial assessment on this patient.**

2. **What questions will you ask initially and why?**

As you attempt to obtain a history from the patient, she makes occasional attempts to speak but produces nothing that makes any sense. Your partner obtains a baseline set of vitals, which are blood pressure 108/68, pulse 96, respirations 18, skin slightly pale and moist, and pupils equal and reactive to light. During the pulse check, your partner discovers a Medic-Alert bracelet indicating that the patient is a diabetic and takes insulin injections. The supervisor states that she was just fine an hour ago when she came in to work.

1. What is most likely this person's problem? How will this patient progress if left untreated?

2. How will you treat this patient and why?

You are dispatched for an unknown problem at a residence. You arrive at a safe scene and find a woman in her 50s at the door waving you in. "Thank you for coming so quickly," she says. "He just sits there. I don't understand what is going on."

She explains that her husband was fine earlier in the day. He was watching the game on TV when she last saw him about two hours ago. She was gardening. "He was fine. We were going out to dinner later this evening."

You approach the patient who is aware of your presence but does not speak. After introducing yourself, he continues to stare at you as you say, "Sir, I am from the ambulance. Can you hear me?" After a few moments, he seems to nod slightly that he can hear you.

1. How would you perform an initial assessment?

2. The patient obviously has difficulty communicating. How will this affect the emergency care you provide?

The patient appears to be breathing adequately. You notice a bit of drool on the side of his mouth, but the patient does not appear to need suctioning. His pulse is present and appears normal, and there is no external bleeding. You notice that his face does not seem even. His cheek and mouth on the right side seem to be sagging.

1. In response to your findings in the preceding paragraph, what questions would you ask the patient's wife?

2. What elements of a physical exam would you perform?

The wife tells you that her husband was fine just two hours ago. He has had no medical problems to speak of. He went to the doctor recently and other than high cholesterol, he was in good health. He had no prior facial drooping or difficulty speaking.

1. Is this definitely a stroke?

2. What transport priority is this patient?

3. On what decisions would you base your choice of receiving hospitals?

Active Exploration

Assessing and treating the "medical" patient can be one of the EMT-B's most challenging propositions. Trauma calls provide many clues, such as mechanism of injury, thus giving the EMT-B a good place to begin when both assessing patients and treating their injuries. The absence of an MOI and the challenge of dealing with a patient who has an altered mental status can make both the assessment and the indicated emergency care somewhat difficult. It is on the medical call that the EMT-B must be extra thorough in obtaining a good history and performing a detailed physical exam as most often the most important clues are difficult to find.

The following activities will help you develop your assessment skills when dealing with the medical patient.

Activity 1: What's Wrong With Me?

This activity is particularly good at helping you learn the specific signs and symptoms of specific medical problems.

1. Using 3 × 5 cards, identify specific medical complaints and place their names on one side of the card. For example, hypoglycemia, hyperglycemia, epilepsy, status epilepticus, generalized tonic-clonic seizure (grand-mal seizure), absence seizure, and stroke.
2. Using your Emergency Care textbook and any other resources you may want to use, make a list on the other side of the card of the signs and symptoms of each of the medical complaints that you have identified.
3. Sit back-to-back with a fellow student. Student #1 will select one of the medical complaints and quickly scan the signs and symptoms on the card. When he is ready, student #2 must begin asking questions that will ultimately lead to the discovery of student #1's medical problem.

Just as valuable as the question-and-answer segment is the inevitable discussion that will ensue when student #2 disagrees with how student #1 presented the scenario. This almost always happens and leads to a better understanding on everyone's part regarding the typical and atypical presentation of various medical conditions.

Activity 2: My Lips are Sealed

The conscious stroke patient who is both physically impaired and also often unable to communicate verbally can be one of the most challenging patients that you will encounter. There is a tremendous amount of frustration and fear associated with being unable to communicate with those around you. This next activity will help you develop an understanding of what it is like from the patient's perspective and help you learn to communicate in a whole new way as a care provider.

1. Pair up with a fellow student and decide in advance who will play the role of the patient and who will play the role of the EMT-B.

2. The student who will be playing the patient must take a few minutes to think of a scenario involving a possible stroke. It may be helpful to refer to the text and to write out some signs and symptoms just to get them clear. Do not let the "EMT-B" see what you are writing or know in advance how you will be presenting to the caregiver.

3. Once the "patient" is ready, the "EMT-B" must enter the scene and begin treating the patient and attempting to obtain as detailed a history as possible. The only catch is that the "patient" must remain responsive but may not provide any verbal feedback. It is up to the "EMT-B" to find an alternative method by which to communicate with the "patient" in order to obtain as complete a history as possible.

This can be a fun and frustrating activity. For a little friendly competition, have a third student observe the entire sequence and document the history as it is obtained. The roles then get reversed and the winner is the "EMT-B" who is able to get the most history in a predetermined amount of time.

RETRO REVIEW

1. When applying a sphygmomanometer, it should be placed _____.
   A. on the patient's abdomen
   B. over the railing of the wheeled gurney
   C. on the patient's index finger (if no nail polish is present)
   D. over the brachial artery

2. Nitroglycerin patches should be removed prior to defibrillation because they can _____.
   A. cause fatal overdoses
   B. interfere with the placement of the electrode pad
   C. produce nitrochlorine fumes
   D. cause arcing between the pads or paddles

3. _____ airways should be used on patients whose gag reflexes are still active.
   A. Oropharyngeal   B. Inverted
   C. Nasopharyngeal   D. Hyperextended

THINKING AND LINKING

CHAPTER TOPIC	HOW IT RELATES TO YOU AND OTHER COURSE AREAS
Hypoglycemia	You are going to see a wide range of behaviors among patients who are hypoglycemic (more on behavioral issues and their causes in Chapter 23). You should not just assume drug use, intoxication, seizure disorders, or behavioral problems when approaching patients—try to find out quickly whether there is a history of diabetes (Chapters 8 and 9).
Seizure disorders	Some seizure patients may have head or spine injuries—either as the cause of the seizure or as a result of it. You should bring spinal-immobilization equipment (Chapter 29) when responding to a seizure call. Also, if the seizure was the result of an injury, you should anticipate possible scene-safety issues (Chapters 2 and 7).
Stroke and aphasia	You will sometimes need to rely heavily on your interpersonal communication skills (Chapter 13) when dealing with stroke patients and their families. The effects of a stroke can cause tremendous confusion, frustration, and even anger. Remember that many stroke calls will involve elderly patients who sometimes require unique approaches and specific care (Chapter 32).

CHAPTER 20

Allergic Reactions

CHAPTER SUMMARY

The body's immune system naturally reacts to any foreign substance. If this reaction is more profound than normal, the patient may have an allergic reaction. Many substances can cause an allergic reaction. A severe allergic reaction that causes respiratory distress and hypotension is known as anaphylaxis or anaphylactic shock.

People do not have allergic reactions the first time they are exposed to the substance that causes the reaction (allergen). After the initial exposure, the immune system creates antibodies to fight the allergen. The second time the person is exposed, the allergen reacts with the antibody, and the body releases chemicals that make the blood vessels dilate, tissues swell, and bronchioles constrict.

The following are causes of allergic reactions:

- Insect bites—usually cause rapid and severe reactions
- Food—reaction onset tends to be slower than insect bites, with the exception of peanuts
- Plants
- Medications
- Dust, chemicals, makeup, and so on

People who have had multiple surgeries may be allergic to latex. Healthcare professionals may also develop sensitivity to latex from wearing exam gloves repeatedly.

Most severe reactions take place immediately, but some may not develop for 30 minutes or so. Mild reactions can progress very quickly to severe reactions. Any patient with a history of an allergic reaction should be monitored very closely, even if no immediate reaction is present. It only takes a matter of minutes for tissues to swell and for the patient's airway to become obstructed.

Signs and symptoms of allergic reactions or anaphylaxis can include:

- Itching
- Hives
- Flushing
- Swelling of the face, neck, hands, feet, or tongue
- Warm, tingling feeling in face, mouth, chest, or hands and feet
- Tightness in throat or chest
- Coughing
- Increased respiratory rate
- Noisy breathing
- Hoarseness or loss of voice
- Stridor
- Wheezing
- Increased heart rate
- Decreased blood pressure
- Watery eyes
- Headache
- Runny nose
- Feelings of impending doom
- Altered mental status
- Nausea or vomiting
- Changes in vital signs

Any of the above signs or symptoms can be associated with an allergic reaction. For anaphylaxis to exist, the patient must have either respiratory distress or signs and symptoms of shock.

If a patient has come into contact with a substance that caused an allergic reaction in the past, suspect an allergic reaction if itching, hives, respiratory distress, or hypoperfusion are present. Keep in mind that it may be the patient's second exposure to a substance; therefore, this would be the first time that he has developed an allergic reaction.

Perform your initial assessment and correct any life-threats found. Ensure a patent airway and apply high-flow oxygen with a nonrebreather mask. Assist ventilations if breathing is inadequate. You may assist the patient with his prescribed epinephrine auto-injector if all the following apply:

- The patient has come into contact with a substance that caused an allergic reaction in the past
- The patient has respiratory distress or has signs and symptoms of hypoperfusion
- The patient has a prescribed epinephrine auto-injector
- Medical-direction orders have been given

Document the administration of the auto-injector and transport the patient. Typical auto-injectors only deliver a single dose of epinephrine. If the patient has additional injectors, bring them in the ambulance in case additional doses need to be given during transport. You would need to contact medical direction before additional doses could be administered.

Treat for shock and prepare for immediate transport those patients who do not have their auto-injectors with them or have never had one prescribed. Call for an ALS intercept.

The auto-injector is a spring-loaded syringe with a single dose of epinephrine. Before contacting medical direction, observe the syringe for its expiration date, ensure that it has been prescribed for your patient, and that the liquid is not cloudy. Press the syringe into the lateral thigh muscle midway between the waist and the knee. Hold it in place until the entire dose is injected. Epinephrine is a hormone that will help constrict the blood vessels and relax the bronchioles. Reassess your patient after 2 minutes.

Epinephrine is a very powerful medication. It makes the heart work harder. This can be potentially dangerous for patients who have heart conditions or high blood pressure. That is why it is so important that EMTs only administer epinephrine auto-injectors to patients who have had them prescribed by their physician. Epinephrine auto-injectors come in two doses: adult and pediatric.

MED MINUTE

Although anaphylactic reactions are relatively uncommon, when they do occur, death may result within minutes; therefore, it is imperative that patients with a history of significant allergic reactions or anaphylaxis have the appropriate medications available to them. This table gives examples of common drugs in each category. Dozens of medications may be available with similar effects.

CLASS OF MEDICATION	MEDICATION NAME(S)	MECHANISM OF ACTION
Beta agonist	Epinephrine EpiPen® auto-injector	A normally occurring chemical within the body that causes increased strength of cardiac contraction, constriction of blood vessels, and dilation of the bronchioles to improve the blood pressure and ventilations of the patient in anaphylactic shock.
Histamine blockers	Diphenhydramine (Benadryl)—H1	H1 blocks the release of histamine 1, which causes bronchoconstriction and vasodilation.
	Cimetadine (Tagamet)—H2 Famotidine (Pepcid AC)	H2 blocks the release of histamine 2, which causes an increase in stomach-acid secretion, and an increase in capillary permeability.
Corticosteroids	Prednisolone (Prelone) Prednisone (Sterapred) Dexamethasone (Decadron)	Decrease inflammation of the skin and within the airways, while restoring the integrity of the membranes of the blood vessels to prevent capillary-fluid leakage.
Bronchodilators	Albuterol sulfate (Proventil) Xopenex (levalbuterol HCl) Atrovent (ipratropium bromide) Combivent (combines albuterol sulfate and ipratropium bromide)	Reduce airway inflammation and mucus secretion in the lungs for patients with allergy-induced bronchoconstriction.

PATHOPHYSIOLOGY PEARLS

It is important to realize that there is a difference between an allergic reaction and true anaphylaxis. An allergic reaction is generally localized and includes signs and symptoms consistent with hypersensitivity to a specific agent. Signs and symptoms of an allergic reaction may include itching, redness, and hives. An anaphylactic reaction is much more severe and one that involves a more systemic reaction including some degree of respiratory or hemodynamic compromise.

During an anaphylactic reaction, a cascade of chemical reactions occurs within the body. As a patient is exposed to an allergen (the agent that initiates the immune response), histamine is released. Histamine is released because the body interprets the allergen as a foreign substance within the body. Histamine is one of the chemicals predominantly responsible for repairing tissue and protecting the patient from further injury or illness.

Histamine causes blood-vessel dilation and constriction of the bronchiole airways. When histamine is released, the blood vessels dilate to promote greater flow of oxygenated blood into the inflamed tissues, and vessels also dilate to more effectively remove damaged tissues and waste products from the blood. Histamine causes bronchoconstriction in an attempt to promote clearance of foreign material from inside the lungs. As foreign materials enter the lungs, the patient will produce large quantities of mucus for the purpose of trapping the foreign material so it does not spread. The narrowed airways will make it easier for the patient to remove the additional mucus and the foreign material from the lungs through forceful coughing in tight airways.

In addition to histamine, there are several other chemicals that are released during an anaphylactic reaction. The additional chemicals released include the following:

CHEMICAL	FUNCTION	FUNCTION
Kinins	Increased blood-vessel permeability	Increased blood-vessel dilation
Prostoglandins	Coronary-vessel constriction	Attraction of immune cells
Leukotrienes	Coronary-vessel constriction	Bronchial constriction
Heparin	Decreased blood viscosity	

Sources

Tintinalli JE, Kelen GD. et al., Emergency Medicine, A Comprehensive Study Guide, 5th Edition, McGraw-Hill, 2000.
Rosen P, Barkin RM, et al., Emergency Medicine Concepts and Clinical Practice, 5th Edition. Mosby, 2002.

REVIEW QUESTIONS

SHORT ANSWER

1. What effect does injected epinephrine have on the body?

2. Why is there never an allergic reaction after an individual's first exposure to an allergen?

MULTIPLE CHOICE

1. Unlike most other food-source allergies, reactions to _____ can be very rapid.
   - **A.** peanuts
   - **B.** flour products
   - **C.** milk
   - **D.** eggs

2. Epinephrine injections can sometime be dangerous in patients who suffer from _____.
   - **A.** COPD
   - **B.** colitis
   - **C.** diabetes
   - **D.** hypertension

3. A patient is not in anaphylaxis unless either _____ or the signs and symptoms of shock are present.
   - **A.** an altered mental status
   - **B.** respiratory distress
   - **C.** an impending sense of doom
   - **D.** respiratory arrest

4. Why do infants rarely develop anaphylaxis?
   - **A.** They are not generally exposed to allergens.
   - **B.** Infants have a natural defense to allergens.
   - **C.** Their immune systems are too underdeveloped.
   - **D.** Infants *do* regularly develop anaphylaxis.

5. Healthcare professionals are among a segment of the population that is growing increasingly allergic to _____.
   - **A.** iodine
   - **B.** alcohol
   - **C.** latex
   - **D.** plastics

SCENARIO QUESTIONS

You are at a local park for your niece's eighth birthday party. As you are talking to some friends, one of them swats his neck and exclaims, "Ouch! What was that?"

"A bee, but don't worry … you killed it," somebody says. The individual who has been stung looks at you with panic in his eyes and says, "I'm really allergic to bees." He starts scratching and you see hives beginning to appear on his arms. He hands you his car keys and hurriedly tells you that he keeps an EpiPen® in his glove box. You notice that his face and hands are beginning to swell.

1. What should you do?
   - **A.** Retrieve the epinephrine injector, help the patient to administer it, and call 911.
   - **B.** Send one of the other individuals to retrieve the EpiPen® while you call for EMS and monitor the patient.
   - **C.** Call for emergency services, help the patient to lie down, and monitor his respirations.
   - **D.** Have the patient walk with you to his vehicle to keep his circulation rapid.

2. After examining the epinephrine auto-injector and determining that it is prescribed to the patient and is not expired, you should _____.

   A. hand it to the patient and remind him how to use it

   B. tell the patient to be still while you inject the epinephrine

   C. hold on to it while determining whether the patient's condition will worsen

   D. have the patient place his hand on the device while you trigger it

3. The patient should firmly press the epinephrine auto-injector to his _____ to activate it.

   A. bicep   B. calf

   C. neck   D. thigh

You are dispatched to the county fair for a woman who is having trouble breathing. You are quickly led to the 56-year-old patient, who is sitting on a bench and laboring to breathe. Her eyes, lips, and hands appear swollen, and her skin is covered with red blotches. The woman's husband tells you that she tried a bite of his seafood plate at lunch, 15 or 20 minutes before her illness began. You ask the patient whether she is allergic to anything and she shakes her head and hoarsely whispers "No." The patient's husband then says, "This is only the second time in our 35 years of marriage that I've been able to talk her into trying seafood. Something tells me that she ain't gonna try it again!"

1. You should immediately administer _____ to this patient.

   A. epinephrine   B. activated charcoal

   C. oxygen   D. milk or water

2. The best option for saving this patient's life is to _____.

   A. request an ALS intercept

   B. utilize a nasopharyngeal airway

   C. complete a SAMPLE history

   D. insert an endotracheal tube

3. Why should you suspect that this patient is suffering from anaphylactic shock?

   A. The patient presents with generalized swelling after being exposed to a potential allergen.

   B. This is only the second time that the patient has eaten a potential allergen.

   C. The patient developed hives soon after consuming a common allergen.

   D. The patient is having respiratory difficulty after exposure to a potential allergen.

CASE STUDIES

CASE STUDY 1   MY THROAT IS GETTING BIG

You are dispatched to the local water-slide park for a difficulty in breathing call. Upon your arrival, you find an approximately 13-year-old girl lying on the grass crying. She is in moderate distress and says that her throat is "getting big." She states also that she is having trouble breathing. An adult at the scene states that she thinks she may have been stung by a bee a few minutes earlier. Someone has run to the other side of the park to get the girl's mother.

1. On the basis of what you know so far, what questions will you want to ask this girl?

2. How will you begin treatment for this girl?

As you are getting vital signs, the mother arrives and wants to know what is going on. You inform her of what you know and she states that her daughter is indeed allergic to bee stings and that she has her medication in her purse. She hands you an EpiPen® auto-injector from her purse.

1. What will you need to confirm before you can administer the medication?

2. How will you administer the medication? Outline your steps.

CASE STUDY 2   I THINK I AM HAVING AN ALLERGIC REACTION

You are dispatched for an allergic reaction to a medication. En route you think about the serious—even fatal—consequences of anaphylaxis and are prepared to act.

When you approach the scene and ensure that it is safe, you find a 34-year-old woman who is sitting in a chair holding a bucket into which she has just vomited. She tells you she thinks she may be allergic to a painkiller she was given yesterday after some minor surgery.

1. What would you look for in your initial assessment?

2. What questions would you ask specifically to determine the extent of the allergic reaction?

3. What observations could you make initially to evaluate the seriousness of the allergic reaction?

The patient tells you that she took the medication twice last night and did not notice any problems. She took another dose this morning and began to vomit. She denies sensations of swelling in the airway or difficulty breathing. She does not have hives or swelling in any part of her body. Her vital signs are pulse 88, strong, and regular; respirations 18 and adequate; blood pressure 116/76; pupils equal and reactive to light; and skin warm and moist.

1. **On the basis of the above information, is this patient experiencing anaphylaxis?**

2. **What treatment would you provide this patient?**

3. **Does this patient require transport?**

Active Exploration

It is probably safe to say that most of us know either directly or through a friend someone who has a severe allergy to something. That "something" could be food, medication, or possibly bee stings. Therefore, the likelihood of encountering a person experiencing a severe allergic reaction is quite good.

Severe allergies are life-threatening and quite often the survival of the patient depends on quick recognition by those at the scene and a quick response by the EMTs or paramedics responding to the scene.

The following exercises will help you increase your ability to recognize a severe allergic reaction and provide the needed emergency care as quickly as possible.

Activity 1: Legal Update

Many states are just now recognizing the life-threatening nature of severe allergic reactions and the life-saving ability of the drug epinephrine. When given soon enough, epinephrine can slow the onset of a severe allergic reaction and buy precious time for more advanced care.

In response to this growing awareness, many states have enacted new legislation that allows EMT-Bs and school officials to administer epinephrine under certain circumstances.

For this activity, you are to conduct a little research and find out whether your state or jurisdiction allows the administration of epinephrine by EMT-Bs and other lesser-trained people such as school personnel.

Find the answers to the following questions as they pertain to your state or jurisdiction:

1. Are there new laws (in the past 5 years) that have addressed the use of epinephrine?

2. Are EMT-Bs allowed to assist with the administration of epinephrine?

3. If so, under what circumstances?

4. Are EMT-Bs allowed to carry and administer epinephrine by standing order?

5. Do the laws allow for other nonmedical personnel, such as in schools, to administer epinephrine?

It is important to compare your findings with those of the others in your class and of your instructor. Laws and regulations can change without some ever finding out about it.

If you have time, do a little research to find out what other states have enacted similar legislation.

Activity 2: Who's Allergic to What

This next activity will give you an interesting perspective as to how many people in your immediate circle have some form of allergy.

Interview at least ten people and ask them the following questions. You can begin with people in your class but must include several friends outside of class as well:

1. Do you have a known allergy? If so, to what?

2. When was the last time you had a reaction to the substance?

3. What was the reaction like? How did it make you feel?

4. Did you receive treatment for the reaction or did it just go away?

5. What treatment did you receive and how long did it take for you to get better?

6. Do you carry epinephrine with you now? If so, when was the last time you checked the expiration date?

You might be surprised at the number of people who state they have some type of allergic reaction to something. You might also find that many of these people do not carry epinephrine and, if they do, many do not even realize it has expired.

One last question to find the answer to: How long does the typical dose of epinephrine last?

RETRO REVIEW

1. You have a 22-year-old male patient who is responsive and pleasant but complaining of "radiating" pain in both upper quadrants of the abdomen. As you treat and transport this patient, how often should you reassess his vital signs?

   A. Every 15 minutes.   **B.** Every 10 minutes.
   C. Every 5 minutes.   **D.** Once is sufficient.

2. Handguns cause _____ velocity wounds.

   A. high   **B.** low
   C. terminal   **D.** medium

3. Repeating your initial assessment of a patient would include all of the following, except for _____.

   A. checking mental status
   B. reassessing scene safety
   C. reestablishing patient priorities
   D. monitoring skin color

THINKING AND LINKING

CHAPTER TOPIC	HOW IT RELATES TO YOU AND OTHER COURSE AREAS
Allergens	Your patient may deny having any allergies and yet still be suffering from the signs and symptoms of an allergic reaction. Make sure you complete a detailed medical assessment (Chapter 11) and do not hesitate to contact medical direction if the patient's condition deteriorates. Remember to continuously monitor the patient's airway, breathing, and heart rate (Chapter 12) and be prepared for respiratory problems (Chapter 16).
Epinephrine	You should always be prepared for cardiac emergencies (Chapter 17) when assisting a patient with an epinephrine auto-injector (Chapter 15). Although the prescribing physician most likely examined the patient before authorizing the prescription, you will have no way of knowing whether the patient developed high blood pressure or some other circulatory problem since that time.
Anaphylaxis	If your patient develops anaphylaxis and does not have epinephrine (or the dose was ineffective), the patient will most likely need ALS care. Contact ALS early if it is available in your area. Appendix A: ALS Assist Skills (in your Emergency Care textbook) will help you help the ALS providers.

Poisoning and Overdose Emergencies

CHAPTER SUMMARY

Sooner or later, as an EMT-B, you will encounter a patient who has over-dosed or been exposed to some form of poison. How will you know? Will you have the knowledge to treat the patient for whatever toxic substance he was exposed to? Checking the scene for empty pill bottles or containers can yield valuable clues, but poisoning and overdose emergencies may require a dependence on on-line medical direction like few other types of calls will.

Any substance that can harm the body is called a poison. Some poisons can cause serious enough problems to create a medical emergency. The vast majority of poisonings are accidental and involve children gaining access to medications, cosmetics, and pesticides.

Poisoning can also be the result of natural toxins. Certain mushrooms, houseplants, and holiday plants, like mistletoe or holly berries, can be poisonous if eaten. Bacterial contaminants in food can also produce deadly toxins.

While people react differently to different poisons, the most severe reactions to poisoning are usually found among the chronically ill or elderly.

How do poisons actually damage the body? That depends on the type of poisonous substance. Corrosive poisons can destroy skin or other body tissues, while poisonous gases can cause suffocation by displacing oxygen in the air. Systemic poisons can cause reactions such as nausea, vomiting, depression or overstimulation of the nervous system, as well as prevent the red blood cells from carrying oxygen.

Poisons are classified by how they enter the body. *Ingested* poisons are swallowed (rat poison, improperly prepared food, and so on), *inhaled* poisons are breathed in (carbon monoxide, insect spray), *absorbed* poisons are taken into the body through contact with unbroken skin (insecticides, agricultural chemicals), and *injected* poisons are inserted through the skin (illicit drugs, snake bites).

When dealing with a case of ingested poison, the EMT-B must gather information quickly. You will need to determine the following information: the substance ingested, how much time has passed, the amount ingested, whether the patient regularly ingests the substance, and what interventions, if any, have been taken by the patient, family, or bystanders. It will also be helpful to the on-line physician if you know the patient's weight and what effects the patient is experiencing.

In some situations, on-line medical direction will instruct you to administer activated charcoal to a patient with an ingested poison. Activated charcoal is processed specifically to absorb certain poisons, decreasing the amount of poison that can be absorbed into a patient's body. Activated charcoal should *not* be used if the patient has an altered mental status; cannot swallow; or has ingested acids, alkalis, or gasoline.

Never force a patient to swallow activated charcoal. If the patient refuses, notify medical direction and continue your ongoing assessment and treatment.

Another option in the treatment of certain ingested poisons is *dilution*. Medical direction may order you to have the patient drink two glasses of either water or milk—half to one glass for pediatric patients. This may be used in situations in which medical direction or poison control believes the patient does not require transport.

Treatment of a patient who has ingested poison includes correction of any immediate life-threatening problems; performing a focused history and physical exam (including SAMPLE history); assessing baseline vitals; consulting medical direction; transporting the patient with any labels, vials, or containers; and performing ongoing assessments.

You may find that, due to their natural curiosity, children may swallow substances that an adult would never think of swallowing—bleach and lye to name just two. Obtain the child's weight and an estimate of the amount of substance that has been ingested—always assuming the largest quantity possible—and follow the instructions of the on-line physician.

When dealing with an inhaled poison, always ensure that the scene is safe prior to entering it. If you are not trained or equipped to do this, you must wait until the appropriate steps have been taken to make the scene safe for your entry. Before contacting medical direction regarding an inhaled poison, get the exact name of the substance, determine when (and for how long) the exposure occurred, see whether any interventions have been taken, and find out what effects the patient is experiencing.

Treatment for a patient who has inhaled a poison should include movement to a safe location, correction of any life-threatening problems, and respiratory support with a high concentration of oxygen. You will also want to complete a focused history and physical exam, along with a SAMPLE history and a set of vitals. Take all labels, vials, and containers with you as you transport the patient to the hospital and do not neglect the ongoing assessment.

Carbon monoxide, a colorless, odorless, and tasteless byproduct of inefficient combustion, is the most commonly inhaled poison. It can be produced by items such as automobiles, wood-burning stoves, or malfunctioning furnaces and heaters. If your patient presents with vague, flu-like symptoms (headache, nausea, dizziness, breathing difficulty, and so on) and has been in an enclosed space, suspect carbon-monoxide poisoning—especially if more than one person has similar symptoms. Patients with carbon-monoxide poisoning will usually improve once outside and on being given supplemental oxygen, but they must still be evaluated by a physician as soon as possible.

If your patient is suffering from an absorbed poison, the first thing to remember is that poisons absorbed by your patient can also be absorbed by *you*. Take necessary precautions prior to providing emergency care to the patient. As with other types of poisons, you will want to quickly ascertain the exact name of the substance, when the patient was exposed, how much of the substance was involved, for how long the exposure continued, what interventions were taken, and what effects the patient is experiencing.

Emergency care of this patient is identical to other poison exposures (resolve any life-threats; perform a focused history, physical exam, and SAMPLE history; transport with all labels, vials, or containers; and continue ongoing assessments) except that you will need to brush any powdered substances and flush any liquid substances from the patient. A patient's eyes, if contaminated, should be flushed with water or saline for at least 20 minutes.

Never attempt to "neutralize" an acid or alkali with diluted vinegar or baking soda in water. This can potentially cause more harm than it would prevent. Instead, flush the area with copious amounts of low-pressure water.

If you are called to assist a patient with an injected poison, you should quickly determine the route of entry, the exact substance (and estimated amount) injected, the time of injection, the patient's weight, any interventions already performed, and the effects that the patient is experiencing. Also, make sure you assess and document the effects of any treatment that you provide.

Although not always recognized as a "poisoning" issue, it is appropriate to include alcohol and substance abuse in this chapter. Many EMT-Bs do not take alcohol-abusing patients seriously, perhaps due to the patient's unusual behavior, occasional lack of personal hygiene, or frequency of contact with EMS personnel. It is easy to become callous toward these individuals, but you are not there to judge them. As an EMT-B, you are there to provide the best emergency care possible to each person, regardless of circumstances.

Patients who abuse alcohol often have the potential for many other ailments and injuries, such as trauma from falls, blood-sugar irregularities, poor nutrition, gastrointestinal bleeding, and so on. Since calls involving intoxicated patients are unpredictable and can be volatile, do not hesitate to request law-enforcement assistance.

When providing emergency care for an alcohol-abusing patient, make sure that you conduct a complete assessment in order to identify any medical emergencies. Also, do not forget that medical conditions such as diabetes, epilepsy, head injuries, high fevers, and hypoxia may make the patient appear intoxicated when he is *not*.

An alcoholic patient may also be suffering from withdrawal and exhibiting a condition known as the DTs (delirium tremens), which causes seizures, sweating, trembling, anxiety, and hallucinations. Alcohol withdrawal can be fatal. All patients with seizures or DTs must be transported to a hospital as soon as possible.

When treating the alcohol-abusing patient, use gloves, masks, and protective eyewear since vomiting is common. Always stay alert for airway and respiratory problems and assess the patient's mental status regularly. Also, monitor vital signs, protect the patient from self-injury, stay alert for seizures, and transport if necessary. Remember that an intoxicated patient *cannot* make an informed refusal of treatment or transport.

The term "substance abuse" means that a chemical substance is being taken for reasons other than medical necessity. The most commonly abused substances are classified as uppers (stimulants that excite the user), downers (depressants that affect the user's central nervous system), narcotics (which produce a stupor or sleep), hallucinogens (which induce excitement and distortion of perception), and volatile chemicals (which produce an initial "rush" followed by depression of the central nervous system). As an EMT-B, you will not need to remember all of the particular drugs and their specific reactions—it will be sufficient to recognize drug overdoses and be familiar with the drug classifications.

Since reactions to drugs can be very similar to other illnesses and injuries, the EMT-B should never assume that just drug abuse is a patient's sole problem. It is not uncommon to have illnesses and injuries also present with drug-abusing patients, so stay alert! You will also occasionally encounter a patient experiencing withdrawal from drugs. The signs and symptoms can include shaking, anxiety, nausea, confusion, irritability, profuse sweating, and possibly even hallucinations.

The emergency care that you provide a drug-abusing patient will be the same regardless of the drug—unless medical direction tells you differently. Once you have determined that the scene is safe and put on your personal protective equipment (gloves, mask, and eye protection because, like with alcohol abuse, vomiting is common), you should perform an initial assessment. Resolve any life-threatening problems and stay alert for airway or breathing issues. Treat the patient for shock, monitor the level of consciousness, assess for signs of injury (particularly the head), look for fresh needle marks (called "tracks") indicating injected drugs, and prevent the patient from hurting himself or others. You should transport as soon as possible, stay in contact with medical direction, and continue to reassure the patient. Stay alert for seizures and vomiting.

Due to the violent nature of drugs and drug abusers, always be prepared to protect yourself and, if necessary, get away from the scene until law enforcement arrives. You must consciously protect yourself from the drugs also—many hallucinogens can be absorbed through the skin, and it is common for intravenous-drug abusers to carry used syringes. *Always* take proper BSI precautions, and even though it seems perfectly acceptable in movies, *never* touch or taste a suspected illicit substance.

MED MINUTE

There are many types of overdoses, some intentional and some accidental. This table gives examples of common drugs in each category. Many other medications may be available with similar effects.

CLASS OF MEDICATION	MEDICATION NAME(S)	MECHANISM OF ACTION
Stimulant	Cocaine Methamphetamine	Central-nervous-system stimulants. Increase heart rate and blood pressure. Increase psychological arousal.
	Methylphenidate (Ritalin)	Ritalin is commonly used in attention-deficit disorders but can be abused as a stimulant.
Depressants Analgesics (pain relievers) (Including narcotics and opiates)	Heroin OxyContin Propoxyphene (Darvon) Oxycocone (Percocet) Hydrocodone (Vicodin)	Depress the central nervous system. When used therapeutically, these medications reduce pain and coughing. Used in excess, they can cause unconsciousness, respiratory arrest, and death.
Hallucinogens	Lysergic acid diethlyamide (LSD or acid)	Causes changes in sensation, mood alteration, and in higher doses, hallucinations.

PATHOPHYSIOLOGY PEARLS

Normal nerve cells are constantly producing chemical messengers designed to transmit a signal from one nerve to another. When a nerve is stimulated, these chemicals are released and a signal is sent across the nerve synapse, or gap between the nerves and the opposite nerve cell. This nerve stimulation completes the action and the impulse is carried out.

In poisonings, specifically organophosphate (chemical substances originally produced by the reaction of alcohols and phosphoric acid) poisonings, the chemical messengers (acetylcholine) are disabled and the movement of the chemical messenger across the nerve synapse is disrupted. Organophosphates irreversibly bind to and deactivate acetylcholinesterase. Acetylcholinesterase is designed to remove the acetylcholine from the end of the nerve, thus freeing up the nerve. An accumulation of acetylcholine at the nerve synapse or gap between the nerves, causes overstimulation of the nerve, followed by exhaustion and disruption of nerve transmission. Herein lies the problem: if the organophosphate remains in contact or bonded to the acetylcholinesterase for 24 hours or more, the acetylcholinesterase is destroyed, and the patient will either have a long-term disability or he will die.

The effects of the accumulation of acetylcholine on the end of the nerve lead to skeletal-muscle cell depolarization, or contraction, and result in rapid violent, uncontrolled muscle contractions known as fasciculations. You will also observe muscle weakness, hypertension, and tachycardia. Additionally, there will also be smooth-muscle contractions in organs of the body and a reduction in cardiovascular rhythm conduction, leading to bradycardia and/or ventricular dysrhythmias.

The accumulation of acetylcholine will cause the following symptoms in patients poisoned by organophosphates:

Salivation (drooling)
Lacrimation (tearing of the eyes)
Urination
Defecation
Gastroenteritis (GI upset)
Emesis (vomiting)

The SLUDGE acronym is commonly used to identify organophosphate poisonings.

Organophosphates were originally developed as insecticides and later used as chemical weapons ("nerve agents") during World War II.

The nerve agents used by military groups are most commonly organophosphates. Sarin is an organophosphate and is best known because of its use during a terrorist attack in a Tokyo subway in 1995.

Sources

Toxicity, Organophosphate and Carbamate on emedicine.com
http://www.emedicine.com/emerg/topic346.htm
Walter FG, Cholenesterase Inhibitors in AHLS Provider Manual, 2ⁿᵈ Edition,
Arizona Board of Regents, 2000, 231–243
Organophosphates in e-medicine.com
http://www.emedicine.com/neuro/topic286.htm

REVIEW QUESTIONS

SHORT ANSWER

1. Why is syrup of ipecac rarely used today?

2. What three signs make up the "opiate triad"?

MULTIPLE CHOICE

1. The most commonly injected poisons include snake or insect venom and _____.
   A. sea-anemone acid   **B.** sodium nitrate
   C. tetanus   **D.** illicit drugs

2. _____ are substances that provide an initial "rush" followed by a depressant effect on the nervous system.
   A. Volatile chemicals   **B.** Downers
   C. Hallucinogens   **D.** Amphetamines

3. What treatment is normally advised for patients who have ingested a mild poison that does not, according to on-line medical direction, warrant care at a medical facility?

   A. Administration of activated charcoal.

   B. Dilution with water or milk.

   C. Flushing with water or saline for at least 20 minutes.

   D. High-concentration oxygen via a nonrebreather mask.

4. If you are treating a drug abuser who is becoming increasingly aggressive, you should _____.

   A. restrain him to the ambulance stretcher

   B. continue talking to him calmly as you complete the treatment

   C. leave the scene and remain in a safe place until law enforcement arrives

   D. use body language and vocal inflexion to express your authority

5. Activated charcoal is manufactured to have more _____ than ordinary charcoal.

   A. volume   B. expandability

   C. surface area   D. ions

Scenario Questions

You arrive at a residence on the east side of town where the police have broken up a party. One of the guests, a 19-year-old female, was found unresponsive in a bathroom. The patient presents with moist skin, constricted pupils, shallow respirations, and responds only with groans when you shout at her.

1. This patient is displaying the signs of a _____ overdose.

   A. volatile-chemical   B. downer

   C. narcotic   D. hallucinogenic

2. During your physical exam of this patient, you would make an extra effort to look for _____.

   A. a decreased pulse

   B. track marks

   C. cyanosis

   D. aphasia

3. What PPE should you use when treating this patient?

   A. Latex exam gloves, a mask, and protective eyewear.

   B. A gown, puncture-resistant gloves, and goggles.

   C. Latex exam gloves.

   D. A HEPA mask and latex or vinyl exam gloves.

You answer a call from a day-care center where a child has apparently consumed some type of household chemical. You and your partner arrive and find the patient, a 3-year-old girl, crying and completely inconsolable. One of the teachers hands you a nearly empty bottle of liquid drain cleaner and tells you that it had been only half full prior to the child finding it. You observe a large amount of the substance on the child's clothing and spilled on the floor. "And because of the instructions on the bottle," the teacher says, "we gave her a dose of ipecac about ... oh, about 10 minutes ago now."

1. The first step in treating this child would be to _____.
    A. have her drink several glasses of milk
    B. contact on-line medical direction
    C. remove her clothing and begin flushing her skin
    D. administer activated charcoal

2. What should you, as an EMT-B, be most concerned about regarding this patient?
    A. Bleeding from stomach trauma caused by the drain cleaner.
    B. Cardiac compromise due to the substance entering the patient's blood stream.
    C. Permanent tissue damage to the patient's digestive tract.
    D. Aspiration of the caustic liquid.

3. On the basis of this scenario, you should assume that _____.
    A. the child spilled all of the drain cleaner and did not actually ingest any of it
    B. the emergency-care instructions on the bottle of drain cleaner are wrong
    C. the day-care center will be fined by Child Protective Services
    D. the child is apparently immune to the effects of ipecac

You are dispatched to an apartment complex early one winter morning after a child called emergency services to report that he could not wake his father. When you arrive, the child—who appears very pale and uncoordinated—leads you to his father's bedroom. You find the patient, an approximately 35- to 40-year-old male, unresponsive, cyanotic, and breathing irregularly. You unzip your airway equipment bag as your partner obtains the patient's baseline vital signs. You turn to the child to gather as much of a SAMPLE history as you can and see the boy unresponsive on the floor.

1. In this situation, you should have a high index of suspicion for _____.
    A. influenza
    B. carbon-monoxide poisoning
    C. domestic abuse
    D. food poisoning

2. You should immediately _____.
    A. contact on-line medical direction
    B. instruct your partner to assess the child
    C. move both patients out of the building
    D. exit the apartment and contact law enforcement

3. _____ is the EMT-B's intervention of choice for carbon-monoxide poisoning.
    A. Adrenaline
    B. Potassium chloride
    C. Albuterol
    D. Oxygen

CASE STUDIES

CASE STUDY 1   MY CHILD TOOK SOME PILLS

You are dispatched to a possible overdose at a residence just outside of town. Upon your arrival, you are met out front by one of the firefighters already at the scene who advises you that inside the house there is a 2-year-old boy who got into his mother's purse and may have taken some of her medication. Inside the house, you find everyone crowded around the little boy in the back bedroom. The mother states that when she got out of the shower, she found her son with her purse on the floor and one of her medication bottles was open. The boy is sitting upright in his mother's arms and appears to be alert.

1. How will you proceed with your initial assessment of this patient?

2. How will you evaluate whether and how much of the medication the child has eaten?

The mother tells you that she pulled several small pieces of pill out of his mouth just as soon as she saw him. She states that he was alone for no more than 20 minutes while she was in the shower.

   In looking at the pill container, you see that the prescription was filled six days ago for a total of 20 pills. The recommended dose on the bottle states to take one pill twice a day as needed for pain. There are eight pills remaining in the bottle.

1. If all the pills were taken as prescribed, how many pills should have been in the bottle when it was opened by the child?

2. What additional information would you want to get from the mother before transport?

CASE STUDY 2   DUDE, MY ROOMMATE WON'T WAKE UP

You are dispatched for an unresponsive person in an apartment not far from the station. It is in a decent part of town. You approach carefully anyway, and a police officer arrives as you approach the door. It is a third-floor walk-up. You enter together and find a person on the living-room floor. His color is so poor you do not even think he is alive. His roommate says he woke up and found the patient there on the floor.

1. What additional information would you look for in the size-up of this call?

2. What actions should you take based on your size-up?

After donning gloves and eye protection, you approach the patient while your partner prepares airway equipment. You do note some weak, gasping respiratory effort and a very weak and slow radial pulse. The patient is unresponsive to both verbal and painful stimulus. There is no obvious bleeding or apparent trauma. His roommate states that the patient had outpatient surgery on his feet and was taking a painkiller of some sort that was given to him by a friend. He said they were "oxy something."

1. **How do you proceed with the initial assessment?**

2. **What happens after the initial assessment in a patient this critical when there are only two of you?**

You are able to maintain the patient's airway patency and provide ventilations as you move to the ambulance for a priority transport. ALS is not available in your area, and you proceed to the hospital.

1. **You note that the patient has pinpoint pupils. What might this indicate?**

2. **Would any of the interventions carried on an ambulance be beneficial to this patient?**

3. **Where would you turn to for medical direction with this patient?**

Active Exploration

While poisonings and overdoses affect all age groups, it is important to know that according to the Drug and Poison Information Center (DPIC) of the Cincinnati Children's Medical Center, 79 percent of all poison-control-center cases involve children, with 64 percent involving children under the age of five. What this tells us is that we must play a bigger role in terms of prevention than is currently the case.

It is difficult to prevent the intentional overdose of a depressed adult who makes an attempt to take his own life. What we can do is become better informed as to how different common medications can affect the body and how best to treat the results in the field. The following activities will help you toward these ends.

Activity 1: Hands and Knees

This first activity will help give you an appreciation of what a typical toddler might see as he makes his way around your home or apartment. It will also help you develop an understanding of how easy it can be for a curious toddler to get into trouble in the average household.

Grab a pen and notepad and get down on your hands and knees and begin crawling around your house. Begin in any room you wish and make your way slowly through every room. Move slowly and be on the lookout for as many signs of danger as possible. Take careful notes and write down as many potential problems as you can find.

Once you have compiled your list, go back through it and attempt to find a solution for each of the potential dangers or problems on your list. Can they be easily prevented? Compare your list of hazards with that of a fellow student. How do the lists compare? Did he identify something that you missed? Discuss how each of you might "childproof" your homes and prevent an accidental poisoning or overdose from occurring.

Activity 2: Oops, I Forgot

Accidental overdoses are quite common in the elderly. They may wake up in the morning and, just like clockwork, take their daily dose of prescribed medications. A few hours later, they cannot remember whether they took their meds or not and, "just in case," they take another dose of their medications. Now this may not result in an immediate overdose, but if it happens several days in a row, it certainly could.

Go to the medicine chest or cabinet in your home and select three to five prescription medications at random. If you do not have any prescription medications in your home, ask to see those of someone who does.

Record the names of the medications and their strengths. Also make note of the recommended dose that is on the label. Now, armed with your list, we want you to research the effects of these medications should someone overdose on them. You may use the Internet or a reference book called a Physician's Desk Reference (PDR). Look up the medication and its effects if it is taken in too high a dose.

If you have time, visit a local pharmacy and ask the pharmacist what might happen if someone took too many of each of the medications. Would the onset of signs and symptoms be rapid or slow?

Understanding how medications can affect the body when taken in varying doses will help you identify potential overdose patients as well as better understand what your patient is experiencing. All of this will lead to better emergency care on your part.

1. A diabetic patient who suddenly begins sweating profusely and displaying abnormal behavior is most likely suffering from _____.

    A. hyperglycemia   **B.** glucose acidosis

    C. hypoglycemia   **D.** diabetes mellitus

2. Which of the following questions would *not* be part of a SAMPLE history?

    A. Who is your doctor?

    B. Have you had anything to drink?

    C. What do you think caused the pain?

    D. What do you take Diazepam for?

3. EMT-Bs carry activated charcoal, _____, and oxygen on their ambulances.

    A. aspirin   **B.** epinephrine

    C. glucose   **D.** nitroglycerin

THINKING AND LINKING

CHAPTER TOPIC	HOW IT RELATES TO YOU AND OTHER COURSE AREAS
Inhaled poisons	Whenever you are responding to an emergency involving possible inhaled poisons, your first priority is your own safety (Chapter 2). Always perform a diligent scene size-up (Chapter 7) and call in appropriately trained personnel if you feel that the scene is unsafe to enter (Chapter 35). Do not forget that a patient suffering from carbon-monoxide poisoning will likely have an inaccurate oxygen-saturation reading on the pulse oximeter (Chapter 9)—so do not make patient-treatment decisions on the basis of it.
Drug abuse	Always watch out for hidden syringes when providing emergency care to intravenous-drug-abusing patients, and if you get poked by a needle, follow your agency's policies for reporting the event (Chapter 14). You will find that many drug abusers will tell you where they hide their syringes (sometimes called "rigs" or "setups") if you just ask them in a respectful manner (review interpersonal communication skills in Chapter 13).
Hallucinogens	If you are dispatched for a patient who may be under the influence of hallucinogens such as PCP (commonly called "angel dust" or "hog"), request law-enforcement assistance (Chapter 2). Many hallucinogens (PCP in particular) can cause patients to be extremely violent and yet have no concept of the damage that they are causing their own bodies—a very dangerous combination.

	If you are conducting a physical exam (Chapter 10) on a patient who has been under the influence of PCP, carefully consider all mechanisms of injury (Chapter 7) and palpate well. Not only is it possible that the patient will not be able to tell you where any injuries are but the patient may also still be using broken limbs "normally."
Alcohol abuse	If your alcoholic patient has suffered even a minor head injury (falling down, walking into a stationary object, etc.), it is a good idea to transport him. Alcoholics are prone to subdural hematomas (Chapter 29), and allowing law enforcement to cart the patient down to the "drunk tank" could prove to be a very poor patient-treatment decision (Chapter 3).

22

Environmental Emergencies

CHAPTER SUMMARY

It is important to understand how the environment will affect your job as an EMT-B. You will encounter patients who are in need of emergency care as a direct result of their environment (snake bites, frostbite, heat stroke, and so on) as well as patients whose medical conditions are being complicated *by* their environment—such as a trauma patient's loss of body heat through conduction. It will be up to you to determine the patient's emergency-care needs and to discern between an environmental cause and an environmental complication.

In cold environments, we can easily lose body heat quicker than we can generate it. The body will actively combat heat loss—but eventually there will only be enough energy to maintain heat in the body's core. This can allow the destruction of exposed tissues (such as skin and extremities) and shut down body functions.

The body loses heat in a number of ways. *Conduction* drains body heat through direct contact with other objects, whereas *convection* will pull the heat away when air currents pass over the body. Radiation, evaporation, and respiration are also ways that our bodies lose heat.

If an individual's entire body loses sufficient heat, he will develop a condition known as hypothermia. This occurs when the person is no longer able to maintain a sufficient core temperature. Patients with injuries, chronic illnesses, and certain other conditions (such as shock, burns, head or spinal injuries, and diabetes) will suffer the effects of heat loss much quicker than healthy individuals. You will notice this among the elderly and very young also.

It is important to maintain an awareness of the patient's environment. At times, it will be obvious that the patient is slipping into hypothermia and yet at other times, you may be looking at so many other factors that you will completely miss it. Some situations (e.g. an intoxicated patient wandering outdoors, an overdose patient who is sweating heavily in a cool environment, a patient who has experienced near-drowning) will warrant your suspicion of hypothermia, even if other factors take your attention.

Injured patients who cannot be immediately removed from a cold environment (like those awaiting extrication from an automobile) must be kept warm with anything on hand that will prevent heat loss.

When assessing a patient for hypothermia, consider air temperature, wind/water chill factor, age, type of clothing worn, injuries, activity during exposure, and the possibility of drug or alcohol use. The signs and symptoms of hypothermia include shivering, numbness, muscle rigidity, drowsiness, loss of motor function, decreased level of consciousness, and a cool abdominal-skin temperature. Also determine whether the patient is oriented to person, place, and time.

There are two ways to rewarm a hypothermic patient, passively or actively. Passive rewarming allows the body to warm itself and active rewarming means that you help it by applying heat sources. You will find the hypothermic patient in one of two conditions. He will either be alert and responding appropriately (in which case you will actively rewarm him with heat packs, warm air, and so on) or he will be unresponsive or not responding appropriately. In this case, you would ensure a patent airway, provide oxygen, and cover the patient with blankets.

When handling a hypothermic patient, you *must* be very careful—treat the person as gently as you would if he had an unstabilized spinal injury. Rough treatment can cause tissue damage and, more seriously, cooled blood from the extremities can be forced into the body's core with tragic results (such as severe heart problems). If you actively rewarm the patient, use *central rewarming*—apply heat to the lateral chest, neck, armpits, and groin. Avoid rewarming the limbs first as this can result in shock. To prevent most of the problems associated with the rewarming process, you should leave the lower extremities exposed as you warm the torso.

If the patient is unresponsive or not responding appropriately, he may have *severe* hypothermia. *Do not* actively rewarm this patient. Instead, remove him from the cold environment and prevent further heat loss (with blankets, and so on) while you provide high-concentration oxygen (warmed and humidified, if possible) and rapid transportation. In cases of extreme hypothermia, the patient might have no discernable vital signs and a core body temperature below 80°F. These patients may still be alive—*do not* assume death, even if 30 minutes or more have passed since loss of discernable vitals. If you cannot find a carotid pulse after 30 to 45 seconds, begin CPR and apply the AED. (Follow local protocols.)

Direct contact with low temperatures (objects, air, water, and so on) can also affect specific areas of the body (most commonly ears, nose, face, hands, feet, and toes). This is known as *local cooling*. Localized cold injuries are either superficial (characterized by the reddening or, in the case of dark-skinned patients, lightening of the skin accompanied by numbness) or deep, in which case all sensation is lost and the skin appears white and waxy.

Superficial cold injuries, also known as *frostnip*, can be treated by removing the patient from the cold environment and warming the affected area— make sure not to rub, massage, or re-expose the affected area to the cold. Affected extremities should be splinted and covered. Tingling or burning during treatment of superficial cold injuries is normal. If the condition does not respond to treatment (or the skin appears white and waxy), you should begin treating for a deep cold injury.

Cold injuries that are deep (*frostbite* or *freezing*) occur when superficial cold injuries go untreated. Deep cold injuries affect not only the skin but also muscles, deep blood vessels, bones, and organs. The skin appearance ranges from waxy and white to blue and blistered and might feel hard just on the surface or all of the way through the affected part. The patient should be treated with high-concentration oxygen and rapidly transported with the affected area covered and protected. *Never massage or rub a frost-bitten area*. Ice crystals in the tissues can cause severe damage. Do not let the patient walk on or use the affected part.

Actively rewarming frostbitten or frozen parts is generally not recommended due to the potential for permanent damage. You should always consult local protocols or contact medical direction in these situations. If transportation will be delayed and you are unable to reach medical direction, you can actively rewarm the affected part by submersing it in warm water (100° to 105°F)—being careful not to let it touch the sides or bottom of the water container—and stirring the water gently. The patient complaining of pain is a positive sign. Once the affected part no longer feels frozen, and the color is either red or blue, you should remove it from the water, dry it gently, and cover it with a dry, sterile dressing (between the fingers and toes, too). You should then keep the entire patient warm, while making sure that the blankets are not weighing on the affected part, and transport as soon as possible with the effected limb slightly elevated.

Our bodies create heat from a series of never-ending internal chemical processes and any heat that is not necessary to maintain our body temperature must be released to the environment around us. When this does not happen, an abnormally high body temperature—or *hyperthermia*—will result. Hyperthermia can be fatal if allowed to progress untreated.

When assessing the hyperthermic patient, do not overlook the potential for non-heat-related illnesses and injuries. Pre-existing conditions, such as dehydration, diabetes, fever, fatigue, and obesity, can hasten the effects of heat, as can the consumption of alcohol and other drugs. Always consider hyperthermic conditions more serious among elderly or pediatric patients, as neither has effective thermoregulation ability.

Initially, after a prolonged exposure to excessive heat, the patient may present with pale, moist skin that feels normal or cool. Due to heavy perspiration and subsequent water consumption, salts are flushed from the system and may result in painful muscle cramps (*heat cramps*) and eventually a form of shock known as *heat exhaustion*.

Potential heat-emergency patients with moist, pale skin that is normal or cool and who are also suffering from signs and symptoms such as weakness, shallow breathing, heavy perspiration, and weak pulse should be moved to a cool environment and placed on oxygen at 15 lpm. You should also loosen the patient's clothing, place him in a supine position with his legs raised, allow small sips of water unless nausea ensues, place wet towels over muscle cramps, and transport.

Heat-emergency patients with hot skin, whether it is dry or moist, are experiencing a true emergency sometimes known as *heat stroke*. If you observe rapid, shallow breathing; a full, rapid pulse; little or no perspiration; and dilated pupils, you should immediately move the patient to a cool environment; remove all clothing; apply cool packs to the neck, armpits, and groin; and keep his skin wet with a towel or sponge. You should also administer oxygen at 15 lpm via a nonrebreather mask and transport immediately. If you are treating a pediatric patient, cool the skin using lukewarm water instead of cold water.

There are many types of accidents and injuries that can occur in or around water other than just drowning or near-drowning. Boating and water skiing and diving accidents can cause fractured bones, bleeding, soft-tissue injuries, and airway obstructions, among other things. It is imperative that you not attempt a water rescue unless you have been specifically trained to do so. There are dangers inherent in water rescues, even at shallow depths, that can quickly convert you from being a rescuer to being a patient.

When you encounter patients in situations relating to water, you should always be alert for airway obstruction; cardiac arrest; head, neck, and internal injuries; hypothermia; evidence of substance abuse; and drowning or near-drowning. What is the difference between drowning and near-drowning? Drowning occurs when resuscitative efforts fail to prevent biological death as the direct result of water submersion, and a near-drowning occurs when those efforts succeed. Biological death resulting from water submersion can sometimes be delayed for more than 30 minutes if the water is cold enough.

In near-drowning cases, you may encounter excessive water in the lungs, or swollen tissues along the patient's airway, which reduces the effectiveness of rescue breathing or artificial ventilations. The force with which you will have to ventilate the patient in this situation can easily cause gastric distention. If you must reduce this distention, ensure that suction is available, turn the patient onto his left side and apply firm pressure to the epigastric area of his abdomen.

It is common to find head and spinal injuries in patients in situations relating to water—whether from diving or being struck by a boat, jet ski, surfboard, or similar objects. All such patients who are unconscious should be assumed to have head and/or spinal injuries. Do not overlook the fact that a medical emergency such as cardiac arrest or seizure may have caused the patient to fall into the water in the first place. With patients found in respiratory or cardiac arrest, you will need to begin resuscitation before spinal immobilization can be done. You should try, to the best of your ability, to keep the patient's head and neck rigid and in a midline position. Do not attempt water rescues (including resuscitation and immobilization with a spine board) unless you have been trained to do so. It is also important to keep in mind that many water-related patients will be susceptible to hypothermia. For this reason, you should always cover the patient to maintain warmth and treat for shock. Near-drowning patients requiring rescue breathing or CPR should be transported as soon as possible, keeping in mind that the receiving facility will need as much information as possible about the situation (e.g. fresh or salt water, cold or warm water, and so on).

Another important element of our environment is made up of the creatures that live in it. Many insects, snakes, and marine animals are venomous—able to inject toxins— and will be the cause of calls to EMS. Insect stings, spider bites, scorpion stings, snakebites, and marine-organism stings or punctures are going to be the most common agents of injected toxins.

Insect stings and bites (from wasps, hornets, bees, ants, and so on) can be painful but are harmless to 95 percent of the population of the United States. The remaining 5 percent, however, will have an allergic reaction— some even developing life-threatening anaphylactic shock. There are only two spiders whose bites can create medical emergencies in humans: the black widow and the brown recluse (also known as the fiddleback spider). Scorpion stings are common in the southwest of the United States but are rarely fatal to humans. In fact, only the rare *Centroroides exilcauda* scorpion is dangerous to humans—and then usually causing respiratory distress or failure only in children.

When assessing a patient with an insect bite or sting, it is essential to gather information from the patient and any bystanders or witnesses. Obtain any information that you can about the source of poisoning (type of insect, and so on). The signs and symptoms of an insect bite or sting include numbness in a body part, redness, difficulty in breathing, abnormal pulse, chills, vomiting, excessive saliva production, and anaphylaxis.

When it comes to treatment, are you required to know all the different insects, spiders, and scorpions and how to counter their poisons? Of course not. If you are familiar with a local insect or spider and know that it is not poisonous to humans, you would simply watch for anaphylaxis in your patient. If you do not recognize the offending organism, urge the patient to be transported to the hospital for evaluation—even bringing the insect or spider if you can quickly and safely do so.

Emergency care for the patient with an injected toxin is fairly straightforward. Begin by treating for shock (even if the patient does not appear to be suffering from shock), call medical direction if your EMS system is not familiar with the organism, quickly remove the stinger or venom sac, remove any jewelry on the affected body part, apply constricting bands above and below the injection site (if allowed by local protocols), and keep the limb immobilized to prevent the spread of the toxin.

Always look for medical-ID devices—they may indicate allergies to certain stings or bites and the potential that a patient is carrying his medication for anaphylaxis.

Nearly 50,000 people in the United States are bitten by snakes annually—but these bites result in fewer than ten deaths. More people die from bee and wasp stings each year! Also, unless anaphylactic shock develops, snakebite fatalities develop slowly—usually over one to two days. Even with these relatively mild statistics, bites from known poisonous snakes (rattlesnakes, copperheads, water moccasins, and so on) should be treated very seriously. You never know whether you are being called to treat one of this year's "fewer than ten deaths." Stay calm to keep your patient calm—it will prevent the venom from moving quickly.

Unless you *personally* know that the involved snake is *not* poisonous, treat every snakebite as if venom were injected. The signs and symptoms of snakebite may include a noticeable bite mark, swelling around the bite, rapid pulse, labored breathing, dim or blurred vision, and seizures. If the snake is dead, transport it in a sealed container for hospital-evaluation purposes. Never transport a live snake in an ambulance—even if it has been captured in a container. Arrange for someone else to bring the snake to the emergency department. Also, if the snake has not been captured at the scene, do not attempt to catch it or approach it in order to observe its markings. Another ambulance crew may end up transporting *you*. Instead, make a mental note of the snake's appearance and describe it to the receiving facility.

Emergency care for a snakebite victim includes contacting medical direction, treating for shock, cleaning the bite area with soap and water, removing jewelry on the affected body part, splinting the extremity and keeping it at or below heart level, applying constricting bands above and below the bite to restrict the flow of lymph—if ordered to do so by medical direction—and monitoring vitals carefully during transport. Never place ice packs on the wound site or cut into the bite and suction or squeeze venom unless you are ordered to do so by a physician—and even then, use a suction cup, never your mouth.

Individuals can be poisoned by marine animals in a variety of ways: from eating improperly prepared seafood or poisonous organisms, to being stung or punctured. Patients may develop a reaction very similar to anaphylaxis after consuming spoiled or contaminated seafood—treat as anaphylaxis. The consumption of poisonous marine life (puffer fish, paralytic shellfish, and so on) is very rare in the United States due to nonavailability. If you do respond to a patient who may have ingested a poisonous sea organism, contact medical direction immediately and be prepared for vomiting, convulsions, and respiratory arrest.

Venomous sea creatures such as jelly fish, sea nettles, Portuguese man-of-wars, and hydra can cause sting injuries. Just as with insect stings, most of these injuries are painful but harmless—and can be soothed by rinsing the area with vinegar or rubbing alcohol. There are individuals, however, who will develop allergic reactions and even anaphylactic shock when stung by these ocean life forms—treat identically to other cases of anaphylaxis. If the patient is stung near the eyes or lips, a physician's attention is required.

Another painful sea-related injury is a puncture wound—usually caused when the patient has stepped on or grabbed a stingray, sea urchin, or other spiny marine animal. Although soaking the injury in nonscalding hot water for 30 minutes will break down the venom, you should not delay transport. This patient will need to be seen by a doctor and possibly given a tetanus shot. Always be alert for the signs of an allergic reaction or development of anaphylaxis.

When documenting environmental injuries, do not neglect to include temperatures, wind chill factors, and so on. Also note how long the patient was exposed to the injuring conditions. With bite and sting cases, it is important to include witness descriptions of the offending organism (size, color, and so on). Also, always continuously document the patient's mental status and ongoing vital signs.

MED MINUTE

Environmental emergencies include a wide range of problems from heat and cold emergencies to bites, stings, and exposure to substances such as poison ivy and poison oak. There are few prescription medications specifically for these situations.

In situations in which a patient who is allergic to poison ivy, poison oak, and other similar substances is exposed to these plants, topical agents such as calamine lotion may be used. You may also use prescription topical and ingested steroids (see Chapter 20—Allergic Reactions). In other injuries (e.g. recovery from cold exposure), you may use analgesic (pain-relieving) medications.

PATHOPHYSIOLOGY PEARLS

Patients experiencing high-altitude pulmonary edema (HAPE) will not have any signs or symptoms of heart failure other than pulmonary edema. Pulmonary edema caused by HAPE will generally be resolved completely a short time after descent.

Although hypoxia is said to be the primary contributor to high-altitude illness, current science believes that major leaks within the pulmonary capillaries begin developing as the patient ascends and are the real culprits in the development of HAPE.

As a patient begins to climb, the atmosphere has a much lower concentration of all gases, including oxygen. As the available oxygen levels decrease, the patient will begin to suffer from hypoxia. It is also believed that increased intracapillary pressure forces the cells of the capillaries apart, allowing protein leakage. When the proteins leak, the capillary is no longer able to keep fluid contained, and pulmonary edema occurs. After the patient returns to an altitude where atmospheric pressure is near normal, the pressure inside the pulmonary artery is reduced and the capillary cells fall together again, stopping the leakage of fluid into the lungs. When fluid stops leaking into the lungs, the patient no longer has pulmonary edema and the patient's heart can effectively pump the fluid within the lungs back into systemic circulation. Therefore, when the HAPE patient descends, you will see an almost immediate and complete recovery.

Clinical signs of HAPE include shortness of breath while at rest, which becomes more intense with physical exertion, a dry cough, which may progress to a productive cough of frothy yellow or pink fluid, and tachycardia followed by cyanosis in the acutely ill patient.

The HAPE patient is treated first and foremost by a change in altitude. Remember that if the patient truly has HAPE, he should return to a normal physiologic state after returning to normal altitude. If the patient for some reason does not resolve the pulmonary edema, you should perform a thorough assessment to determine whether there is another cause for the pulmonary edema. When managing unresolved HAPE, you should focus on providing better oxygenation and ventilation. You can accomplish this quite easily and successfully by bag-valve-mask ventilation.

Sources

Rosen P, Barkin RM, et al., Emergency Medicine Concepts and Clinical Practice, *5th Edition, Mosby, 2002*

Tintinalli JE, Kelen GD. et al., Emergency Medicine, A Comprehensive Study Guide, *5th Edition, McGraw-Hill, 2000*

Semonin-Holleran R, Air and Surface Patient Transport Principles and Practice, *3rd edition, Mosby, 2003*

Hall JB, Schmidt GA, Wood LDH, Principles of Critical Care, *McGraw-Hill, 1992*

REVIEW QUESTIONS

SHORT ANSWER

1. Why would you avoid warming a hypothermic patient too quickly?

2. What poisonous snakes are native to the United States?

1. When currents of air pass over a body and carry away heat, it is called
   _____.

   A. radiation   **B.** convection

   C. evaporation   **D.** transduction

2. Why should you never massage or rub a frozen part of a patient's body?

   A. Reintroduction of circulation can cause severe shock.

   B. The body part can easily be cracked or broken.

   C. Microscopic ice crystals can cause serious tissue damage.

   D. Blood vessels can constrict, decreasing blood flow to the affected area.

3. Humidity in a hot environment can slow the evaporation of perspiration
   and quickly cause _____.

   A. hyperthermia   **B.** toxemia

   C. hypothermia   **D.** edema

4. Gases entering the bloodstream from a damaged lung is called a(n)
   _____.

   A. pulmonary thrombus   **B.** arterial gas embolism

   C. hyperbaric anomaly   **D.** Deuser's embolus

5. The best device for an ice rescue is probably a _____.

   A. ladder

   B. rope with a loop tied at one end

   C. cold-water submersion suit

   D. flat-bottomed aluminum boat

SCENARIO QUESTIONS

You respond to a 4 A.M. "man down" call on 168th Street. As you arrive, you
are motioned over to a gutter by the police officer who found the man. The
patient is a 58-year-old very cold but responsive male who complains of severe pain in his right leg. You cut open the patient's wet pants and find an
open fracture just superior to the knee. The patient tells you that he had left a
bar over on 157th Street at about 2 A.M. and started walking home. The patient
had slipped on ice and fallen onto a curb, near where he was found, and
knew immediately that he had "broken" his leg. He then waited for "an hour
or so" for someone to find him before attempting to get back to his feet. It was
at that point that the patient's injury became an open fracture and he fell to
the ground again.

1. How should this patient be prepared for transport?

   A. Splint the injured leg, place the patient in the shock position, and
   cover him with blankets.

   B. Remove all of the patient's clothing, splint his leg, and transport him
   with all but his lower extremities wrapped in heated blankets.

   C. Splint the injured leg and wrap the patient with hot packs and
   blankets.

   D. Secure the patient to a spine board and cover him loosely with foil-
   type emergency blankets.

2. On the basis of this patient's situation, he would have been losing body
   heat through convection and _____.

   A. radiation   **B.** reduction

   C. evaporation   **D.** conduction

3. _____ is(are) the safest prehospital method(s) to return a hypothermic patient's body temperature to normal.

   A. Hot packs warming the torso (core)   **B.** Extremity massage
   C. Heated interchange   **D.** Controlled insulation

Your unit is dispatched to the pier for some sort of scuba-diving accident. You meet the incoming boat and find that the patient is a 27-year-old woman who is responsive and complaining of pain accompanied by swelling on the right side of her face. The crew tells you that she had been diving all morning, conducting studies of deep-sea coral beds. The patient had been preparing to return to the surface when an eel startled her, causing her to jerk her head to the side. She had then hit the right side of her face on a sea anemone that was on a coral shelf. The patient tells you that she is allergic to sea-anemone stings, and she had rushed to the surface in case she needed her epinephrine auto-injector—which she, so far, has not.

1. In order to relieve the pain of the stings, you should _____.

   A. apply a cold compress to the patient's face
   B. rinse her cheek with warm, nonscalding water
   C. have the patient utilize her epinephrine auto-injector
   D. rinse the affected area with rubbing alcohol

2. In addition to monitoring the patient for signs of anaphylaxis, you should also suspect the possibility of _____.

   A. internal injuries   **B.** hypoperfusion
   C. decompression sickness   **D.** hypoxia

3. Medical direction may order you to take this patient directly to a(n) _____.

   A. hyperbaric-trauma-care center
   B. marine-allergen-exposure clinic
   C. emergency-anaphylactic-response center
   D. marine-hyperbole treatment facility

It turns out to be 102°F on the day of your city's annual marathon. Not surprisingly, about one hour into the race, you are approached at your aid station by one of the runners. The man, in his early 20s, presents with rapid, shallow breathing, dilated pupils, and hot, dry skin.

1. You should immediately recognize that this patient is suffering from _____.

   A. heat cramps   **B.** heat diffusion
   C. heat stroke   **D.** heat exhaustion

2. How should you treat this patient?

   A. Place him in the air-conditioned ambulance; remove his clothes; apply cool packs to his neck, armpits, and groin; keep his skin wet; administer high-concentration oxygen; and transport immediately.
   B. Move him into the shade, keep his skin wet and fanned aggressively, administer oxygen; and have him drink plenty of water.
   C. Place him in the air-conditioned ambulance, pour water over his skin for 5–10 minutes, apply cold packs to his wrists and ankles, administer high-concentration oxygen, and transport if he does not improve.
   D. Have the patient sit in the back of the air-conditioned ambulance, administer oxygen by nonrebreather mask at 15 lpm, supply plenty of cold water for the patient to drink, and monitor his vital signs.

3. This severely hyperthermic patient is not perspiring because _____.

   A. his body has been depleted of all fluids

   B. the temperature-regulating components in his brain have begun to shut down

   C. the high ambient temperature causes excessive evaporation

   D. his body is reacting to the loss of salt and fluid

CASE STUDIES

CASE STUDY 1   THIS TRAILER IS BOILING!

It is midsummer and your region has been experiencing a record heat wave with temperatures well over 100 for the past several days. You are dispatched to an unresponsive person in a local mobile-home park. Upon your arrival, you are met by a nice man who tells you he came to get his friend for their weekly game of bridge and found him unresponsive and lying on his couch. Upon entering the mobile home, you find an approximately 70-year-old male who appears unresponsive and is lying on the couch. Your initial assessment finds his breathing to be rapid and shallow and his pulse is 104 and slightly weak. His skin is very hot to the touch and dry. As you tap and shout, he is somewhat responsive to your verbal stimulus.

1. Given what you know so far, what is likely to be this man's problem?

2. Given that his ABCs are intact, how would you begin treating this patient?

You start to undress the man so that you can begin to cool him while your partner gets the stretcher. He is moaning softly and moving his arms in response to your actions. Before your partner returns with the stretcher, the man has what appears to be a generalized tonic-clonic seizure.

1. What is the most likely cause of this man's convulsive activity? What should you do for it?

2. How will you attempt to cool this man as you transport, and is oxygen therapy appropriate?

You are called for a "missing elderly man" at 14323 Ridge Terrace. It is February and you were hoping to have a slow day *inside* the station, since it is quite cold. You arrive to find that a 74-year-old man with Alzheimer's disease had wandered out to the screened porch and sat down for an unknown time. His visibly shaken son is unsure how long he had been out there but estimated it could have been for 1 to 2 hours. It is 9°F with a wind chill of −1. Your observations of the man are that he seems to be conscious, is wearing only pajamas, his skin is a bit pale and cool, and he is not shivering. He is now in the living room.

1. **How long do you believe the patient was out in the cold?**

2. **How would you perform an initial assessment?**

The patient appears to be breathing adequately and is not injured. He does not speak, which his son feels is a slight decline from his normal mental status. His vital signs are pulse 66, respirations 12, pupils equal and reactive to light, and blood pressure 170 over 92. He has a history of diabetes and high blood pressure and had a heart attack several years ago.

1. **How severe is the patient's hypothermia?**

2. **What complicating factors have you identified?**

The patient is prepared for transport. He is wrapped in a blanket, placed on the stretcher, and moved to the ambulance.

1. **What treatment should the patient receive?**

2. **What is the difference between active and passive rewarming?**

Active Exploration

The topic of "Environmental Emergencies" is a very comprehensive one. It includes the obvious heat- and cold-related problems as well as water emergencies and the assortment of bites and stings that people get when enjoying life in the outdoors. Each of us lives and works in different parts of the nation; therefore, the specific environmental emergencies that we are likely to encounter will be vastly different. While you will not be expected to become an expert in all areas relating to environmental emergencies, you should become knowledgeable in those aspects that you are most likely to encounter in your region.

The following activities will help you with your understanding of some of the basic principles relating to environmental emergencies.

Activity 1: Face First

The human body is an amazing machine, and one of its most amazing aspects is its ability to adapt to the environment in an attempt to sustain life. For this next activity, you will need a large bowl of ice water and a fellow student to assist you.

1. Begin by having your partner take your resting pulse and record it on a piece of paper.
2. Next, you will need to take two or three deep breaths and then place your face deep into the bowl of ice water.
3. Have your partner wait approximately 1 minute before taking your pulse again. If possible, record the pulse every 30 seconds until you can no longer hold your breath and must come up for air.

What did your partner notice about the pulse of the "patient?" There should have been an obvious decrease in the pulse rate following submersion in the ice water.

This is caused by something known as the "mammalian diving reflex" and it is stimulated during cold-water immersion. In an attempt to reduce the amount of oxygen consumed during cold-water submersion, the body slows the heart rate and metabolism. This helps explain how some people can withstand long periods of submersion in cold water with little or no residual damage. This reflex seems to be most active at birth and its efficiency reduces with age.

An alternative method of doing this activity is to have the "patient" hooked up to a cardiac monitor, making it easier to see and record the changes in heart rate.

Activity 2: Stings for a Bite

No matter where you live, there is a strong likelihood that you share the environment with some small animal or insect that has the potential for creating havoc in your life. This next activity involves identifying two such creatures and learning how they affect the human body should one become infected by their venom.

1. Identify at least two creatures that inhabit your region that are venomous to some degree. If you are not aware of any, ask your instructor or other people in your life who might know. A park ranger or someone who teaches wilderness survival should be of some help.

2. Using the Internet or the local library, conduct some research to determine what signs and symptoms the creatures cause in someone who is bitten or stung. How are most people affected by the venom and how long does it take to develop signs and symptoms after being bitten or stung?

3. What is the most appropriate treatment for the specific bite or sting?

4. Compare your findings with those of your fellow students. Did your research resemble that of the other students? Were your findings consistent with theirs?

For your own safety, it is a good idea to know the common habitats of the most dangerous creatures in your region. Knowing this will help you avoid becoming a patient yourself.

RETRO REVIEW

1. Not making eye contact with the person to whom you are speaking usually indicates _____.
   - **A.** respect
   - **B.** anger
   - **C.** unease
   - **D.** interest

2. Epinephrine can be fatal in patients with _____.
   - **A.** muscular dystrophy
   - **B.** hypertension
   - **C.** epilepsy
   - **D.** sulfa allergies

3. A(n) _____ should never be used for patients with a suspected spinal injury.
   - **A.** stair chair
   - **B.** short spine board
   - **C.** basket stretcher
   - **D.** emergency move

THINKING AND LINKING

CHAPTER TOPIC	HOW IT RELATES TO YOU AND OTHER COURSE AREAS
Convection	As you are treating your patient in a cold environment (outside during winter, in a refrigerated factory, and so on), remember to take care of yourself also (Chapter 2). You will be just as susceptible to heat loss as your patient is.
Ambient temperature	When you arrive to provide emergency care to an elderly patient (Chapter 32), make assessing the general ambient temperature in the residence part of your scene size-up (Chapter 7). Many older people lose the ability to effectively feel the temperature around them—possibly causing or complicating medical conditions with excessively high or low temperatures.
Near-drowning	You should assess near-drowning patients thoroughly (Chapters 10 and 11)—it may not always be obvious what medical or trauma condition initially led to the submersion. Do not leave the ambulance without the equipment to provide ventilations, oxygen, and suctioning (Chapter 6).
Bites and stings	If your patient has been bitten or stung by an insect, always ask whether he has had allergic reactions in the past (Chapter 20). If there is anaphylaxis in the patient's history, you should determine whether the patient has an epinephrine auto-injector available (Chapter 15). If the patient has a history of anaphylactic shock or is beginning to experience respiratory difficulty, attempt to coordinate an ALS intercept (Chapter 13). Also, see Chapter 37 to better understand the steps that ALS personnel will take to assist the patient.

23

Behavioral Emergencies

CHAPTER SUMMARY

You will respond to many behavioral emergencies as an EMT-B. Many things can initiate a behavioral emergency including stress, mental illness, and drug and alcohol abuse. Your priority in these emergencies is safety. You will approach these patients cautiously, and you may require police assistance.

The following are traumatic and medical conditions that may affect a person's behavior:

- Hypoglycemia
- Hypoxia
- Hypoperfusion
- Stroke
- Head injury
- Mind-altering substances
- Hypothermia
- Hyperthermia

When patients are faced with a stressful situation, they may exhibit normal stress reactions. Generally, your unhurried, caring approach can give them the time to gain control of their emotions. If the patient does not calm down and you cannot determine a physical cause for the behavior, you must assume that the behavior may be caused by a psychiatric problem.

There are some general rules to keep in mind when dealing with a patient experiencing a behavioral emergency. Be sure to introduce yourself and make sure that the patient understands your role in the situation. Assure him that you want to help him. Listen intently to what he wants to tell you. Always ask him for permission before attempting anything that would invade his personal space, such as taking vital signs. Be alert for sudden changes in behavior and take appropriate safety precautions.

Common signs and symptoms of a patient experiencing a behavioral emergency include:

- Panic or anxiety
- Poor hygiene, unusual appearance
- Agitation
- Unusual speech patterns
- Unusual behavior or thought patterns
- Suicidal or self-destructive behavior
- Violent or aggressive behavior directed toward others

When responding to a threatened suicide, pay particular attention to personal safety. There is an increased potential for the scene to be unsafe. Law enforcement must secure the scene prior to the arrival of EMS.

Certain factors are associated with the risk of a person attempting suicide. Some or all of these factors may be present in such a patient.

- Depression
- High stress levels
- Emotional trauma
- Age—high rates between 15 and 25 and then again over 40 years of age
- Alcohol and drug abuse
- Verbal threats of suicide
- Suicide plan
- Previous threats or attempts
- Sudden improvement from a depression

All suicidal patients need to be transported. You may need police assistance in order to accomplish this.

For all patients experiencing a behavioral emergency, care should consist of:

- A careful scene size-up
- An initial assessment and treating of life-threats
- If possible, a focused history and physical exam
- An ongoing assessment

Remember that the more reassured you can make your patient feel, the further you will get in your assessment process.

When dealing with aggressive or hostile patients, keep the following safety precautions in mind:

- Have law enforcement secure the scene
- Do not separate yourself from your partner or others who could help
- Have an escape route; do not let the patient get between you and the exit
- Be observant for any weapons
- Be alert for sudden changes in behavior

Reasonable force and restraint may be necessary to keep a patient from hurting himself or someone else. In most locations, law enforcement can order restraint and transport, but they must assist in the process. The restraints must be humane and safe. Be sure you have adequate help to restrain the patient and have a plan. One person should talk to and reassure the patient through the procedure. Do not impact the patient's airway while restraining him. All restrained patients need to be monitored closely. Document the reason for restraint thoroughly.

MED MINUTE

This table gives examples of common drugs in each category. Many other medications may be available with similar effects.

CLASS OF MEDICATION	MEDICATION NAME(S)	MECHANISM OF ACTION
Anxiolytic (antianxiety)	Alprazolam (Xanax)	Benzodiazepine/central-nervous-system depressant
Antipsychotic	Chlorpromazine (Thorazine) Fluphenazine (Prolixin) Risperidone (Risperdal)	Reduce or eliminate symptoms of schizophrenia and psychoses through actions on specific receptors in the brain.
Antidepressants • MAO inhibitors	Isocarboxazid (Marplan) Phenelzine (Nardil)	There are many types of antidepressants. Most act on the central nervous system and on one or more chemicals (neurotransmitters) in the brain.
• Selective-serotonin-reuptake-inhibitors (SSRI)	Fluoxetine (Prozac) Sertraline (Zoloft) Paroxetine (Paxil)	
• Tricyclic antidepressants	Imipramine (Tofranil) Amitriptyline (Elavil)	Because these act on the brain, overdoses often result in serious illness or death.
Antimanic (used in bipolar disorder—previously called manic-depressive illness)	Lithium (Eskalith, Lithotabs)	Inhibits neurotransmitters involved in creating manic (elated) states.

PATHOPHYSIOLOGY PEARLS

Behavioral emergencies always present a number of challenges to the EMT-B, not the least of which is patient restraint. A problem that is sometimes encountered by EMS providers and law-enforcement personnel is positional asphyxia or, more simply, suffocating a person by impeding his ability to breathe. There have been several documented cases of positional asphyxia while a patient was in either police or EMS custody.

A review of the normal physiology of breathing is helpful in understanding the work of breathing and the impact that body position can have on breathing. Generally speaking, a healthy person uses both the intercostal muscles and the diaphragm to breathe. When a person is in any position other than upright, the movement and subsequent lift of the chest created by the intercostal and accessory muscles is limited and the patient can only breathe by using the diaphragm.

The ultimate goal of restraining a patient is to minimize his body movements in an attempt to protect both the patient and EMT. The problem with completely restraining a patient is that compression of the shoulders and chest onto any surface will significantly reduce chest-wall expansion. Furthermore, compression of the patient's lower body will limit or completely stop movement of the diaphragm or muscles of the abdomen and essentially paralyze the patient's breathing.

No one will argue with a decision to restrain a patient for the protection of the patient or others; the question is how restraint will be accomplished. Restraining a patient facedown is never acceptable and may lead to positional asphyxia. Gone are the days of sandwiching a patient between two backboards and transporting him facedown. It is imperative that the EMT-B identify patients in need of restraint and proactively determine the most appropriate method for accomplishing the restraint.

Sources

Bledsoe BE, Porter RS, Cherry RA, Paramedic Care: Principles and Practice, Volume 3. Medical Emergencies, Prentice Hall, 2001

REVIEW QUESTIONS

SHORT ANSWER

1. Why can a sudden improvement from depression be a cause for concern?

2. What are the characteristics of an aggressive or hostile patient?

MULTIPLE CHOICE

1. _____ can cause restlessness, confusion, cyanosis, and an altered mental status.
   A. Strokes
   B. Lack of oxygen
   C. Excessive heat
   D. Hypoglycemia

2. What could be the result of improperly restraining a patient?
   A. Civil liability
   B. Positional asphyxia
   C. Criminal charges
   D. All of the above

3. What might cause a patient to present with erratic behavior, fainting, seizures, profuse perspiration, drooling, and a rapid pulse but normal blood pressure?
   A. Hypoperfusion
   B. Alcohol poisoning
   C. Low blood sugar
   D. Head trauma

SCENARIO QUESTIONS

You are responding to an individual who called 911 complaining of a headache. The patient, a 22-year-old male, meets you on the street as you arrive and climbs into the back of the ambulance. The patient then makes himself comfortable on the stretcher and refuses to answer any questions other than the one regarding his age. As you press him for more information, he looks at you angrily and says, "Don't push me; you don't know what I'm capable of."

1. At this point you should _____.
    A. have your partner assist you in restraining the patient
    B. order the patient to exit the ambulance
    C. indicate to your partner to contact law enforcement
    D. inform the patient that if he does not cooperate he will be restrained

2. What should you do if this patient then physically attacks you?
    A. Quickly exit the ambulance and run to a safe location.
    B. Defend yourself with your fists and attempt to subdue the patient.
    C. Attempt to force him out of the ambulance.
    D. Restrain the patient with soft restraints or roller gauze.

You are dispatched to a local high school for an "ill student." The school nurse meets you in the parking lot and begins leading you and your partner across campus. "I think that she might be sick," the nurse begins. "But she won't let me see her, so I figured that you may have more luck." The nurse informs you that the patient, who is 16 years old, has consistent behavioral problems at school and that her boyfriend apparently broke up with her the previous day. She leads you to a student rest room and tells you which stall the girl is in. You approach the closed stall door and identify yourself. The girl responds with sobs and yells for you to leave her alone. You explain that you are just there to help her and she responds, "Well, you're too late then." Your partner quietly instructs the nurse to request law-enforcement assistance.

1. You should avoid _____ with this patient while awaiting law enforcement.
    A. further personal interaction   B. taking an authoritative tone
    C. attempting to build rapport   D. All of the above

2. Which of the following is most appropriate to say to show this patient that you are listening?
    A. "Is this about you and your boyfriend breaking up?"
    B. "I understand that you're upset, but you need to open the door."
    C. "When I was your age, I had many of the same feelings you do."
    D. "Why am I too late to help you?"

CASE STUDIES

CASE STUDY 1   I'LL KEEP AN EYE OUT FOR YOU

You are dispatched to a residence in one of the poorer areas of town for an unknown medical reason. It is just before 5 A.M. when you receive the call. The reporting party states that he heard screaming coming from the house and called 911. To be on the safe side, you ask dispatch whether law enforcement is responding and the dispatcher confirms they are en route. A few minutes later you arrive at the scene and see no law-enforcement personnel. The house is quiet, and there are lights on inside. There is one car parked in the driveway.

1. **What would you do at this point?**

A minute later a patrol officer arrives at the scene. You advise him that the house has remained quiet since you arrived and that you have seen no one. The officer approaches the house and after knocking at the door enters the residence. A minute later he comes back out and waves you and your partner to come inside. At the door, he tells you that there is a man in the kitchen with a pretty bad eye injury, that the scene looks safe, and that there is no one else in the house that he can see. You approach the man as he is sitting with his face in his hands at the kitchen table. You introduce yourself and ask for permission to help him. He begins to sob and repeat the words, "Why, why, why?" When you ask what happened to his eye, he tells you that he pulled it out with his bare hands. He continues to cry and ask why. He then orders everyone out of the house and tells you he wants to be alone.

1. **How should you proceed at this point? Can this man refuse emergency care?**

Further questioning reveals that the man's girlfriend left him recently and he felt it was his fault. For that reason, he decided to injure himself as punishment. He begins to warm up to your presence and allows you to take a set of vital signs and place a sterile dressing over his damaged eye. Then, suddenly he jumps up and orders everyone to leave. He states that he must suffer and does not want anyone to help and again orders everyone from the house.

1. **In your mind, is this man competent to refuse emergency care? How will you proceed?**

CASE STUDY 2	I DON'T KNOW WHO THIS GUY IS, BUT SOMETHING IS WRONG

Your ambulance is called to a local church at the request of the police. The pastor found a person sleeping in the church. When the pastor began to speak with the man who identified himself as "God," he recognized the need for the police.

You arrive to find a somewhat unkempt man in his mid-30s sitting in a pew and rocking back and forth. He appears conscious, makes eye contact, and is in no apparent distress.

1. **What are your initial thoughts after the police tell you the man thinks he is God?**

2. **How would you perform your initial assessment?**

The patient is breathing adequately and does not appear to have any visible injuries. He remains hesitant and leans away when you come close. You try to ask him questions, and he just rocks back and forth. Another EMT attempts to check his pulse, and the patient slides farther down the bench away from her.

1. **Is there anything you can do to convince the patient to answer your questions?**

The police say, "OK, this is a psych patient, and he can't stay here. Just get him to the hospital. You don't need to do any of this stuff." You still have not exchanged any meaningful words with the patient.

1. Who in your community has the authority to force a patient to go to the hospital against his will?

2. If the patient will not cooperate with you or verbally consent to go—or resists totally—whose responsibility is it to make the decision to and subsequently restrain the patient?

Active Exploration

Patients experiencing a behavioral emergency can be some of the most challenging and dangerous for the EMT-B. As our lives become increasingly complex and stress begins to play a bigger part, the chances of experiencing a behavioral incident increase. In most cases, these are normal people responding to abnormal situations out of fear and panic. Being able to recognize such a situation before it explodes and knowing how to respond when it does will help you provide better emergency care for these patients and help you remain safe as a care provider.

Activity 1: Here to Help

Like a Hazmat team or a heavy extrication team, most communities have the resources to manage and treat people experiencing a behavioral emergency. It takes training and experience to appropriately assess and manage these patients. This is training and experience most EMT-Bs just do not have. Therefore, you must rely on the expert resources in your local community. The following activity will help you discover what resources are available in your community to help provide these patients with the emergency care they deserve.

1. Contact other healthcare professionals whom you know and ask them what mental-health resources are available in your area.
2. What services do these resources provide? Are they just counselors, or is there an inpatient treatment facility in your area?
3. Contact at least one mental-health resource in your community and ask what services it provides for patients experiencing a behavioral emergency.

The larger the population is, the more resources will be available. A good place to begin is in the local phone book under "Mental Health." As an EMT-B, you will eventually encounter someone with a behavioral emergency. Knowing what you can do at the scene and knowing the resources available for later will ensure that the patient gets the help he needs in a timely manner.

Activity 2: Acting Out

One of the best ways to get better at talking with an emotionally unstable person or one who has a mental illness is through role playing. While it is not easy for everyone to play the character of someone with a behavioral emergency, there are at least a few in every class who are willing and quite able to do so.

Discuss this with some of your fellow students and identify someone who would be willing to play the role of a patient with an emotional or behavioral problem. Have him think up a scenario that you must respond to.

Practice talking to this person with at least one other fellow student observing. If you have a video camera, taping the interaction is very helpful in revealing both good and bad approaches to these patients. Otherwise, following each scenario or interaction, discuss with both the observer and the patient the pros and cons of your approach or response.

Some of the major aspects of a good response are good eye contact and a very empathetic voice and manner. Pay attention to your body language as well during your interaction.

RETRO REVIEW

1. When blood escapes from damaged inner layers of a blood vessel and begins to collect in the outer layers, it is called a(n) _____.
   A. thrombus
   B. bolus
   C. aneurysm
   D. hemodissection

2. A good medical radio report has _____ parts.
   A. four
   B. eight
   C. two
   D. twelve

3. A severely exaggerated immune-system response to a foreign substance is more commonly called _____.
   A. rheumatism
   B. anaphylaxis
   C. HIV
   D. hemophilia

THINKING AND LINKING

CHAPTER TOPIC	HOW IT RELATES TO YOU AND OTHER COURSE AREAS
Situational stress	The sight of soft-tissue injuries such as cuts, avulsions, and amputations (which you will cover in depth in Chapter 27) and open, angulated fractures (Chapter 28) will cause tremendous fear in many of your patients. You will help the situation quite a bit by maintaining a calm, professional demeanor (Chapter 1).
Suicide	While working in EMS, you will undoubtedly encounter individuals who have attempted or committed suicide. While these can be psychologically difficult calls (Chapter 2), they can also be physically dangerous. Gather as much information as possible from dispatch (Chapter 13) prior to entering the scene and do not forget about scene safety. Gases, poisons, and firearms (Chapters 21 and 27) can all, obviously, pose a threat to you and your crew.

Always remember to use proper PPE (Chapter 2) at suicide scenes—you will not know what drugs or poisons might be present. |
| Refusal of treatment | You may get more treatment refusals from behavioral-emergency patients than any other type of patient. Contact medical direction (Chapter 13) or law enforcement for these patients—they definitely need emergency care and *you* may be liable if you do not persist (Chapter 3) and ensure that they get it.

Always keep yourself (and your coworkers) in safe positions when dealing with a behavioral-emergency patient (Chapter 2)—the potential for sudden violence can be very high. |

24

Obstetrics and Gynecological Emergencies

CHAPTER SUMMARY

You may be called upon to assist with a birth during your career as an EMT-B. The key word is assist; remember that the mother does the majority of the work. It is a very natural process that typically does not present with any complications. Reviewing the process regularly will keep your skills tuned and allow you to be confident when the actual event happens.

The fetus develops in the uterus during pregnancy. The placenta, which is implanted in the uterine wall, supplies the fetus with nutrients while also removing waste products. The placenta is attached to the fetus by the umbilical cord. Surrounding the fetus is the amniotic sac that contains fluid that helps protect the fetus and provides a constant temperature.

During delivery, the cervix must dilate from 2 to 10 cm so that the fetus can pass from the uterus into the vagina. Crowning happens when the baby starts to emerge from the vaginal opening. The baby is typically headfirst, or in a cephalic presentation. If the legs or buttocks deliver first, it is called a breech presentation.

Labor has three stages:

- First stage—start of regular contractions until the cervix is fully dilated
- Second stage—from full dilation of the cervix to the time the baby is born
- Third stage—from the time the baby is born until the afterbirth is delivered

Labor contractions start during the first stage of labor and come in shorter intervals as labor progresses. They may be as close as 3 minutes or less apart when delivery is near.

The contractions also become longer in duration as labor progresses, typically 30 seconds to 1 minute per contraction. As an EMT-B, you should time the duration and frequency of the contractions. When contractions last 30 seconds to 1 minute, and are 2 to 3 minutes apart, delivery of the baby may be imminent. The woman may also state she has the urge to move her bowels as the baby moves down the birth canal and presses on her rectum.

Usually, the amniotic sac will break during labor and the contents will either trickle or gush out of the vagina. This is one reason that taking full BSI precautions is very important during a delivery. The fluid should be clear. A greenish or yellow brown color may indicate the presence of meconium staining that can indicate fetal distress. Expect bloody discharge during childbirth, but any amount greater than 500 cc should raise concern.

As an EMT, you will decide whether you have time to transport the mother or whether you should attempt the delivery at the scene. Ask the expectant mother the following questions:

- Name, age, and expected due date.
- Is this her first delivery?
- How long has she been in labor?
- How far apart are her contractions?
- Has her "water" broken?
- Does she feel like she needs to move her bowels?
- Examine for crowning, keeping the patient's privacy in mind.

Remember that any third-trimester patient you transport should be propped on her left side to displace the fetus off the large blood vessels.

If the baby is presenting cephalically, then consider it a normal delivery and assist the mother with the delivery. Look to see if the umbilical cord is around the baby's neck during delivery and gently remove it. Suction the baby's mouth and then nose with a bulb syringe once the head is delivered. Support the baby's head and body while the delivery is completed. All babies, especially premature infants, need to be kept warm after delivery.

Once the baby is born, he needs to be assessed for adequate breathing and circulation. Usually suctioning, drying, and warming will stimulate a newborn who is not breathing on his own. If breathing does not begin within 30 seconds, then you must start resuscitation measures. A newborn's respiratory rate should be 40 to 60 breaths per minute, and his heart rate should be at least 100 beats per minute. If his heart rate is less than 100 beats per minute, provide artificial ventilations for 30 seconds and reassess. If the heart rate is less than 60 beats per minute, then chest compressions and artificial ventilations must be performed. Supplemental blow by oxygen may be needed for newborns who have central cyanosis but adequate respiratory and heart rates.

In a normal delivery, the umbilical cord may be cut once the cord has stopped pulsating and the baby is breathing on its own. The placenta is usually delivered within a few minutes after the baby is born. Save the afterbirth tissues for a physician to examine to determine whether the entire placenta has been expelled.

Keep in mind that you really have two patients, the baby and the mother. Assist the mother in delivering the placenta, controlling vaginal bleeding by massaging the uterus after delivery if necessary, and generally make her comfortable. Assess the mother for any early signs of shock and treat accordingly.

Occasionally you will be faced with complications such as a breech presentation, a limb presentation, or a prolapsed umbilical cord. You may have to insert several gloved fingers into the vagina to help keep the baby from putting pressure on the umbilical cord and cutting off its own circulation. All of these situations require high-flow oxygen for the mother and rapid transport. Multiple births may be normal deliveries but make sure that you have adequate resources to provide emergency care for both infants and the mother.

There are several emergencies that can occur in pregnancy prior to childbirth.

- **Placenta previa**—the placenta has implanted too low in the uterus, close to the cervix, and can cause significant bleeding.
- **Abruptio placentae**—the placenta separates from the uterine wall, and can cause significant bleeding.
- **Ectopic pregnancy**—when the egg implants in an area other than the uterine wall.

All the above conditions can cause hypoperfusion. The patient should be transported rapidly and be treated for shock.

Other complications include:

- Eclampsia—seizures late in pregnancy due to high blood pressure
- Excessive weight gain
- Swelling of hands, feet, and face
- Miscarriage
- Trauma to the pregnant female

There are several emergencies that can occur related to the female reproductive system:

- Vaginal bleeding not related to menstrual cycle or trauma
- Trauma to the external genitalia

When sexual assault is the cause of trauma to the genitalia, both medical and psychological emergency care must be given. Law enforcement must also be notified.

MED MINUTE

Pregnancy does not routinely involve the use of many drugs because of the risk of developmental complications in an underdeveloped fetus. The female patient with the potential of becoming pregnant may use oral contraceptives to prevent pregnancy, while the pregnant patient often takes prenatal vitamin supplements to promote health in the fetus. This table gives examples of common drugs in each category. Dozens of medications may be available with similar effects.

CLASS OF MEDICATION	MEDICATION NAME(S)	MECHANISM OF ACTION
Oral contraceptives	Estrogen–Progestin combinations (Avaine, Brevicon, Demulen, Enpresse, Microgestin, Ortho-Novum, Ortho-Cept, and Ortho-Tri-Cyclen)	Used to prevent conception and to treat menstrual irregularity.
Prenatal vitamins	Folic acid (Folvite)	Vitamin supplements to ensure adequate nutrition of the fetus while in utero.
	Prenatabs	
	Natafort	

PATHOPHYSIOLOGY PEARLS

One of the things that should concern you most in a pregnant patient and that you as an EMT-B can identify is an elevated blood pressure. An important and normal physiologic characteristic common in pregnancy is a maternal blood pressure that is lower than the patient's normal blood pressure. Therefore, when hypertension occurs in the pregnant patient, it should always be monitored closely and assumed to be abnormal until proven otherwise.

In discussing hypertension and pregnancy, it is critical to at least mention pre-eclampsia. Although this is not the primary focus of this pearl, it is a significant problem that occurs during pregnancy at around the same time that the HELLP syndrome does, roughly in the last three months of pregnancy.

Many of the occurrences of hypertension in pregnancy are said to be the result of maternal vasospasm. Pregnancy-induced hypertension (PIH) is most commonly seen in a first pregnancy or in patients with a history of clinical hypertension or nongestational diabetes.

A very severe form of PIH is known as HELLP syndrome. HELLP syndrome occurs rarely, but when it does, it should be considered a very serious finding. HELLP syndrome typically has a rapid onset and is most commonly seen in the last three months of pregnancy and may even develop shortly after delivery of the fetus.

HELLP stands for Hemolysis (breakdown of red blood cells—RBCs), Elevated Liver enzyme levels and a Low Platelet count. These are the hallmark problems that occur in women with this syndrome. These patients will have bleeding problems, liver problems, and blood pressure problems that are potentially life threatening to themselves and the baby. The fragmentation of RBCs may actually cause the patient to progress from pre-eclampsia to the development of multisystem organ failure and death because of vessel occlusion by the fragmented RBCs.

Patients with HELLP syndrome typically complain of generalized weakness, epigastric pain, and nausea and vomiting or flulike symptoms. Unfortunately, these patients often show very few signs of pre-eclampsia. Once diagnosed, management of HELLP syndrome is the same as for the patient diagnosed with severe pre-eclampsia: delivery of the fetus.

Sources

Rosen P, Barkin RM, et al., Emergency Medicine Concepts and Clinical Practice, 5th Edition, Mosby, 2002
Tintinalli JE, Kelen GD, et al., Emergency Medicine, A Comprehensive Study Guide, 5th Edition, McGraw-Hill, 2000
O'Hara-Padden M, "American Family Physician," September 1, 1999, American Academy of Family Physicians.

REVIEW QUESTIONS

SHORT ANSWER

1. Why should you always have suction equipment ready when transporting a pregnant trauma patient?

2. What causes supine hypotensive syndrome?

MULTIPLE CHOICE

1. *Abruptio placentae* is the medical term for _____.
   A. breaking the "bag of waters"
   B. premature placental separation
   C. delivery of the "afterbirth"
   D. a rupture of the uterus

2. Full dilation of the cervix occurs in the _____ stage of labor.
   A. first
   B. third
   C. second
   D. effacement

3. A cephalic presentation means that _____.
   A. the newborn is suffering from a severe buildup of cranial fluid
   B. the mother is supine with her pelvis elevated
   C. the baby is birthing in the normal, head-first manner
   D. the umbilical cord is wrapped around the infant's neck

4. Meconium staining of the amniotic fluid is an indication of _____.
   A. a placental infection
   B. gestational diabetes
   C. uterine perforation
   D. fetal distress

5. What is a very late sign of an ectopic pregnancy?
   A. Acute abdominal pain
   B. Low blood pressure
   C. Vaginal bleeding
   D. Irregular pulse

SCENARIO QUESTIONS

You respond to a head-on vehicle collision and are directed to one of the drivers, who turns out to be eight months pregnant. The rescue squad has extricated her from the vehicle and turned her over to your care. She is complaining of severe abdominal pain and is nearly hysterical, worrying about the condition of her baby.

1. How should this patient be transported?
   A. Secured to a long spine board that is tilted to the left.
   B. In the Trendelenburg position.
   C. In a vest-type extrication device that is loosened at the torso.
   D. Secured to a long spine board that is propped with pillows under the patient's left side.

2. How can you best support this patient emotionally?
   A. Let her know that everything is going to be fine.
   B. Hold her hand and listen quietly while she expresses her concerns.
   C. Reassure her that the baby is well protected in the uterus.
   D. All of the above.

3. How much blood volume can this patient potentially lose before exhibiting signs of shock?
   A. 55–60 percent
   B. 20–25 percent
   C. 40–45 percent
   D. 30–35 percent

You are dispatched to a bank where one of the employees is bleeding. You are quickly ushered into the rest room where you find the patient, a 22-year-old woman, in tears and holding sanitary pads to her genital area. Several pads, soaked with blood, are discarded on the floor. During your assessment of the patient, she tells you that she is not menstruating and that she knows "for a fact" that she is not pregnant. There is no evidence of trauma.

1. What are the proper steps you should take to provide emergency care for this patient?

   A. Take BSI precautions, assure an adequate airway, assess for signs of shock, administer high-concentration oxygen, and transport immediately.

   B. Take BSI precautions, attempt to stop the bleeding with direct pressure, treat for shock, administer high-concentration oxygen, and transport rapidly.

   C. Take BSI precautions, assure an adequate airway, evaluate for shock, provide supplemental oxygen with a nasal cannula, and transport.

   D. Take BSI precautions, ensure a patent airway, monitor for, and react to, signs of shock, and wait for an ALS intercept.

2. The most serious potential complication for this patient is _____ shock.

   A. toxic

   B. psychogenic

   C. hemorrhagic

   D. compensated

3. What is the most effective way to determine the cause of this patient's hemorrhaging?

   A. Vaginal palpation with a gloved hand.

   B. It is not possible and should not be attempted.

   C. Extensive questioning during the SAMPLE history.

   D. Visual inspection by an EMT-B of the same gender.

You are called to a residence for a woman who is in labor. You arrive to find a 27-year-old mother of three who states that her waters have broken and her contractions are about four minutes apart. She is surrounded by her two oldest children, her husband, and the neighbor who notified EMS. Upon visual inspection, you observe that the umbilical cord is protruding from the vaginal opening. The patient tells you that she will be ready to go with you as soon as she uses the bathroom to move her bowels.

1. Why should you deny the patient's request to use the bathroom?

   A. With a prolapsed-cord situation, the patient's straining to move her bowels could result in a stroke.

   B. You should not deny the request, but you should make sure that the patient holds the umbilical cord in place with a saline soaked gauze pad.

   C. Because the potential for a bacterial infection is too great.

   D. With this patient's birthing history and current contractions, it is possible that she might deliver the baby into the toilet.

2. Which of the following is the most important step in providing emergency care for this mother and child?

   A. Asking the two children and the neighbor to leave the room.

   B. Inserting several gloved fingers into the vagina and keeping the baby from pressing on the cord.

   C. Gently pushing the umbilical cord back into the vagina.

   D. Using the equipment from a sterile OB kit to cut and tie the cord.

3. In what position should this patient be placed for transport?

   A. There will not be enough time to transport.

   B. On her side with her knees together.

   C. With her head down and her buttocks raised with a pillow.

   D. In the position of most comfort.

CASE STUDIES

CASE STUDY 1   I CAN'T BELIEVE I'M GOING TO HAVE MY BABY IN A TENT!

You are dispatched to a possible "woman in labor" at a campground about 20 minutes outside of town. Upon your arrival, you are met by a park ranger who tells you there is a pregnant woman in labor at one of the campsites. He leads you and your partner to the site. A few yards away you can hear a woman screaming in pain. As you enter the campsite, you can hear a man from inside a tent attempting to comfort the woman, with little success. You announce your arrival and poke your head inside the tent. You are surprised to see three small children in addition to the mother and the man. The man steps out of the tent and insists that you get his girlfriend to the hospital because "she is going to have the baby right here if you don't get moving."

1. How will you begin to take control of the scene at this time?

2. What clues are there in the environment that may help during your assessment of the woman?

The ranger takes the boyfriend and the three children off to the side and begins to get a history. Meanwhile you have determined that the woman is 36 weeks along and that her contractions are 3 minutes apart. Her last two children were delivered early and the labor lasted just 2 hours with the last child. Your partner places her on some oxygen and gets a set of baseline vitals while you continue with your assessment. Upon observing the vagina, you see what appears to be crowning.

1. Do you have time to transport or will you stay and attempt to deliver at the scene? What factors lead you to this decision?

2. How do you accurately time contractions for a woman in labor?

Your ambulance is called for "vaginal bleeding" at 554E West Creekside Drive. As you respond, you realize that you have not had a call for vaginal bleeding since you got your EMT certification.

You arrive at the residence and ensure that the scene is safe. Since the call involves bleeding, you don gloves and ensure that you have eyewear available. You find the patient lying in bed. She appears conscious and is covered by blankets.

1. **What other observations should you make as you approach and begin your initial assessment?**

2. **Is it possible to develop shock from vaginal bleeding?**

The patient responds to you and is alert and oriented. You do not identify any problems during the initial assessment. Your partner places the patient on oxygen by nonrebreather mask as you continue to talk to the patient. She tells you that she began bleeding yesterday and thought that her period had just started very early. The bleeding became more severe by yesterday evening and into this morning.

1. **How would you determine the extent of bleeding?**

2. **What additional questions should you ask during the history?**

3. **What type of physical examination should you perform?**

The patient does not believe she is pregnant. She does not take birth-control pills or any other medications. She has abdominal pain that is described as "crampy" and across her lower abdomen. She has never experienced this type of pain or bleeding before.

1. **Is there any treatment you can perform or any manual way of stopping the bleeding?**

Active Exploration

Obstetrics is the medical specialty that deals specifically with the care of women during and after childbirth, while gynecology is the specialty dealing with the care of women in general and more specifically the diagnosis and treatment of problems pertaining to the reproductive organs.

As EMT-Bs, it is only a matter of time before you encounter the female patient with "abdominal pain" or the call for the "woman in labor." Because these types of calls make up a relatively small percentage of the total call volume, it is easy to become overwhelmed by an otherwise straightforward patient.

Even though most of these types of calls do not involve trauma, a thorough and accurate history is essential. The following activities will assist you in learning to provide emergency care for these patients.

Activity 1: What's in the Kit?

Most EMT-Bs are familiar with an OB kit in that they know one exists. Yet they may not have spent any time getting to know one. The time to become familiar with the contents of such a kit is *not* on the scene of a possible delivery.

For this activity, you must borrow a sample OB kit from your instructor and, along with a fellow classmate, identify and discuss each of the elements of the kit. If you are not sure what an item is used for, ask another student or your instructor.

To take this activity one step further, use one of the training manikins in class to set up a mock delivery scene, placing the drapes and towels as you would during a real field delivery.

Activity 2: What Was It Like for You?

For this activity, we want you to interview a couple who has had a child in the recent past. The more recent the better: that way the mother's recollection of all the small details will be better. Prepare a list of questions ahead of time and arrange to meet for a short time so that you can ask your questions and gain some insight into what a delivery is like from both the mother's and father's perspectives.

If possible, it may even be appropriate to team up with one of your fellow classmates and conduct the interview together. Ask the parents to take you back through the experience as they remember it, from prenatal care to the beginning of contractions (the first stage) to the delivery of the placenta (if the mother even remembers that part) to coming home with the new baby for the first time.

Gather as much detail about the experience from both sides as you can. Keep in mind that you want to ask questions from an EMS perspective and perhaps gain some insight into how you might be better able to care for both the mother and father if such an event happens outside the hospital.

RETRO REVIEW

1. You are called to assist a local homeless man who is sweating profusely, trembling, and arguing with people only he can see. You have dealt with this particular patient countless times before but have never seen him act this way. You also notice, surprisingly, that he does not smell like alcohol. You should suspect _____.

   A. meningitis   **B.** delirium tremens

   C. neuropathy   **D.** hypothermia

2. The connective tissue that holds a muscle to the bone is called (a) _____.

   A. ligament   **B.** cartilage

   C. tendon   **D.** manubrium

3. Each box on a PCR is known as a _____.

   A. data set   **B.** data capsule

   C. data range   **D.** data element

THINKING AND LINKING

CHAPTER TOPIC	HOW IT RELATES TO YOU AND OTHER COURSE AREAS
Crowning	Your patient will most likely be uncomfortable with you (whether male or female) visually inspecting her vagina. This is another situation where your professional demeanor (Chapter 1) and effective communication skills (Chapter 13) can significantly reduce the patient's stress. Also remember that crowning and childbirth can occasionally cause bowel movements. You will want to ensure proper PPE (Chapter 2) and have extra linen or towels on hand to prevent contamination.
Bleeding	Blood loss following a delivery will usually be substantial but normal and controllable with basic techniques (sanitary pads, massaging the uterus, and so on). You should still be very alert for the signs of shock (covered in Chapter 26) and make sure you have your airway, oxygen, and suction equipment (Chapter 6) close by.
Ectopic pregnancy	You should suspect that any female patient (of childbearing age) with abdominal pain (Chapter 18) may be experiencing an ectopic pregnancy. You will need to transport immediately (Chapter 32) and treat for shock en route (Chapter 26).
Trauma and pregnancy	When you are responding to large trauma incidents (vehicle collisions, and so on) and you find a pregnant patient, anticipate the elevated potential for internal injuries (Chapter 27) and be prepared to treat for shock (Chapter 26).

25

Putting It Together
for the Medical Patient

CHAPTER SUMMARY

Medical patients can be more challenging than trauma patients because the specific signs and symptoms exhibited by the patient could be caused by several different underlying problems. Remember that your training as an EMT-B will guide you in your assessment of a medical patient whether he has a single complaint or multiple complaints. Some patients may have chief complaints that you have no specific treatment for, but your assessment process is always the same. For all patients, you will asses their airway, breathing, and circulation and treat any life-threats. You will make a priority decision regarding transport of your patient and whether an ALS intercept would be beneficial. You will then determine whether you have any interventions that would help your patient. Medical direction is always available if you need guidance for a particularly challenging patient or situation.

PATHOPHYSIOLOGY PEARLS

Did you ever hear the terms cardiac wheezing or cardiac asthma being used? Is this a heart problem or a breathing problem?

Cardiac asthma is not asthma, but it does mimic asthma. A patient with cardiac wheezing will obviously have wheezing, but the wheezing will typically be isolated to the left side of the patient's chest, he will have shortness of breath, and he may also have a cough. Cardiac asthma is actually a precursor to a sudden attack of congestive heart failure.

In asthma, wheezing is caused by inflammation of the airways and constriction of the bronchial smooth muscle around the airways. In cardiac asthma, wheezing, as previously mentioned, begins on the left side of the chest because the left side of the heart has begun to fail and cannot eject the blood it is receiving from the right side of the heart. As the left side of the heart fails, back pressure is built up within the lungs and fluid begins to leak into the alveoli. As this fluid begins to accumulate, wheezing and shortness of breath occur.

The treatment for asthma does not work on cardiac asthma and can actually worsen a patient's condition. Treatment of cardiac asthma involves the identification of the disease process through obtaining an accurate medical history; the administration of oxygen; the monitoring of vital signs, including oxygen saturation using pulse oximetry; and the administration of medications. Medications used to treat asthma include inhaling treatments and in some cases epinephrine. Breathing treatments and epinephrine, if given to a patient with CHF, will likely worsen the patient's condition and may precede death. Remember that the more the heart works, the more oxygen it needs. These medications will make the heart work harder by stimulating stronger and faster contractions of the heart.

The most important treatment for CHF is ensuring that the patient has an open, patent airway; administering high concentrations of oxygen; providing ventilatory support; and if necessary, administering medication. The medications used to treat the CHF patient are primarily those that reduce the amount of work the heart has to do (the exact opposite of the asthma treatment) and those that help draw fluid away from the patient's lungs.

The most important aspect of assessing these patients is to treat the patients on the basis of the way they present and to perform a complete history and physical exam. The patient's past medical history should also help determine the proper path to follow in the management of a wheezing patient.

Sources

Rosen P, Barkin RM, et al., Emergency Medicine Concepts and Clinical Practice, *5th Edition, Mosby, 2002*
Tintinalli JE, Kelen GD, et al., Emergency Medicine, A Comprehensive Study Guide, *5th Edition, McGraw-Hill, 2000*

REVIEW QUESTIONS

SHORT ANSWER

1. What should you do if unusual circumstances are making it difficult to assess the medical patient's condition?

2. What are the five basic decisions that an EMT-B must make when assessing a medical patient?

MULTIPLE CHOICE

1. What should you do if your patient tells you that he is suffering from a disease that you have never heard of?

   A. Ask the staff at the receiving facility about it when you arrive.

   B. Ask the patient to explain the disease.

   C. Look it up in Gray's Pocket Guide.

   D. Act as if you know what the condition is to prevent the patient from losing confidence in your abilities.

2. As an EMT-B, look for and treat the problems for which you have
_____.

    A. medications   **B.** experience

    C. equipment   **D.** treatments

3. What should you do if a medical patient is complaining of a severe headache?

    A. Administer aspirin (if your EMS system allows it to be stocked on your ambulance).

    B. Cover the patient's eyes with a dark cloth or folded towel.

    C. Monitor the ABCs and transport.

    D. Administer oxygen at 6 lpm and begin palpating for a possible cause.

SCENARIO QUESTIONS

You arrive at a college dorm room for an apparent drug overdose. The patient, a 19-year-old male student, is responsive to your voice but is unable to keep his eyes open or speak. You notice a prescription sedative bottle on the floor and a nearly empty bottle of vodka on the nightstand. The student who called 911 tells you that the patient's sister had just died in an auto crash the day before and that he had been very despondent.

1. After securing the airway and ensuring adequate respirations and circulation, what should you do next?

    A. Administer activated charcoal.

    B. Place him in the recovery position and prepare a suction unit.

    C. Transport the patient with the pill and alcohol bottles.

    D. Obtain baseline vital signs.

2. What is the best method of determining the maximum number of sedative pills that the patient is likely to have ingested?

    A. Multiply the daily prescription amount by the number of days since the prescription was filled, add that amount to the number of pills currently left in the bottle, and subtract that sum from the originally prescribed quantity of pills.

    B. Add the number of pills left in the bottle to the original quantity, and then multiply that number by the amount of pills prescribed daily.

    C. Simply subtract the number of pills left in the bottle from the originally filled quantity.

    D. Subtract the number of pills left in the bottle from the original quantity, add the number of days that have passed since the prescription was filled to that figure, and subtract it from the quantity that appears on the label.

3. How should you obtain a SAMPLE history on this patient?

    A. Keep rousing the patient and asking him "yes" or "no" questions.

    B. Try to get the SAMPLE information from the student who knows the patient.

    C. Forego the SAMPLE history and just prepare the patient for transport.

    D. Attempt to contact the patient's family.

You arrive at a residence after being called by a child who reports that her mother is "sick." A young girl leads you to the living room where you find a 30- to 35-year-old woman sprawled on the floor and crying in pain. You immediately ask whether she fell and she tells you, through clenched teeth, that she got down on the floor due to unbearable general body pain. She continues, in rapid bursts of pained speech, that she has terminal spinal cancer and is currently taking morphine and diazepam. She begs you to help her with the pain.

1. How would you begin treating this patient?
   A. Help her to self-administer any prescribed medications.
   B. Administer oxygen with a nonrebreather mask at 15 lp m and transport immediately.
   C. Complete an initial assessment.
   D. Contact medical direction and ask for advice.

2. What can you do to assist this patient with her pain level?
   A. Calmly continue to reassure her.
   B. Instruct the young girl to place a diazepam tablet into her mother's mouth.
   C. Nothing. Simply prepare her for transport.
   D. Encourage her to take more of the prescribed morphine.

3. This is one type of call where you, as an EMT-B, will have to depend on _____.
   A. your pharmacology knowledge
   B. medical direction
   C. unconventional treatments
   D. your partner

CASE STUDIES

CASE STUDY 1   MEDICAL OR TRAUMA—THAT IS THE QUESTION

It is 10 A.M. and you are called to an assisted-living facility for a person who has had a fall. Upon your arrival, you are directed to the back-patio area where you find an approximately 80-year-old female lying on her side at the bottom of a small set of steps. She is responsive and moaning loudly. Her ABCs appear stable, and the person helping the woman states that she was found here approximately 20 minutes ago and that no one saw her fall.

1. What should be the focus of your initial line of questioning for this patient?

2. Why is it important to determine whether the patient remembers why she may have fallen?

Through questioning the patient, you have determined that she does not remember falling, just that she felt dizzy. She then remembers being on the ground and having pain in her hip. Her vitals are stable except for an obviously irregular pulse. She states that she takes several medications but cannot remember what they are. You ask someone to retrieve her medications for you.

1. What information can be found on the typical prescription-medication bottle?

2. Will you want to take vitals on this patient every 5 or 15 minutes?

Your ambulance is called for a report of general body weakness at 2401 Cross Court. Your EMS system uses a dispatch system that assigns priority according to patient complaint and other factors. This call is priority 2—no lights or sirens.

Nonetheless, you still respond promptly and with safety in mind. You arrive at the scene to find it safe with a relative greeting you at the door, saying, "He's in here." You walk to the couch and find a 56-year-old man lying on the couch. His color is normal, he appears to be breathing deeply and adequately, and is oriented as you begin to speak to him.

1. **What is your general impression of this patient?**

2. **What BSI precautions should you take?**

The man tells you that he feels "weak." He has no energy and has not had for the past month or so. But now he just feels like he cannot get off the couch. You ask him whether he has any pain or injury. He replies, "No."

1. **How do you assess a patient without a specific medical or traumatic complaint?**

You find that the patient continues to deny pain or injury. He denies taking medications and reports that his only history is prostate cancer six years ago. He had his prostate removed and has had no problems since then. His vital signs are pulse 82, strong and regular; respirations 12, nonlabored and adequate; blood pressure 110/78; pupils equal and reactive to light; skin warm and dry; and oxygen saturation 99 percent. The patient reports that he has been to his personal physician because of the fatigue. A complete physical including EKG did not reveal abnormalities.

1. **Could this patient have a psychiatric history? Could he be depressed? Faking symptoms?**

2. **Does this patient need oxygen?**

You transfer the patient to your stretcher and transport the patient to the hospital. His vitals remain unchanged. You turn him over to the hospital staff and complete your documentation.

Active Exploration

The typical medical patient offers many challenges that trauma patients typically do not. First of all, there are no mechanisms of injury to offer clues or open wounds to keep you busy. You should see most medical complaints as an opportunity to practice good history-taking skills and to remain as open and objective as possible. The important thing is to resist the urge to come to a definite conclusion or to diagnose the patient's problem. Your job is to develop and use a standardized approach to your assessment and gather as many facts as possible.

The following activities will help you develop your assessment skills and your understanding of the importance of a good history.

Activity 1: Which Way Do I Go—Medical?

You will see presented below a series of short vignettes of medical patients. These are not full case studies but more basic first impressions of various patients. Your job will be to quickly decide the most appropriate assessment path for each patient. You will remember from Chapter 11, "Assessment of the Medical Patient," that there are essentially two possible assessment paths you can take for any medical patient: the rapid medical assessment and the focused medical assessment. If necessary, please review these two paths in Chapter 11 of your textbook before proceeding with this activity.

1. A 63-year-old female who was complaining of a severe headache before becoming unresponsive.

2. A 44-year-old male who is complaining of severe substernal chest pain. This patient has a history of heart problems and takes nitro. He is responsive and in moderate distress.

3. A 13-year-old female who is just waking up following what was described as a full-body seizure.

4. A 26-year-old male who collapsed while playing basketball in a church gymnasium. The patient is unresponsive upon your arrival.

5. A 92-year-old female who suddenly was unable to speak. She appears responsive but is unable to follow simple commands or respond verbally. She is alert and looking around.

6. A 63-year-old female who was complaining of a severe headache before becoming unresponsive.

Activity 2: What's in a Name?

The more you know about the medications that you may encounter in the field, the better an EMT you will be. This activity will have you investigate four commonly encountered medications in a slightly unique way. Using the Internet, do a search for MSDS. This will pull up several sites that offer access to "material safety data sheets" for just about any chemical under the sun.

Once you have located one of these sites, conduct a search for an MSDS for the following medications:

- Activated charcoal
- Epinephrine
- Oral glucose
- Nitroglycerin

Study these MSDS sheets and learn what you can about each of these medications.

RETRO REVIEW

1. Constricting bands should be placed above and below a snakebite to restrict the flow of _____.

   A. blood   **B.** plasma

   C. lymph   **D.** platelets

2. You are dispatched to a dorm room at the local university for an individual who is "not acting right." The campus police department has secured the scene and you are escorted to the patient's location. You find a 19-year-old male student who seems dazed, tells you that his head feels "numb," and who has some swelling of the membranes in his nose and mouth. You should suspect _____.

   A. cerebral meningitis   **B.** ethanol poisoning

   C. substantive dehydration   **D.** volatile-chemical abuse

3. Which of the following is *not* considered an abdominal organ?

   A. Pancreas   **B.** Liver

   C. Spleen   **D.** Gall bladder

THINKING AND LINKING

CHAPTER TOPIC	HOW IT RELATES TO YOU AND OTHER COURSE AREAS
Multiple medical complaints	You may find yourself providing emergency care for a patient in respiratory distress who is developing anaphylaxis following a bee sting (Chapter 20) and who has a history of COPD and asthma (Chapter 16). Since you are not trained (or expected) to make emergency-care decisions based on the subtleties of each condition, you should stick to the basics: Airway, Breathing, and Circulation. Remember to pass along all of a patient's medical history (Chapter 9) and complaints to advanced care via radio reports, verbal reports, and written reports (Chapters 13 and 14). Although much of the information may mean little to you, it might drastically change the way the patient is cared for at the receiving facility.
Spinal astrocytoma?	You will regularly encounter patients with diseases or conditions that you have never heard of. As long as you ask the patient in the right way (Chapter 13), he will usually be willing to explain it. Do not hesitate to contact medical direction (also in Chapter 13) for guidance when you are unsure how a patient's pre-existing condition relates to his current complaint (Chapter 8).
Home medical equipment	When responding to medical patients in their homes, you will encounter many different types of medical devices—from supplemental-oxygen-delivery systems (Chapter 6) to life-support equipment and specialized beds. Always ask about equipment that you are unfamiliar with—somebody in the home will most likely be a good source of information about it. When moving patients from specialized beds or chairs (pneumatic, vacuum forming, silicone, and so on), do not forget to use proper lifting techniques (Chapter 5).

26

Bleeding and Shock

CHAPTER SUMMARY

As an EMT-B, it is critical that you quickly identify serious trauma and shock. The patient's outcome will depend on many factors, including early identification, appropriate emergency care, and rapid transport to a trauma center.

The circulatory system is made up of the heart, blood vessels, and the blood. All three of these must be adequately functioning to properly perfuse the patient. Perfusion is the adequate circulation of blood to supply the cells and tissues with oxygen and nutrients. The heart is the pump of the system and circulates the blood through the body via three major types of blood vessels. These vessels are known as arteries, capillaries, and veins. The body holds a specific amount of blood. If hemorrhaging occurs and enough blood volume is lost, hypoperfusion will occur. The brain, spinal cord, and kidneys are the most sensitive to inadequate perfusion. Hemorrhaging can either be external or internal.

Take adequate BSI precautions while treating a patient with external bleeding. The bleeding may present in one of the three following ways:

- **Arterial**—bright red, rapid, spurting, profuse
- **Venous**—dark red, steady flow
- **Capillary**—medium red, oozing, easily controlled

You should determine the severity of an external bleed on the basis of the amount of blood lost and the patient's condition. For an adult, you should consider a blood loss of approximately 1 liter as serious, while for an infant, you should consider a blood loss of 150cc as serious. If any patient has signs of shock, regardless of the amount of blood lost, you should consider it as serious. Control any external bleeding with the following procedures:

- Direct pressure/pressure dressing
- Elevation
- Pressure points

- Splinting
- Cold applications
- PASG (pneumatic anti-shock garment)—following local protocols and/or with advice from medical direction
- Tourniquet—*only as a last resort* for life-threats

There are special considerations when managing nosebleeds and bleeding from fractured skulls.

The extent of an internal bleed can be just as serious but not as obvious as an external bleed. If the internal organs are damaged, they can lose a large amount of blood very quickly. Sharp bone ends from broken extremities can damage large blood vessels, causing a significant blood loss. You should determine which patients have the potential for bleeding internally by performing a thorough history and physical exam as well as by establishing the mechanism of injury. Mechanisms of blunt and penetrating trauma that may cause internal bleeding include:

- Falls
- Motor-vehicle or motorcycle crashes
- Automobile vs. pedestrian collisions
- Blast injuries
- Gunshot wounds
- Stabbings
- Impaled objects

Signs of internal bleeding include:

- Injuries to the outside of the body
- Bruising
- Swollen, painful, or deformed extremities
- Bleeding from a body orifice
- Rigid, tender, distended abdomen
- Vomiting dark or bright red blood
- Blood in the stools, dark or bright red
- Signs and symptoms of shock—remember that falling blood pressure is a *late* sign

Managing the patient with internal bleeding includes treatment for shock and rapid transport.

Shock may develop if any one of the following occurs:

- The heart pumps inadequately.
- Blood volume is lost.
- The blood vessels dilate, creating a larger container for the heart to pump the blood through.

The severity of shock is determined by these categories:

- **Compensated**—The body attempts to compensate for the decrease in perfusion by increasing the heart rate and respiratory rate.
- **Decompensated**—The body can no longer compensate to maintain adequate perfusion or blood pressure.
- **Irreversible**—The organ systems are no longer perfused. Patients die due to damaged organs.

Signs and symptoms of shock include:

- Altered mental status
- Pale, cool, clammy skin
- Nausea and vomiting
- Changes in vital signs (increased pulse and respirations, decreased blood pressure [late sign])
- Other signs—thirst, dilated pupils, cyanosis around lips and nail beds

Infants and children compensate much longer than adults do. It is crucial you suspect shock early and treat it aggressively in infants and children.

Patients in shock must be given high-flow oxygen to supplement the oxygen being delivered to the tissues. Rapid transportation is one of the most effective treatments. Your goal is not to be at the scene of a crash longer than 10 minutes (the platinum 10 minutes) and to have your patient on the operating table within in 1 hour (the golden hour) of the crash occurring. In addition to rapid transport, you should:

- Manage the airway and provide assisted ventilations/CPR if necessary
- Control any external bleeding
- Elevate the legs 8 to 12 inches if no head/spinal injury is suspected
- Splint any suspected bone injuries—using a longboard splints the body as a unit
- Maintain patient's body heat

MED MINUTE

There are many drugs that may hide the effects of developing shock. You will read in this chapter that signs of shock increase with elevated pulse and respirations, anxiety, and changes in skin color. There are medications that will prevent the pulse from rising. These medications (listed below) may lead you to believe a patient is stable when shock is developing. This table gives examples of common drugs in each category. Many other medications may be available with similar effects.

CLASS OF MEDICATION	MEDICATION NAME(S)	MECHANISM OF ACTION
Beta blockers	Atenolol (Tenormin) Labetalol (Normodyne)	Used for hypertension. Block the actions of the sympathetic nervous system. May keep the pulse low during shock.
Calcium-channel blockers	Diltiazem (Cardizem) Amlodipine (Norvasc)	Used to slow the heart rate and reduce blood pressure. May keep the pulse low during shock.

PATHOPHYSIOLOGY PEARLS

Earlier in your studies, you learned that blood is made up of plasma and formed elements. Let us take a closer look at these microscopic miracles that make up the formed elements.

Red blood cells (RBCs, or erythrocytes) look like small disks with concave sides. This concave appearance is due to the cells neither having a nucleus nor several other common cellular structures. RBCs contain hemoglobin that transports oxygen to the body tissues and picks up carbon dioxide, a requirement for maintaining adequate tissue perfusion. RBCs have a rough trip through the body and only last about 120 days and are then broken down in the liver.

White blood cells (WBCs, or leukocytes) come in five different types. While each type performs a different function, they are all involved in defending the body and functioning as part of the immune system. We will briefly look at each type.

- Neutrophils—primary function is to fight bacterial infection.
- Eosinophils—primary function is to fight allergens and parasites.
- Basophils—primary function is to release histamine (a vasodilator) and heparin (an anticoagulant).
- Monocytes—only remain in circulation for about 24 hours before moving into the peripheral tissues. Monocytes in the tissues are called macrophages. As the name implies, these cells function by engulfing and then destroying invaders or damaged cells.
- Lymphocytes have a very large nucleus and move from the bloodstream to the tissues, and then back to the bloodstream. The various lymphocytes that function to defend us against invaders (these are T-cells or T-lymphocytes), produce and distribute antibodies (these are B-cells or B-lymphocytes), and destroy abnormal tissue (these are NK-cells or Natural Killer cells).

Platelets (or thrombocytes) are not truly individual cells but are fragments of cells. These smallest of the formed elements play a vital role in hemostasis (the cessation of bleeding/clotting).

Together, these microscopic miracles provide vital perfusion to the body's tissues, protect against invaders, destroy damaged cells, and help control bleeding. Any disruption in these normal processes (such as hypoperfusion or shock) could have dire consequences.

REVIEW QUESTIONS

SHORT ANSWER

1. How can shock occur in patients with no internal or external blood loss?

2. What is the EMT-B's best clue to the possibility of internal bleeding?

MULTIPLE CHOICE

1. You should not use the PASG if the patient presents with cardiogenic shock or _____.
   - **A.** pelvic injuries
   - **B.** any abdominal injuries
   - **C.** abnormal lung sounds
   - **D.** distal bleeding

2. *Petechiae* are small round purplish spots caused by _____.
   - **A.** capillary bleeding
   - **B.** hypotension
   - **C.** bacteria
   - **D.** severe blunt trauma

3. Epistaxis can be caused by hypertension or a severe blow to the patient's
   _____.

   A. abdomen   **B.** nose

   C. pelvis   **D.** lower back

4. A sudden loss of _____ of blood is considered serious in an average
   adult.

   A. 1/2 liter   **B.** 250 cc

   C. 3/4 liter   **D.** 1,000 cc

5. Children can maintain a normal blood pressure until approximately
   _____ of their blood volume is gone.

   A. 25 percent   **B.** 75 percent

   C. 50 percent   **D.** 90 percent

SCENARIO QUESTIONS

Your unit is dispatched at 1436 hours to a cabinet shop for an employee who is not feeling well. Upon your arrival, you are led to the patient, a 33-year-old male, who is lying on the couch in the company break room. The patient has pale, cool, clammy skin and a rapid pulse. He tells you that just before going to lunch at noon, he had been using the table saw and it had kicked back a piece of wood into his abdomen. You lift his shirt and see a large purple bruise in his left upper quadrant.

1. The most appropriate emergency care for this patient is to _____.

   A. cover him with a blanket, place him in the Trendelenburg position, and transport as soon as possible

   B. administer oxygen with a nonrebreather mask at 15 lpm, place the patient flat on the gurney with his legs raised 8 to 12 inches, keep him warm, and transport immediately

   C. apply a nasal cannula with the oxygen set at 6 lpm, secure a bulky dressing to the patient's abdomen, raise his legs 8 to 12 inches, and transport immediately

   D. administer oxygen with a nonrebreather mask at 15 lpm, place the patient in the Trendelenburg position, and transport immediately

2. This patient may have sustained an injury to his _____.

   A. spleen   **B.** appendix

   C. aorta   **D.** gallbladder

3. When does this patient's *golden hour* begin?

   A. As soon as you arrive.

   B. 60 minutes after the injury.

   C. When the patient arrives at the hospital.

   D. At the moment of injury.

You and your partner are standing in line to pick up dinner when a call from another EMT-B comes across your portable radio. He is panicked and requesting immediate medical assistance at his location. You know that his unit was dispatched to a traffic crash only minutes from your location, so you tell dispatch that you will respond. Upon your arrival, you find that a car had swerved off the roadway and crashed into the back of the other ambulance. One of your fellow EMT-Bs had been crushed between the two vehicles. He is responsive but keeps trying to hit you while shouting incoherently. Both of his legs were severed just above the knees and you and your partner are able to move him to the ground. You try pushing dressings onto his injuries while your partner leans on the appropriate pressure points, but the bleeding does not stop. The injured EMT-B is becoming unresponsive.

1. It is imperative that you immediately _____.
   A. administer high-concentration oxygen
   B. apply a tourniquet to each leg
   C. assist your partner in pushing on the pressure points
   D. transport the patient

2. Once the blood loss is controlled, the two most important things that you, as an EMT-B, can do are _____.
   A. administer oxygen at 15 lpm with a nonrebreather mask and provide immediate transportation
   B. administer high-concentration oxygen and provide intravenous saline
   C. apply a nonrebreather mask and administer high-concentration oxygen
   D. place the patient in the Trendelenburg position and transport immediately

3. You would use the _____ pressure points in this situation.
   A. aortic   B. distal
   C. femoral   D. superior

4. This call would most likely result in _____.
   A. death to the patient
   B. your resignation from EMS
   C. an investigation into the injured EMT-B's actions
   D. a critical-incident-stress debriefing

You arrive for a severe-bleeding call at a supermarket butcher shop. The patient, a 46-year-old male, had been preparing meat when the knife slipped and sliced into his right forearm. The patient's coworker is holding a blood-soaked towel over the injury, and you observe blood on the floor, display cases, and one wall. "Man, it was shooting everywhere!" the coworker tells you. "But I put a tourniquet on and that stopped most of it." You find the patient responsive and complaining vigorously that he "made such a stupid mistake." Other than a slightly elevated pulse, the patient appears stable.

1. If, after examining the wound, you feel that the tourniquet is not necessary, you should _____.
   A. contact medical direction for advice
   B. remove the tourniquet while holding direct pressure on the wound
   C. document your finding and leave the tourniquet in place
   D. elevate the extremity, hold a sterile dressing on the wound, and cut the tourniquet

2. After applying a pressure dressing to the wound, you should frequently _____.
   A. tighten the bandage
   B. replace the blood-soaked dressings
   C. check for a distal pulse
   D. apply pressure to the brachial artery

3. You should transport this patient in _____.
   A. a position of comfort   B. the semi-Fowler's position
   C. the recovery position   D. the shock position

CASE STUDIES

CASE STUDY 1   DID ANYONE GET THE LICENSE NUMBER OF THAT HORSE?

You are dispatched to a local horse-training stable on the other side of town. The call came in for a "man kicked by a horse." Upon your arrival, you are directed to a bench beneath a tree where some people are gathered around a man lying on the bench. As you approach, you see an approximately 40-year-old male in moderate distress. He is guarding his abdomen and moaning in pain. He also appears pale. You are told by one of the bystanders that the patient was in the process of replacing shoes on one of the horses when the horse stepped forward and delivered a kick directly to his abdomen, sending him falling back on the ground. At first the man states he just had the wind knocked out of him, but shortly after he tried to get back to work, he complained of feeling really light-headed, and needed to lie down. That is when they called 911.

1. How would you go about evaluating the MOI in this case?

2. What other concern might you have before initiating treatment for this patient?

Witnesses describe him as having been thrown back several feet and landing on his buttocks in the dirt. They tell you that he never lost consciousness, and only had some difficulty breathing immediately following the kick but no other problems. You obtain a set of baseline vitals and record them as follows: BP 110/90, pulse 108 weak and regular, respirations 22 and somewhat labored. His skin is pale, warm, and sweaty. Your assessment of his abdomen reveals moderate tenderness in the epigastric region with some guarding and rigidity.

1. Is oxygen therapy indicated for this patient and, if so, how much and by which device?

2. How often will you want to take vitals on this patient and, if he is indeed going into shock, how are his vitals likely to change during transport?

CASE STUDY 2   HURRY. PLEASE HURRY. HE CUT HIMSELF BADLY!

You are called to a sidewalk in a residential neighborhood for a male patient with a reported laceration. You recognize the area but are concerned that the laceration may be a result of violence. After checking with the dispatcher, you find that the injury was caused by a hedge trimmer.

    You arrive at the scene to find a man sitting on his lawn with a bloody towel applied to his left forearm. The towel is soaked red as is much of the white painter's pants he is wearing.

1. What do your observations tell you?

2. What are the parts of the size-up and what do they tell you?

The hedge trimmer has a safety that shut the device off automatically after the man dropped it. Your partner unplugs it anyway for additional safety. The man is in a considerable amount of pain as he tells you of the "huge" laceration to his left forearm. He has an open airway and is breathing a bit rapidly but adequately. He has a thick bath towel over the wound, which is soaked through with blood. You note some excess blood dripping onto the ground. It is a relatively cool day, but the patient looks pale and sweaty.

1. How would you complete the initial assessment?

2. Should you remove the towel to assess the wound and bleeding?

3. What priority would you give this patient?

The wound is deep and continues to bleed. It will require bleeding control because it is too big to stop easily on its own. The blood is dark red and flowing steadily. You are concerned about blood loss and shock.

1. How would you control the bleeding from the patient's arm?

2. What signs and symptoms would you see that indicate developing shock?

Active Exploration

As you have already learned from reading the chapter in your Emergency Care textbook, trauma is the leading cause of death in the United States of persons between the ages of 1 and 44. As an EMT-B, you are likely to respond to many calls involving trauma. These calls require quick action on the part of the EMT-B in terms of assessment and emergency care and often require rapid transport to an appropriate receiving hospital capable of managing severe trauma.

The following activities will help you develop your trauma-assessment skills.

Activity 1: The Spill Drill

This first activity will help you become better at estimating external blood loss. Like any other skill that you as an EMT-B will learn, it will take practice for you to acquire this skill and stay good at it. You will need a fellow student, a measuring cup, and some red food coloring. Since most fluids in the medical field are measured in milliliters, it will be important to find a measuring cup that has milliliters indicated on the side. Most measuring cups these days have both metric and standard increments on them. Just in case you do not find a metric measuring cup, the following conversions will be of some help:

- One cup equals 250 mL
- Two cups equals 500 mL
- Three cups equals 750 mL
- Four cups equals 1 liter

1. Without letting your partner know the amount, add water to the measuring cup. Put in a few drops of red food coloring to simulate the color of blood.
2. Find a suitable hard floor surface that you can pour the water onto without causing a hazard or staining the surface.
3. Now have your partner examine the spill and guess the amount of liquid spilled onto the floor.

Take turns back and forth, using different quantities of water and guessing the amount. You can complicate things somewhat by pouring the water over the clothing of a person. The fact that clothing absorbs much of the fluid makes it much more difficult to estimate how much was spilled.

Activity 2: You Can Run, But You Cannot Hide

This next activity will help you become better at taking repeated sets of vital signs. This is an especially important skill when you are dealing with victims of trauma. You will need a blood pressure cuff, stethoscope, and a fellow student acting as patient for this activity.

1. To begin, take a complete set of baseline vitals on your partner and record them on a piece of paper.
2. Now have your partner run a predetermined course. It can be several hundred yards or up and down several flights of stairs. The goal is to get the pulse well above the resting rate.
3. Once he returns from the activity, immediately have him lie down and retake his blood pressure, pulse, and respirations. Record them next to the baseline set for comparison.
4. Wait 5 minutes and repeat another set of blood pressure, pulse, and respirations. Record these as well.
5. Repeat the vital signs at least three times or until they return to normal.

This activity will allow you to get practice taking vitals on someone other than a resting simulated "patient." It will also give you practice taking vitals more quickly and comparing each set with the previous sets just as you would with any unstable patient.

RETRO REVIEW

1. Stimulation of the _____ while suctioning the airway can slow a patient's heart rate.

   A. carotid nerve   B. oropharynx
   C. vagus nerve   D. uvula

2. Using _____ means using the force necessary to keep the patient from injuring himself or others.

   A. restraining devices   B. escalating force
   C. defensive tactics   D. reasonable force

3. The common causes of _____ can be grouped into four basic categories: hypovolemic, metabolic, environmental/toxicological, and cardiovascular.

    A. syncope   **B.** apnea

    C. hyperperfusion   **D.** strokes

THINKING AND LINKING

CHAPTER TOPIC	HOW IT RELATES TO YOU AND OTHER COURSE AREAS
Bleeding	Patients with venous bleeding from neck trauma will need immediate emergency care in order to prevent the chance of an air embolus (Chapter 27). It is especially important to take BSI precautions (Chapter 2) when treating an open neck wound because you will initially have to cover the wound(s) with your hand. Also, if you are treating a patient with an open neck wound, you will need to have occlusive dressings readily available (when you reach Chapter 33, you will cover properly stocking the ambulance).
Direct pressure	If your patient is bleeding from a severe head injury (Chapter 29), make sure that you do not use too much pressure to stop the bleeding. Doing so could injure the brain—sometimes driving debris or skull fragments into the brain tissue. You should also assume that a mechanism strong enough to cause severe head injuries could also have injured the patient's neck and spine (Chapter 29 also).
Shock	If your patient's skin becomes pale and clammy and he begins to act restless or frightened, suspect shock. You will then need to administer oxygen (Chapter 6), monitor his mental status (Chapter 8), and elevate his feet—if no spinal injury is suspected (Chapters 5 and 29).

27

Soft-Tissue Injuries

CHAPTER SUMMARY

As an EMT-B, you will often be required to treat patients with soft-tissue injuries. Your professionalism and knowledge will be very important to these patients because open, soft-tissue injuries tend to cause the most stress and can be very frightening to the patient and bystanders. This chapter shows you how to treat for soft-tissue injuries, and, with practice, your proficiency and professionalism will greatly assist in comforting the patient and keeping the trauma scene calm.

Soft-tissue injuries can occur to the skin, fatty (adipose) tissues, muscles, blood vessels, fibrous tissues, membranes, glands, and nerves. Skin, which suffers the most visible soft-tissue injuries, serves several important functions: protection, water balance, temperature regulation, excretion, and impact absorption. Skin consists of three main layers: epidermis, dermis, and subcutaneous.

Soft-tissue injuries are either open (break in the skin) or closed (no break in the skin). Closed, soft-tissue injuries are commonly called *internal injuries*, but they can be more specifically categorized as contusions, hematomas, and closed crush injuries. Many internal injuries can cause profuse bleeding and, as a result, the onset of shock. When treating possible internal injuries, ensure a patent airway and appropriate breathing and administer high-concentration oxygen.

Open wounds, which are classified by appearance or cause, are categorized as abrasions, lacerations, punctures, avulsions, amputations, and open crush injuries. The airway and breathing of the patient with an open injury need to be monitored, as does any bleeding. Control bleeding with direct pressure, elevation, and, if necessary, using arterial pressure points. Watch out for and, proactively, treat for shock.

There are as many facets to the treatment of open wounds as there are categories. Abrasions and lacerations can usually be helped with dressings and direct pressure. Puncture wounds can appear benign but can mask severe internal damage—so treatment will include anticipation of shock, and immediate transport. Reassure patients with puncture wounds, as these can be very frightening. Impaled objects are puncture wounds with the violating object still embedded. *Never remove an impaled object, as this may increase internal bleeding.* Treat an impaled object by controlling any profuse bleeding and packing it with bulky dressings to hold it steady. Finish by securing everything with bandages or cravats.

An object impaled in the cheek presents a unique problem. The rule is to *never remove an impaled object*, and yet an object impaled in the cheek may cause an airway compromise. For this reason, you may remove it on two conditions. One, both ends of the object are free and visible (meaning that it cannot have punctured the cheek and embedded in the jaw) and, two, it can be removed relatively easily.

For an object impaled in a patient's eye, stabilize the object with dressings and bandages and cover both eyes to reduce sympathetic eye movements.

Treat avulsions by cleaning the wound and folding the skin back into its normal position. Then control any bleeding and apply bulky pressure dressings.

Open neck wounds create an altogether different dilemma, not only because there can be profuse bleeding but also because if air is sucked into an open vein, it will create an air embolus that may kill the patient. It is for this reason that open neck wounds are treated immediately with a gloved palm until an occlusive dressing can be prepared and applied.

Chest injuries can be open or closed and take three different forms: blunt trauma, penetrating objects, and compression. Open chest wounds are treated with occlusive dressings, high concentrations of oxygen, and rapid transport. Some of the more common complications of severe chest injuries include pneumothorax, hemothorax, and cardiac tamponade, all of which are not truly treatable at the EMT-B level. If you are treating a patient with one of these serious chest-injury complications, maintain the airway, monitor the breathing, administer high-concentration oxygen, and transport as soon as possible.

Abdominal injuries often present with pain (starting as mild and quickly becoming worse), cramps, nausea, weakness, and thirst. They may also have obvious signs such as lacerations or punctures to the abdomen, pelvis, or lower back. Maintain the patient's airway, be alert for vomiting (possibly even of blood), allow the patient to lie on his back, and flex his legs at the knees to reduce tension on the abdominal muscles. Administer high-concentration oxygen, do not give anything by mouth, treat for shock, and transport as soon as possible.

Burns are classified by agent/source, depth, and severity. The three depths of burn classification are superficial, partial-thickness, and full-thickness burns. Superficial burns are characterized by generalized redness and pain, and partial-thickness burns by intense pain, blisters, and a mottled appearance, while full-thickness burns may appear charred black or brown or even dry and white. The following factors are considered while determining burn severity: source, body regions involved, depth, body surface area (BSA), age of the patient, and whether any other injuries or illnesses are involved. The body surface area involved is determined by the *rule of nines*—a simple formula for determining what percentage of a body is burned—in which adult, child, and infant bodies are divided into percentage-sections that either equal nine or are derivatives of nine.

The agent or source of a burn is considered thermal, chemical, electric, light (usually involving the eyes), or radiation. The standard EMT-B treatment for most burns is to ensure that the burning process has stopped and cover with dry, sterile dressings. Chemicals, however, will need to be brushed off or flushed away prior to dressing. Chemicals in the eyes require extensive flushing as well—at least 20 minutes of constant water or saline flow and immediate transportation.

Always treat burn patients for shock and transport as soon as possible.

Electrical injuries are unique in that electricity will burn where it enters, where it exits, and along the internal path that it follows. The patient who has had an electric shock may experience respiratory difficulty or arrest and irregular heartbeat or even cardiac arrest. *Make sure that all electrical hazards are removed prior to entering the scene.* When treating a patient who has had an electric shock, maintain a patent airway because the shock may cause swelling along the respiratory structures. Provide basic cardiac life support if necessary. Otherwise treat for hypoperfusion (shock); administer high-concentration oxygen; treat for any spinal or musculoskeletal injuries; apply dry, sterile dressings to the burn sites (of which there will always be at least two); and transport as soon as possible.

Dressings cover wounds and bandages hold the dressings in place. Always wear disposable gloves and other barrier devices to prevent contact with any body fluids while dressing open wounds. In order to properly dress an open wound, you must first take BSI precautions and expose the wound by cutting away clothing, and so on. Then, using sterile dressings, cover the entire wound and the surrounding area. Control any bleeding and then utilize bandages to hold the dressings in place.

Never apply bandages too tightly or in a manner that may restrict circulation.

MED MINUTE

When injuries bleed, there are many variables that determine how bad the bleeding will be. These include the depth and location of the wound as well as whether a vein or artery was damaged. One additional factor is whether the patient is taking "blood-thinning" medications. Patients taking these medications (listed in the table below) will bleed more seriously, even from minor wounds. It will be more difficult for the wound to naturally clot. This table gives examples of common drugs in each category. Many other medications may be available with similar effects.

CLASS OF MEDICATION	MEDICATION NAME(S)	MECHANISM OF ACTION
Anticoagulant	Warfarin sodium (Coumadin)	Blocks clotting factors in the blood. Used to treat thrombosis in the legs and as a prevention of thrombosis (clots). Also used for the prevention of TIA (transient ischemic attack) and stroke. Also used as a rodenticide (in rat poison).

Antiplatelet	Acetylsalicylic acid (aspirin)	In addition to its pain- and fever-reducing properties, aspirin inhibits platelet aggregation (clumping or formation). This may prevent formation of clots that could break free and travel to other parts of the body.
		Excess aspirin can lead to severe GI bleeding and impairment of clotting.

PATHOPHYSIOLOGY PEARLS

According to the American Cancer Society, skin cancer is the most common type of all cancers, accounting for nearly half of all the cancers seen in the United States. Over 1,000,000 cases of nonmelanoma (basal or squamous) and over 54,000 cases of melanoma occur annually in the United States. The American Cancer Society estimates there will be 9,600 deaths from skin cancer in 2002 (7,400 from melanoma and 2,200 from basal or squamous).[1]

Basal-cell carcinoma usually develops in sun-exposed body areas such as the face, neck, and hands. It starts in the lower layers of the epidermis. The lesion first appears as a small, shiny bump. As this bump enlarges, it develops a central depression with a beaded edge.

Squamous-cell carcinoma also develops in sun-exposed body areas and starts in the lower layers of the epidermis. This lesion first appears as a raised, reddened, scaly area. As the lesion develops, it forms a concave ulcer with raised edges. This form of carcinoma may metastasize into the lymph nodes, resulting in the spread of carcinoma and possibly in death.

Melanoma carcinoma develops in the melanocytes of the skin. Melanocytes are the cells that contain melanin, the pigment that gives color to the skin. Melanoma is the least common but most dangerous form of skin cancer. Even though it is almost always curable in early stages, it causes the majority of skin cancer deaths.

Persons with any of the following signs and symptoms should consult their physicians for further follow-up:

- Any change on the skin, especially in the size or color of a mole or other darkly pigmented growth or spot, or a new growth.
- Scaliness, oozing, bleeding, or change in the appearance of a bump or nodule.
- The spread of pigmentation beyond its border such as dark coloring that spreads past the edge of a mole or mark.
- A change in sensation, itchiness, tenderness, or pain.

Continual advances in healthcare offer many choices to patients with cancer. The key is to identify the cancer and begin treatment early.

1 *American Cancer Society.* Skin Cancer Facts. *American Cancer Society (April 2002). www.cancer.org/docroot/*

REVIEW QUESTIONS

SHORT ANSWER

1. Besides controlling blood loss, what is the reason for aggressively treating an open neck wound?

2. What is an evisceration?

MULTIPLE CHOICE

1. As a general rule, a dressing should only be bandaged into place over an open wound if _____.
   - **A.** there is the potential for further trauma
   - **B.** the patient needs to be transported
   - **C.** bleeding has been controlled
   - **D.** it has been cleared of all debris

2. Burns are evaluated and classified by source, depth, and _____.
   - **A.** accompanying injuries
   - **B.** character
   - **C.** intensity
   - **D.** severity

3. The major functions of the skin are _____.
   - **A.** protection, water balance, temperature regulation, excretion, and impact absorption
   - **B.** shock absorption, temperature regulation, perspiration, and organ containment
   - **C.** hormone production, general protection, and fever reduction
   - **D.** fluid regulation, temperature control, impact absorption, blood filtration, and mast cell production

4. The major problem caused by electrical shock is not normally _____.
   - **A.** the result of electricity
   - **B.** cardiac in nature
   - **C.** the burn
   - **D.** in the respiratory system

5. Which of the following is *not* an agent or source of burns?
   - **A.** Infrared light
   - **B.** DC current
   - **C.** Chemical bases
   - **D.** Ultraviolet light

SCENARIO QUESTIONS

You are dispatched to a local rodeo arena for a 32-year-old man who was crushed beneath a falling bull. You arrive and find the man unresponsive with a deep purple coloration to his shoulders, neck, and head. He has a very weak pulse, low blood pressure, and good bilateral breath sounds. Once you get him loaded into the ambulance and reassess his vital signs, you find a decreasing pulse pressure.

1. Treatment of this patient would include maintaining an open airway, administering high-concentration oxygen, _____, transporting as soon as possible, and considering an ALS intercept.
   A. creating a flutter valve
   B. treating for shock
   C. providing positive pressure ventilations
   D. relieving chest pressure

2. This patient is most likely suffering from _____.
   A. cardiac tamponade
   B. tension pneumothorax
   C. traumatic asphyxia
   D. both cardiac tamponade and traumatic asphyxia

3. Pulse pressure is _____.
   A. the diastolic reading divided by the pulse rate
   B. another term for blood pressure
   C. the difference between systolic and diastolic readings
   D. the strength of a patient's pulse when palpated

You are treating a woman who had been trapped in a car fire following a collision. The anterior surface of her legs, groin, and lower anterior torso are severely burned and you notice accessory muscle use during respirations as well as singed nares. She is alert and crying but denies any pain from the burns.

1. According to the *rule of nines*, this woman has been burned on approximately _____ percent of her body surface.
   A. 32   B. 28
   C. 48   D. 53

2. In addition to possible respiratory burns and shock, what should you be concerned with when treating this patient?
   A. Hypoperfusion   B. Aortic trauma
   C. Dehydration   D. Spinal injury

3. This woman has most likely suffered _____ burns.
   A. partial-thickness   B. superficial
   C. full-thickness   D. second-degree

You have arrived to provide emergency care for a police officer who was shot during a convenience-store robbery attempt. The scene is secure and the patient, a 48-year-old male, is alert but gasping for air and coughing up blood. You expose his upper body and see an entrance wound just superior to the right nipple and no apparent exit wound. The patient has diminished breath sounds on the right side, a weak pulse, and low blood pressure.

1. What should you do first following the discovery of this patient's chest wound?
   A. Apply an absorbent dressing.
   B. Place your gloved hand over the puncture site.
   C. Conduct a rapid trauma assessment to find any other injuries.
   D. Administer high-concentration oxygen via a nonrebreather mask.

2. This patient is in an extremely critical condition and is displaying the signs of _____.

    A. hemopneumothorax   **B.** cardiac asphyxia

    C. tension pneumothorax   **D.** hemopulmonary perforation

3. This patient's injury is considered to be a(n) _____ puncture wound.

    A. perforating   **B.** occlusive

    C. complicating   **D.** penetrating

C A S E S T U D I E S

CASE STUDY 1	**STABBED IN THE BACK**

You are dispatched to the local fairgrounds for a victim of an assault. You are directed by the on-site security to the far side of the carnival where one police officer is questioning a young man who is seated on the ground and another officer is placing a male adult in handcuffs. The first officer explains that the two men were in a fight and it appears that the man being questioned was stabbed in the back.

    Upon being questioned, the young man states that he was attacked from behind and felt a sharp stabbing pain below his right shoulder blade. He is complaining of pain in his right chest and shortness of breath.

1. **How will you begin your assessment on this patient?**

2. **What additional information will you want before leaving the scene?**

As you are obtaining a baseline set of vital signs, your patient begins complaining of more trouble breathing. He states that he feels tightness in his chest and is having difficulty catching his breath. Upon examining him, you discover a small puncture wound just below his right scapula with just a small amount of blood. You put him on 15 lpm of oxygen by nonrebreather mask and continue with obtaining a baseline set of vitals. Once he is loaded into the ambulance, his breathing continues to become more and more labored, and you can hear a slight hissing sound coming from the small wound on his back each time he takes a breath.

1. **What is likely to be causing his breathing difficulty and how will you treat it?**

2. **What piece of the detailed physical will most likely reveal the most about this patient's condition and what will it reveal?**

You are dispatched to the scene of a structure fire. Upon your arrival, you see a fully involved garage fire that has spread to the attached dwelling. Upon reporting to the scene commander, you are assigned to check out a resident of the house who has sustained burns on his arm. Additional firefighters and apparatus arrive at the scene in an attempt to save the residence.

1. What logistical issues for treatment and transport of this patient will you face at the scene?

2. Will additional EMS units be necessary on the scene?

The patient is sitting on the curb with a blank look on his face. His wife is sitting next to him sobbing. A sooty, but otherwise fine, dog is near them. The burns were sustained by the man as he entered the structure to rescue the dog. You note that his entire lower left arm and hand seem seriously burned and that his clothes seem to be burned to the skin.

1. What have you learned from these observations to form a general impression?

2. How would you complete the initial assessment?

The patient is conscious, alert and oriented. Oxygen is applied by nonrebreather mask. You begin to examine the arm as your partner gets vital signs on the unburned arm. You observe blotchy black-and-white skin, with the man's sweatshirt sticking to his skin in many places. He also has a wedding ring on the ring finger of his burned hand. The burns cover the total lower left arm.

1. What body surface area (BSA) is covered by these burns? What type of burns are these?

2. Would you try to pick the cloth out of the burned tissue? Would you remove the wedding ring?

3. Should the dressings applied to this patient be wet or dry?

Active Exploration

Injuries to soft tissues can be challenging for the new EMT-B for several reasons. First and foremost, just seeing the human body deformed by traumatic injury takes some getting used to. There is no doubt that the question on the minds of most EMT-B students as they begin their EMS career is whether they will be able to "handle" seeing someone with major injuries. As you will quickly discover, there is much more to worry about in most emergencies than the soft-tissue injury, and you will be too busy managing an airway to get too distracted by a badly injured leg.

Being able to quickly recognize the difference between life-threatening and non-life-threatening injuries is important for any EMT-B. Then, you must be able to quickly and efficiently control the bleeding from an open wound with the most appropriate equipment available. The following activities will help you sharpen your bandaging skills so that you will be ready when in the heat of an emergency.

Activity 1: All Bleeding Stops, Eventually

This activity will expose you to two of the most common tools used for the dressing and bandaging of open wounds, the roller gauze and the triangular bandage.

1. Using a fellow student as a patient, have him place a piece of tape anywhere on an arm or leg to simulate an open wound with arterial bleeding.
2. Now, using an appropriate-size dressing and roller gauze, create a pressure bandage as if you were trying to control a difficult arterial bleed.
3. Leaving that dressing in place, duplicate the same dressing on the opposite extremity, only this time you may only use two triangular bandages.
4. Compare the two dressings: Which was easier to apply? Which seems to be doing a better job if it was a difficult arterial bleed? Is one able to provide more pressure than the other? Which one does the "patient" think is better?
5. Switch roles and repeat the process. Pay close attention to your exact technique, how you hold the bandage, and how you wrap it. Try new techniques in an effort to improve on speed and efficiency.

Many new EMT-Bs are too conservative when placing pressure bandages and attempting to control severe bleeding. It is common for an EMT-B to place a bandage that is too loose and is thus less effective. Take note of how tight the bandage is and consider which material might be best for different types of injuries and in different locations.

Activity 2: Guess the BSA

This is an easy yet practical way to quickly learn the skill of estimating body surface area (BSA). Estimating BSA is most commonly done for burn patients, as some facilities can only manage small burns and patients may need to be triaged to a burn center for immediate care.

1. Working in groups of three or four students, have one student shade in specific areas on the "Burn Worksheet" that is provided on page 358.
2. Have the same student then verbally describe to the others the body areas that were shaded in.
3. Keeping their answers confidential, the other students must then estimate the BSA affected according to the verbal description given.
4. Everyone then compares answers to see of they all agree. If they do not, then find out why.

It is a good idea for the student describing the affected BSA to also write a specific percentage for easy comparison with the others. Then, the activity continues until each student in the group has had a chance to be the host.

This exercise also reinforces the use of anatomical vocabulary.

1. In keeping with good body mechanics, you should avoid reaching more than _____ inches in front of your body.
   A. 6 to 8   **B.** 12 to 24
   C. 10 to 14   **D.** 15 to 20

2. Ongoing assessments should be performed on _____ patients.
   A. all   **B.** critical
   C. responsive   **D.** unstable

3. You are dispatched to a residence for a disturbed 18-year-old female who has cut the side of her throat with a kitchen knife. Upon your arrival, you find that the police have safely disposed of the knife and that the patient has a steady flow of dark blood coming from the wound. After discussing the injury with you, the patient refuses to let you touch her but does agree to ride to the hospital in your ambulance. You should _____.
   A. transport her to the hospital for treatment
   B. sit and calmly explain again why the patient should accept your help
   C. ask law enforcement personnel to force the patient to accept treatment
   D. have the patient sign a refusal-of-treatment release form

THINKING AND LINKING

CHAPTER TOPIC	HOW IT RELATES TO YOU AND OTHER COURSE AREAS
Open wounds	The gruesomeness of some open wounds can increase the anxiety felt by your patients and bystanders. Your professional demeanor (Chapter 1) and quick emergency care will help offset this stress and calm the situation. You will also need to take appropriate BSI precautions (Chapter 2) in order to protect yourself and your patient.
	Occasionally, bystanders at a trauma scene will become ill or possibly faint. You will need to ensure that these "new" patients have patent airways (Chapter 6) and anticipate potential head and/or spine injuries (covered in Chapter 29).
Gunshot wounds	You should always wait for law enforcement to check the scene of a shooting prior to entering and providing emergency care (Chapter 2). Violent confrontations are too unpredictable for you to assume that the patient or bystanders can be trusted.
	The impact of a bullet can cause indirect spinal injuries, so it is a good idea to bring the spinal-immobilization equipment with you (again, in Chapter 29).
Electrical burns	When responding to an electricity-related trauma call, remember to always make sure that the scene is safe to enter (Chapter 7). Downed power lines and arcing wires can easily be missed in the quest to provide emergency care.
	Also, always bring your AED and airway kit to the patient's location—electricity can cause both respiratory (Chapter 16) and cardiac (Chapter 17) arrest.

28

Musculoskeletal Injuries

CHAPTER SUMMARY

One of the most common aspects of your job as an EMT-B will be responding to muscle and skeletal injuries. These injuries, which can range from minor to life threatening, can sometimes be so grotesque in appearance that you may be tempted to focus on them and neglect other threats to the patient's life.

The musculoskeletal system is composed of the muscles, bones, tendons, ligaments, cartilage, and joints found throughout the body. Bones provide structure and protection for the body and are formed of dense connective tissue. Bones also store minerals (such as calcium) and some of the larger bones provide the marrow for red-blood-cell production. Bone ends meet at articulation points called *joints*. Bones are classified by appearance, long, short, flat, or irregular, and are covered by a strong, white fibrous material called the *periosteum*—which becomes visible when trauma exposes a bone.

The most common bone injury is a break, or *fracture*—which causes blood loss that leads to swelling in the adjoining tissues and the formation of a blood clot. The still-healthy cells near the fracture site will begin to divide within hours of the break, beginning to repair the bone, tissue, and blood vessels damaged during the injury. The type of fracture, type of bone, and the health and age of the patient will determine whether this repair process takes days or months to complete. It is very important that bones be properly immobilized as quickly as possible after the break so that there is less chance for further tissue damage and improper bone repair.

Muscles (the three types of which are skeletal, smooth, and cardiac) are the fibrous tissues that cause movement of the body parts or organs. They are separated into two categories; voluntary and involuntary. Simply put, voluntary (or skeletal) muscles can be moved by the conscious will of the individual, whereas involuntary (such as smooth or cardiac) muscles complete their functions without conscious direction.

Cartilage, which is smooth and less rigid than bone, can be found on the ends of bones (aiding articulation) and in the more flexible areas of the body (nose, outer ears, and so on). Tendons are bands that connect the muscles to their bone anchors, and ligaments support the joints by holding the bone ends together, providing the joint with a stable range of motion.

There are three types of mechanisms that cause injuries to the musculoskeletal system: direct force (being struck by an object, causing crush and fracture injuries), indirect force (caused by the momentum of an injury to an adjoining body part), and twisting, or rotational force (caused when part of the body rotates and the adjoining part remains firm). Sports injuries and automobile collisions account for many of the musculoskeletal injuries you will see.

As an EMT-B, it is not your job—and should not be your intention—to diagnose a muscle or bone injury. In fact, if there is no deformity present, you will have no way of determining whether the patient's pain and swelling is caused by a sprain (stretching and tearing of ligaments), strain (overstretching of a muscle), dislocation (disruption of a joint), fracture, or just a bruise. You should treat each painful and swollen extremity as a fracture. Although fractures are rarely life threatening, bones are living tissue and will bleed after breaking. Some seemingly simple fractures can cause substantial internal blood loss. For example, consider a simple fracture of the femur—the powerful muscles around the femur tend to contract and spasm after a break. This commonly pulls the two bone ends, causing them to override each other, resulting in tissue damage. Traction splints, designed specifically for this injury, pull the bone ends apart and allow them to realign in a more natural way. This will reduce bleeding, swelling, and pain for the patient.

A closed extremity injury means that the skin has not been broken. An open extremity injury means that either the bone has torn through from the inside or some other object penetrated the skin from the outside. Open fractures are more serious because of the increased risk of infection and because they often must undergo surgery.

Your examination of an injured extremity will require your skills of observation, touch, and hearing. You will look for any deformity or discoloration, feel for anything out of the ordinary, and listen for crepitus—the sound of bone ends rubbing together. Always expose injured areas by removing or cutting away clothing but remain sensitive to the patient's modesty and the environmental conditions that may lead to heat-loss complications. It is *very important* that you not become distracted by a particularly gruesome deformity and neglect to assess for life-threats such as airway or breathing problems. Your physical exams will also be very important because the patient may become so focused on a painful deformity that he cannot pinpoint any other injuries.

The signs and symptoms of musculoskeletal injuries include pain or tenderness, deformity or angulation, crepitus, swelling, bruising, locked joints, nerve or circulatory compromise, and exposed bone ends. After all life-threats have been assessed and cared for (and the patient is relatively stable), any painful, swollen, and deformed extremities must be splinted. Effective splinting will immobilize the adjoining joints and bone ends and prevent further damage to muscles, nerves, and blood vessels. It will also keep a closed fracture from becoming a painful open fracture during transport.

Before splinting, you should attempt to realign, or straighten, any deformed or angulated extremity. This is to ensure circulation to the distal extremity as well as allowing the extremity to fit into a splint. Are you frightened by the thought of straightening a patient's horribly angulated limb? That feeling is not uncommon, but the positives outweigh your potential squeamishness. Realigning a deformed extremity will protect nerves, tissues, and circulation, and after a brief moment of increased pain, will actually decrease the patient's discomfort.

To realign a deformed extremity, your partner should hold the distal end of the extremity while you support the areas above and below the injury site. Your partner will then gently apply manual traction toward the long axis of the extremity, and if no resistance is felt, hold it until you complete the splinting. Usually, joint injuries should be splinted as found unless there is distal cyanosis or lack of pulse, in which case you should gently attempt to realign the extremity—unless resistance is encountered.

Although most EMS units carry rigid, formable, and traction splints, it is not uncommon for the EMT-B to improvise splints for certain situations. You can use pillows, blankets, magazines, lumber, umbrellas, rolled newspaper—nearly anything. Regardless of the splint composition, the steps for splinting are the same. Expose the injury site; assess distal pulse, motor function, and sensation (PMS); align area to be splinted; immobilize the adjacent joints and bone ends; pad the voids; and reassess PMS after the splint is in place. Do not forget to resolve any life-threats prior to splinting, make sure that the splint is neither too loose nor too tight, and apply splints prior to moving the patient—if possible.

Traction splints, used only for femur fractures, come in two varieties: bipolar model (which cradles the leg between two rods) and unipolar model (which supports the leg with a single bar alongside the leg). You should exert traction just enough to realign the leg, and do not use the patient's pain level as a reliable gauge for sufficient tension—the painful muscle spasms associated with a femur fracture will not subside for several minutes after the bone ends are properly realigned. Do not use a traction splint if there is an ankle, knee, or pelvic injury or an avulsion or partial amputation that could be separated by the traction. If there is a chance that the patient will be lifted or moved following placement of the traction splint, do not use the bipolar model—it will lose traction if the pelvis is raised.

So, you are familiar with musculoskeletal anatomy, the assessment of injuries, the general rationale for splinting, and even the concept behind the traction splint. What do you do for *specific* injuries? What if your patient has a shoulder injury or a badly twisted ankle? The following sections cover specific emergency care for specific injuries.

Your patient most likely has a shoulder-girdle injury if he has shoulder pain, has a "dropped" shoulder and is holding his arm against the side of his chest (a possible fracture of the clavicle), or has suffered a severe blow to the back above the scapula. You should check for deformity anywhere around the shoulder girdle. If the head of the humerus can be palpated, or moves in front of the shoulder, this is a sign of an anterior dislocation—which may be caused by a fracture. The first step is to assess distal PMS. If there is PMS abnormality, immobilize the shoulder with a sling and swathe and transport as soon as possible. Do not attempt to reduce any dislocations found and always reassess distal PMS after placement of the sling and swathe. If the dislocation reduces itself ("pops back in"), the patient *must* be seen by a doctor.

Falls, motor-vehicle collisions, and crushing injuries of the lower body can cause pelvic injuries. Suspect an injury to your patient's pelvis if he presents with pelvic, hip, groin, or lower back pain (usually accompanied by obvious deformity); pain when pressure is applied to the pelvic wings or pubic bones; an inability to raise legs while supine (do not test this complaint!); the foot on the injured side turning outward, or unexplained bladder pressure. Do not forget that injuries to the pelvis may also cause serious damage to internal organs, blood vessels, and nerves—the blood loss may be great enough to cause shock. Also, suspect that a back injury may accompany any severe pelvic injury. It may be difficult to differentiate between a fractured pelvis and a fracture of the proximal femur—so when you are unsure, treat as if for a pelvic injury. You should move the patient as little as possible, determine distal PMS, return the patient's lower limbs to the anatomical position and stabilize them, apply a PASG if the patient is hypotensive, assume spinal injury and secure the patient to a spine board, and reassess for distal PMS. Then, transport the patient as soon as possible and monitor vital signs.

Since many EMS systems no longer carry the pneumatic antishock garments, a new alternative for the treatment of a suspected pelvic fracture is the *pelvic wrap*. Some systems suggest that the wrap be used for patients with pelvic deformity or instability, whereas others urge its use if just a mechanism of possible pelvic injury is present.

When the head of the femur is pushed or pulled from its pelvic socket, a hip dislocation occurs—which is difficult to differentiate from a hip fracture as patients will feel "intense pain" with both injuries. A patient with an anterior hip dislocation will usually present with a lower limb that is rotated outward and a flexed hip. The most common hip dislocation, however, is the posterior dislocation, in which the patient's leg will rotate inward and he will usually have a bent knee and a flexed hip. The patient will usually be unable to flex the foot or lift the toes, and there is often a lack of sensation in the limb—an indication that the sciatic nerve has been damaged.

Emergency care for a patient with a dislocated hip includes assessing distal PMS (and contacting medical direction if a deficit is found), securing the patient to a long spine board, immobilizing the leg with pillows or blankets, treating for shock, and transporting. If the dislocation reduces itself during transport, notify the receiving-facility staff. Avoid focusing on only one possible injury—occasionally, hip dislocations are accompanied by femur fractures.

A patient with a hip fracture, which is actually a fracture of the proximal femur head or neck area, can present with localized pain, swelling, discoloration (a potentially late sign), an inability to support weight, and a shortened appearance of the injured limb. Hip fractures are very common among elderly patients due to brittle or weakened bones.

Emergency care of the hip fracture begins with the assessment of distal PMS. You then have three choices for treating the hip: (1) Bind the patient's legs together, support them with pillows or blankets, and place the patient on a long spine board. (2) Secure long, padded splints to the patient—from the armpit down beyond the foot on the outside and from the crotch down beyond the foot on the inside. (3) Apply a PASG if protocols permit it.

If the patient complains of pain and tenderness of the knee and you can see swelling or obvious deformity, a knee injury has occurred. This injury can be a fracture of the distal femur, a dislocation of the knee joint (which, if the distal pulse is absent, should be immediately reported to medical direction), a dislocation or fracture of the patella, or fracture of the proximal tibia and/or fibula. Regardless of the injury's cause, treatment is only based on whether the knee is found bent or straight. If the knee is bent, assess distal PMS, secure padded board splints from the hip to the ankle—perhaps using a pillow to support the knee—and reassess PMS. If the knee is straight, assess distal PMS, immobilize medially and laterally with two padded board splints, pad any voids at the knee and ankle, and reassess PMS. It may be necessary, on the order of medical direction, to gently move the lower leg anteriorly to restore a pulse in a knee dislocation.

An injury to the tibia or fibula will present with pain, swelling, and, occasionally, deformity. You should treat the patient for shock (including the administration of high-concentration oxygen) and immobilize the lower leg—following PMS assessment—with an air splint, two splint boards, or a single splint with an ankle hitch.

It is difficult to differentiate between sprains and fractures with ankle or foot injuries—both present with pain and swelling—so always treat them as if for a fracture. Remember to asses for distal PMS, immobilize appropriately, reassess PMS, treat the patient for shock, and apply an ice pack to reduce pain and swelling.

To provide the most helpful information to the receiving facility (not to mention protecting yourself and your agency) always check and document distal pulses before and after splinting an injury.

MED MINUTE

There are a wide variety of medications, from those that treat the pain and inflammation caused by sudden injury (such as a sprain) to those caused by chronic conditions such as arthritis. These medications are listed in the following table. This table gives examples of common drugs in each category. Many other medications may be available with similar effects.

CLASS OF MEDICATION	MEDICATION NAME(S)	MECHANISM OF ACTION
Nonsteroidal anti-inflammatory drugs Over the counter (OTC)	Ibuprofin (Motrin, Advil)	Anti-inflammatory medication, reduces fever (antipyretic) and pain (analgesic).
	Naproxen (Aleve, Anaprox)	Inhibits cyclooxygenase-1 (COX-1) and prostaglandin to achieve its effect.
Nonsteroidal anti-inflammatory	Celecoxib (Celebrex)	Used to reduce pain and swelling in arthritis patients. Due to a slightly different route of action (COX-2 vs. COX-1 inhibitor), it is believed to have fewer side effects than other NSAIDS.
	Rofecoxib (Vioxx)	
Other NSAIDS	Indomethacin (Indocin)	Also used for arthritis and to affect prostaglandin synthesis.
	Oxaprozin (Daypro)	

PATHOPHYSIOLOGY PEARLS

Every time you move a muscle, it is the culmination of an impressive biological process. An electrical impulse travels down a nerve fiber connected to a muscle. As the impulse reaches the nerve ending, it stimulates the release of a chemical called acetylcholine (ACh). This acetylcholine travels across a microscopic gap (called a synapse) to the ACh receptors on the muscles.

When ACh attaches to these receptors, it causes little gates to open. You might think of the ACh as a key unlocking the gate. As various gates open, a chemical ballet begins. Sodium, normally on the outside of the cell, rushes into the cell. Potassium, normally on the inside of the cell, rushes out of the cell. Then, calcium, also normally on the outside of the cell, rushes into the cell. As this ballet continues, the exchange of sodium, potassium, and calcium causes additional chemical processes, ultimately resulting in the contraction of the muscle fibers. This contraction is an "all or nothing" contraction meaning that if a stronger contraction is needed, more fibers are stimulated.

As the stimulus to contract stops, the release of acetylcholine also stops. Another chemical, called acetylcholinesterase (AChE), is now released to remove the ACh remaining in the synapse. The stopping of ACh release and the release of AChE result in the muscle contraction ceasing. It is the release of acetylcholinesterase that is stopped or reduced by organophosphates (used in some nerve agents), which do not allow muscle relaxation.

Obviously, this is an oversimplified explanation, but the next time you turn a page in your textbook or write your classroom notes, think about the wonders of the human body.

REVIEW QUESTIONS

SHORT ANSWER

1. How was the traction splint developed?

2. What should you do if a patient has no pedal pulse following a knee dislocation?

MULTIPLE CHOICE

1. Splinting a closed, angulated fracture in the position in which it was found is usually ineffective and may cause a(n) _____ during transport.
   A. distal protrusion
   B. hematomic rotation
   C. ischeal tuberosity
   D. open fracture

2. A new alternative to the use of a pneumatic antishock garment in the treatment of pelvic injuries is called a(n) _____.
   A. Ehrsen's pump
   B. iliac compress
   C. pelvic wrap
   D. crest cast

3. _____ fractures are considered very serious because they can result in a three- to four-pint-internal blood loss.
   A. Pelvic
   B. Femur
   C. Humerus
   D. Skull

4. After applying a splint, sling, or any other emergency-immobilizing device, you should always _____.
   A. ask the patient to attempt to move the secured part
   B. check proximal pulse, motor function, and sensation (PMS)
   C. immediately obtain a new set of vital signs
   D. reassess distal circulation, sensation, and motor function

5. Bones are made of _____ tissue.
   A. integumentary
   B. connective
   C. calcified muscle
   D. skeletal

SCENARIO QUESTIONS

You pull up to the skateboard park in your ambulance and immediately see the reason you were called. A girl is sitting on the concrete at the bottom of a staircase with her left leg angulated about 90° from the midthigh. You approach the crying patient, a 14- to 16-year-old girl who is clutching the broken pieces of a skateboard, and see that she has an open femur fracture on her medial thigh, midway between the knee and groin. One end of the broken bone is exposed and dark red blood is dripping slowly from the wound.

1. Barring any complications, you will treat this fracture by _____.
   A. splinting it in place
   B. applying a rigid splint
   C. securing it to the uninjured leg
   D. utilizing a traction splint

2. As you form your general impression of this situation, you should develop a high index of suspicion for _____.
   A. airway compromise and altered mental status
   B. the danger of or the potential for more violence at the scene
   C. head, spinal, and internal injuries
   D. pneumothorax resulting from rib fractures

3. Your first priority in this situation would be to _____.
   A. immobilize the broken leg
   B. complete an initial assessment
   C. administer high-concentration oxygen
   D. perform a focused physical

A group of you are helping a friend move out of his apartment. He has a 37-inch television and, despite your warning, he tries to carry it down the stairs by himself. You hear the loud crash of the television careening down the stairs, followed by shouts for help. You rush to the stairs and find your friend on his back across several steps, wedged between the walls that line the staircase. The sole of his left foot is pressed flat against one wall and his left ankle is unnaturally twisted. The television is in pieces at the foot of the stairs. He tells you that he did not hit his back or head but had "slid" into his current position after stepping on a piece of cardboard. Several other people carefully free the patient from his awkward position as you support his foot and lower leg. His respiratory rate and pulse are normal for the situation.

1. As you treat the patient's twisted, deformed ankle, you should not _____.

   A. assess distal PMS function
   B. try to remove his shoe
   C. attempt to realign his foot
   D. elevate the extremity once stabilized

2. When splinting this injury, you should ideally try to _____.

   A. wrap it first with an elastic bandage
   B. secure it in the flexed position
   C. place a rigid splint anteriorly
   D. immobilize the patient's knee

3. If your friend's ankle becomes swollen and painful while waiting for the ambulance, you should _____.

   A. apply an ice pack
   C. loosen the splint

   B. provide gentle tension
   D. offer him aspirin

It is a clear summer day and your unit is on standby at a college baseball game. You are a fan of the home team and a posting at such an event can be a nice break from your normally hectic call schedule. The batter hits a high fly ball that is caught by the right fielder. Suddenly, the runner on third charges for home and, arriving a fraction of a second before the ball, collides horribly with the catcher. The runner gets up and walks back to his team's cheering dugout, but the catcher stays on the ground. You are called out to home plate and find the player, a 19-year-old male, yelling in pain and clutching the left side of his pelvic area. You ask the patient whether he hurts anywhere other than his hip and he hisses through clenched teeth, "No ... no, please, you gotta help me!"

1. How should you move this patient onto the spine board?

   A. Get two people to assist you and use the extremity lift.
   B. You and your partner can use the clothes drag.
   C. Logroll the patient gently onto his right side.
   D. Use a scoop stretcher with one person at each corner.

2. How would you "package" this patient to prevent further pelvic injury?

   A. Place a folded blanket between the patient's legs from groin to ankles and bind his legs together with wide cravats.
   B. Secure the patient's legs and torso to the long spine board and wrap a *figure eight* strap around his feet.
   C. Slide a folded blanket under the patient's knees and bind his legs together with wide cravats.
   D. Tie a rigid splint from the patient's knee to his chest and secure the splint to the long spine board.

3. This patient may have a hip fracture, which indicates a crack or break in the _____.

   A. iliac crest
   B. proximal femur
   C. inferior acetabulum
   D. lateral ischium

CASE STUDIES

CASE STUDY 1   I HEARD A BIG SNAP!

You are dispatched to a local gym for a possible broken leg. Upon your arrival, you are escorted to a sparring ring on the far side of the main gym. On the mat is a young adult male in obvious pain. A gym employee who identifies himself as an EMT is holding an ice pack on the patient's right lower leg. As you approach, you can see significant deformity to the patient's lower right leg. The gym employee states that the patient was sparring with a partner when they both came up with a powerful turning kick at the same time. Their legs came together right at the shin and they heard a loud snap, and the next thing they saw was the patient on the mat in severe pain. His foot was turned completely around the wrong way. The EMT on the scene advises you that the patient did not hit his head and never lost consciousness, so he does not think there is any chance of spinal injury. The patient's ABCs are all right.

1. **What is your primary concern for this patient?**

2. **How will you determine the circulatory status of his right leg?**

Upon examination of the injury, you find the right leg to be angulated to the right just above the ankle. As you assess the right foot, you are unable to locate either pulse. The patient is able to move his toes slightly but with pain. He can also feel you touch his foot.

1. **Would you attempt to straighten his injured leg or would you splint it in the position you find it in?**

2. **If, once you straighten his injured leg, you still cannot locate a distal pulse, what will you do?**

CASE STUDY 2   I THINK I SPRAINED MY WRIST

You are called to a shopping center for a fall. You arrive to find a laughing man in his 70s holding his wrist while surrounded by his wife, mall security, and a few bystanders. With a giant smile, he greets you and says, "I think I sprained my wrist. It hurts a bit but I can still move it so I don't think it is broken." He rotates his wrist for you and winces a bit while he does it. You discourage him from moving his wrist and perform an initial assessment and find no problems. You now turn to the history and physical exam.

1. **The patient tells you his sprained wrist is his only injury. Do you accept this or investigate further?**

2. **Is the cause of the fall important?**

The patient denies any other injuries. You ask specifically about his elbow, shoulder, and neck. You palpate these areas and find no signs of injury or pain. He did not sustain a head injury. You now turn your attention to his wrist.

1. **How would you examine his wrist? What would you look for?**

Your palpation of the wrist and examination of his distal circulation and sensation do not reveal any abnormalities.

1. **Do you think the wrist is broken?**

2. **Does this patient require treatment for the injury, such as splinting?**

Active Exploration

It will not take long for the average EMT-B working the streets to see a wide variety of musculoskeletal injuries. Some are very minor, manifested only by pain on palpation, while others appear as gross deformities in conjunction with a major mechanism of injury. One of the most important concepts the new EMT-B must learn and understand is that the majority of isolated musculoskeletal injuries are *not* life-threatening. They are certainly painful, and they are often the worst thing that has ever happened to the patient. But you must learn to prioritize these injuries, especially in light of a major MOI. If the major bones are broken and deformed, there is a strong likelihood that the person has other more serious internal injuries.

The following activities will help you develop your skills related to the assessment and treatment of musculoskeletal injuries.

Activity 1: Practice Makes Perfect

When it comes to developing your long-bone- and joint-splinting skills, there is nothing better than good old-fashioned practice. This first activity will have you practicing these skills using only the most basic of materials. You will need a small assortment of supplies that should be easy to gather. Some newspaper, a couple of magazines, some short and long pieces of cardboard, and several triangular bandages should do the trick. You will also need a fellow student to play the role of patient.

Using the following four "rules," take turns with your partner splinting various simulated injuries. Alternate back and forth and change the injury from upper to lower extremity and from long-bone to joint injuries.

1. Check circulation, sensation, and motor function before moving the injury.
2. Immobilize the suspected fracture site.
3. Immobilize the joints above and below the suspected fracture site.
4. Re-evaluate circulation, sensation, and motor function.

Refer to these "rules" as you progress through the splinting process. Carefully evaluate each step of the way to see if what you are doing is really meeting the objective.

29

Injuries to the Head and Spine

CHAPTER SUMMARY

After completing a good assessment and ensuring that the ABCs are satisfactory, what is most important to your patient? The woman who dove headfirst into shallow water … the man whose head hit the windshield during the collision … the boy who was thrown from the horse onto the fence … if they knew what you, as an EMT-B, know, what would they want you to do for them?

The human body's nervous system, which is its control system, is made up of the central nervous system and the peripheral nervous system. The central nervous system, as its name implies, is the control center—the brain and spinal cord. The nerves extending out from the spinal cord, feeling, and responding, make up the peripheral nervous system. A subcategory of the peripheral nervous system is the autonomic nervous system, controlling the functions that are unconscious (digestion, heartbeat, and so on). The brain receives all data and emits all impulses, which are carried through the spinal cord to be distributed as needed. Damage to the spinal cord can block incoming and outgoing messages or even cause impulses to "jump tracks"—fooling both the brain and other parts of the body.

The head consists of the skull and brain, covered in a thin veil of muscle and skin. The cranium is essentially an enclosed case that protects the soft, easily damaged brain, and the front exterior of the cranium holds 14 irregularly shaped bones that form the face. At the base of the skull is an opening through which the spinal cord passes from the brain down into the spinal column. Cerebrospinal fluid circulates over the brain and down through the spinal cord, bathing and protecting the components of the central nervous system.

The spinal column is a stack of 33 irregularly shaped bones called vertebrae that both protect the spinal cord and support the upper half of the body. From superior to inferior, there are 7 cervical (neck) vertebrae, 12 thoracic (rib-supporting) vertebrae, 5 lumbar (midback) vertebrae, 5 sacral (lower-back) vertebrae and 4 coccygeal (tailbone) vertebrae. The sacral and coccygeal vertebrae form the posterior of the pelvis.

Damage to the head will most likely injure the scalp first—which, due to extensive blood vessels, will bleed profusely. Control this with direct pressure, unless there is a depressed skull injury or an open skull injury, in which case you would dress loosely with sterile gauze.

Skull injuries can affect the bones of the cranium and of the face—falling into two basic categories: open and closed. If the cranium has remained intact after a trauma, the injury is considered closed. If the cranium is cracked, split, or broken into pieces, the injury is an open one. Always assume that a scalp injury hides an open head wound.

The brain can be injured either directly or indirectly. An open head wound where the brain tissue is lacerated, punctured, or bruised by broken bone or a foreign object is considered a direct injury. An indirect injury would be a concussion or contusion, where an impact to the skull has transferred its energy to the brain.

The signs and symptoms of a skull fracture and a brain injury can be similar, including visible bone fragments and bits of brain tissue, altered mental status (utilize the Alert Verbal Painful Unresponsive scale for assessment), deep lacerations or hematoma to the scalp, cranial depressions, large swollen spots, unusual cranial shapes, severe head pain, clear fluid flowing from the ears and/or nose, and so on. Since there are so many different, and subjective, indicators of skull and brain injuries, you can simply assume them based on mechanism of injury. Due to similarities in some appearances and behaviors, never just assume alcohol intoxication or drug use in your patient—first rule out the possibility of head injury.

What is the best way to treat a patient with an apparent skull fracture or brain injury? As always, start by taking appropriate BSI precautions. Whenever you are dealing with a head injury, you should assume (and treat for) a spinal injury as well—provide manual stabilization of the head and use the jaw-thrust maneuver to open the airway. If the patient is unconscious, provide the manual stabilization but insert an OPA and be ready with suction—head-injury patients tend to vomit. You should then evaluate the breathing, providing assisted ventilations if required and always providing high-concentration oxygen, and apply a cervical collar. Control any serious bleeding, keep the patient calm and reassured, dress any open wounds, care for shock, and transport promptly. Reassess vitals every 5 minutes.

If you are not sure how badly a head-injury patient is injured, or if the patient is unresponsive, take cervical-spine precautions and properly secure the patient to a long spine board. During transport, the board may be tilted to the side to allow for drainage in the event of vomiting—which can occur without warning with a head injury.

You should not remove objects impaled in the cranium—they should be stabilized with bulky dressings. If the impaled object is too long to allow for transportation, you will need to cut it. Always seek the counsel of medical direction or the emergency physician before cutting an impaled object.

Impacts, if they are strong enough, may cause facial fractures. Bone fragments, blood, blood clots, teeth, and even a separated palate may obstruct the airway following a facial impact. You may also see discoloration, swelling, facial distortion, and mandibular dislocation. Your top priority with facial impacts or fractures is airway control—again, assume spinal injury and take appropriate actions. Do not neglect the possibility of a brain injury accompanying a severe facial impact.

Some brain injuries are caused by internal events such as bleeding or blood clots. The signs and symptoms will be identical to trauma-related brain injuries—only there will be no trauma or MOI.

Spinal injury must be assumed any time there are serious head, neck, back, chest, abdominal, or pelvic injuries. You should always overtreat patients with the potential for spinal injuries because, as the old saying goes, better safe than sorry (*or* sued!). Spinal injuries will usually be in the form of fractures (with and without bone displacement), dislocations, strains, or slipped or compressed disks. Not all spinal injuries will affect spinal nerves. The spine is most often injured by compression, excessive flexion, extension, rotation, diving accidents, motor-vehicle collisions, gunshot wounds, and falls (from either more than three times the patient's height or with enough force to cause open ankle injuries).

Sports are also a common cause of spinal injuries—from in-line skating, to football, skiing, sledding, and diving.

The signs and symptoms of spinal injuries are paralysis of the extremities (the most reliable indication), pain with or without movement, and tenderness along the spine. Any one of these indicators warrants spinal immobilization—but you can also use MOI as your sole deciding factor. Other signs and symptoms of spinal injury are impaired breathing, spinal deformity (*very rare*), priapism, posturing, loss of bowel and bladder control, extremity nerve impairment, neurogenic shock, and soft-tissue damage to the head and neck.

If the patient is conscious when you arrive, determine the MOI, ask questions that will reveal the presence of injury to the spine ("Do you feel tingling anywhere?"), and check for contusions, deformities, lacerations, punctures, penetrations, and swelling. Also, check for the equality of strength in the extremities. If the patient is unresponsive, question bystanders about the MOI and the patient's mental status; inspect for contusions, deformities, lacerations, punctures, penetrations, and swelling; and palpate for tenderness (patient may be responsive to Pain) and deformity. Spend very little time trying to determine spinal injury in unresponsive patients—if there is an MOI, immobilize the patient.

Emergency care for all potential spinal-injury patients should include manual in-line stabilization of the head and neck, assessing the ABCs and completing the rapid trauma assessment, and applying the cervical collar. Then, assess extremity PMS, apply a spinal-immobilization device, and provide high-concentration oxygen with a nonrebreather mask—include artificial ventilations, if necessary. You should then reassess extremity PMS.

Cervical collars are designed to limit movement *when used in conjunction with an immobilization device* such as a long spine board or a vest-type extrication device.

How do you immobilize a patient who is found in the seated position? If there is no need for an emergency move, manually stabilize the patient's head, use an appropriately sized cervical collar, and apply a short spine board or vest-type extrication device—to which you will secure the torso first and the head last. Also, ensure that the torso straps do not interfere with respirations.

If you find that the patient's situation and surroundings will allow for the use of a short spine board, there are several guidelines that are specific to that particular piece of equipment. To start off, you will need to assess the patient's back, shoulder blades, arms, and collarbones prior to applying the device. The EMT-B who is applying the board must angle it so that it slides behind the patient without disturbing the arms of the other rescuer who will be maintaining manual stabilization of the patient's head and neck. The uppermost holes of the board should be level with the patient's shoulders, and the board should not extend beyond the coccyx. You should also never apply a chin strap to the patient (which may prevent him from opening his mouth during vomiting), and do not pad between the cervical collar and the board as this may cause hyperextension of the neck.

If you need to get a supine patient onto a long spine board, the log roll is your best option. The patient should be rolled, with the spine maintained in an in-line position, onto his side—at the direction and count of the rescuer holding the head. Take the opportunity during the roll to assess the posterior of the patient and, once on the board, pad any voids between the patient and the board. In order to immobilize the patient's head, place pillows, foam blocks, rolled blankets, or some other commercially available device on either side of the head and secure in place with tape or Velcro straps. If the patient is pregnant, once she is secured to the board, you should tilt it to the left to minimize compression of the abdominal vessels.

While placing a pediatric patient (less than six years old) onto a spine board, you will need to pad from the patient's shoulders to his feet to compensate for the proportionally large head and to keep it in the neutral position.

You will, as an EMT-B, come across patients who are up and walking around at a crash scene, yet when you evaluate their MOI, it will be obvious that they require immediate spinal immobilization. Since it is possible that the patient simply has not yet dislodged a spinal bone fragment or some other type of injury, having him sit or lie on the ground could be very dangerous. This patient needs to be placed on the spine board while still standing. Since it is impractical, and in some cases dangerous, to try and secure the patient to the board while he is in a standing position, you will need to lay the patient down *on* the board and secure him when supine.

What if, as is the case with many sporting- and motorcycle-related injuries, the patient is found wearing a helmet? The main concern with helmets relates to airway management—can the airway be accessed and protected with the helmet in place? If the helmet fits snugly, if the patient is not in cardiac arrest, if there are no airway or respiratory problems, and if the helmet does not prevent the EMT-B from quickly accessing the airway, it can be left on and secured with the rest of the patient to the spine board. If the helmet must be removed, it is always a two-rescuer procedure.

You will occasionally be dispatched to a vehicle collision and be required to treat a pediatric patient who requires spinal immobilization but is still in a child safety seat. Due to the risks associated with relocating a child from a safety seat to a spine board, you can leave the child in the safety seat unless there is a need for resuscitation, or some other reason for him to be supine. You can pad the voids around the child's body, immobilize him relatively well, and transport, all with the child in the safety seat.

When documenting possible head or spine injuries, always include whether or not the patient lost consciousness and the progression of the patient's mental status.

MED MINUTE

There are not a lot of medications that are given by prescription in the acute phase of head or spine injuries. Many of the medications taken after an injury have been covered in previous chapters. For example:

- Pain medications (e.g. NSAIDS) may be taken for the pain and swelling that may occur after an injury to the spine.
- After a head injury, it is not uncommon for seizures to develop, creating a need for antiseizure medications.
- Open head wounds may require cleaning and stitches. This will create a need for pain medication in the days after the injury and possibly the need for antibiotics to prevent infection.

PATHOPHYSIOLOGY PEARLS

During your training, you may have encountered other students walking the halls reciting things like, "On old Olympus towering tops a Fin and German viewed some hops." But what are they doing? What does this mean? They are trying to remember the names of the 12 cranial nerves. Evaluating these nerves will give you information on the status of the nervous system.

Cranial Nerve I is the **O**lfactory nerve and is responsible for the sense of smell. Impairment to this nerve will cause an impaired sense of smell.

Cranial Nerve II is the **O**ptic nerve and is responsible for vision. Impairment to this nerve will cause a decreased visual field or even blindness.

Cranial Nerve III is the **O**culomotor nerve and is responsible for eye movements, opening of the eyelids, pupil constriction, and focusing. Impairment of this nerve will cause drooping eyelids, dilated pupils, inability to move the eyes in certain directions, double vision, and difficulty in focusing.

Cranial Nerve IV is the **T**rochlear nerve and is responsible for inferior and lateral eyeball movement. Impairment will cause double vision and the inability to rotate the eye inferiorly or laterally.

Cranial Nerve V is the **T**rigeminal nerve and is responsible for the sense of touch, temperature, and pain. There are three divisions that serve various areas and impairment will cause a loss of sensation in the area that is affected. The ophthalmic division serves the upper face, the maxillary division serves the middle face, and the mandibular division serves the lower face and jaw. In addition to loss of sensation, impairment to the mandibular division will cause impaired chewing.

Cranial Nerve VI is the **A**bducens nerve and is responsible for the lateral movement (abduction) of the eye. Impairment will cause an inability to rotate the eye laterally (at rest, eyes normally rotate medially).

Cranial Nerve VII is the **F**acial nerve and is responsible for facial expression; the autonomic control of tear glands, nasal and palatine glands, submandibular and sublingual salivary glands; and for the sense of taste. Impairment will cause the inability to control muscles on the affected side of the face, sagging resulting from loss of muscle tone, and a distorted sense of taste. Degeneration of this nerve causes the condition of Bell's Palsy.

Cranial Nerve VIII is the vestibulocochlear (formerly **A**uditory) nerve and is responsible for hearing and equilibrium. Impairment will cause nerve deafness, dizziness, nausea, vomiting, and loss of balance.

Cranial Nerve IX is the **G**lossopharyngeal nerve and is responsible for swallowing, salivation, the gag reflex, regulation of blood pressure and respirations, and the sensations of touch, pain, and temperature of the external ear. Impairment will cause the inability to sense bitter and sour tastes and impaired swallowing.

Cranial Nerve X is the **V**agus nerve and is responsible for swallowing; speech; regulation of pulmonary, cardiovascular, and gastrointestinal function; and sensations of hunger, fullness, and intestinal discomfort. Impairment will cause hoarseness or loss of voice and impaired swallowing and gastrointestinal motility. If both vagus nerves are damaged, death will result.

Cranial Nerve XI is the accessory (also called **S**pinal accessory) nerve and is responsible for swallowing and the movements of the head, neck, and shoulders. Impairment will cause impaired movement of the head, neck, and shoulders; difficulty in shrugging shoulders on the damaged side; and paralysis of the sternocleidomastoid, making it hard to turn toward the injured side.

Cranial Nerve XII is the **H**ypoglossal nerve and is responsible for the movements of the tongue during speech, food manipulation, and swallowing. Impairment will cause difficulty in speech and swallowing. If both hypoglossal nerves are damaged, the tongue cannot be protruded (stuck out). If only one nerve is damaged, the tongue is deflected toward the damaged side.

The next time you check your patient's pupils or assess a potential stroke patient, you will have a new understanding of the cranial nerves.

REVIEW QUESTIONS

SHORT ANSWER

1. Why is removal of a patient's clothing to check for spinal deformity not recommended?

2. What is a direct brain injury?

MULTIPLE CHOICE

1. The failure of the nervous system to regulate the diameter of blood vessels can lead to _____.
   - **A.** neurogenic shock
   - **B.** psychogenic shock
   - **C.** hypovolemic shock
   - **D.** volumetric shock

2. The term "uptriage" means to _____.
   - **A.** increase priority
   - **B.** stop treating one patient to treat another
   - **C.** overtreat
   - **D.** decrease priority

3. Today's smaller vehicles and contoured seats make it more difficult to use _____ for extrications.
   - **A.** vest-type devices
   - **B.** power tools
   - **C.** cervical collars
   - **D.** short spine boards

4. Closed head injuries will usually only cause hemorrhagic shock in _____ patients.
   - **A.** comatose
   - **B.** infant
   - **C.** diabetic
   - **D.** elderly

5. The _____ spine is usually only damaged by the most severe MOIs.
   A. thoracic   **B.** cervical
   C. lumbar   **D.** temporal

SCENARIO QUESTIONS

You arrive at the scene after an assault. The police have the situation under control and the suspects are in custody. It is your job to treat the man whom the suspects beat with a baseball bat. The patient, a 20- to 25-year-old male, blinks his eyes and makes gurgling noises when you speak loudly to him. He is bleeding profusely from numerous head wounds, has extensive bone-structure deformities around his face and cranium, and his jaw is off center so that his upper and lower teeth do not meet as they should.

1. The gurgling sound should indicate to you that the patient _____.
   A. is trying to speak
   B. needs artificial ventilations
   C. has a brain injury
   D. has a compromised airway

2. This patient should be properly secured to a long spine board and _____.
   A. rotated into a lateral recumbent position
   B. tilted into a modified Trendelenburg position
   C. set flat on the gurney for transport
   D. positioned with his feet 12 to 24 inches below his head

3. While attempting to control bleeding from the head wounds, you should not _____.
   A. dress with loose gauze
   B. allow the blood or cerebrospinal fluid to flow freely from the patient's nose or ears
   C. apply firm direct pressure
   D. leave bone fragments in place

In order to reach an unresponsive passenger, the rescue squad has just completed an emergency extrication of a conscious 42-year-old male from the wreckage of a vehicle. The crew lays the patient on your long spine board and returns to work. Your partner maintains manual, in-line stabilization of the patient's head and neck while you conduct a rapid trauma assessment. You discover that the patient has lost bowel control, is priapismic, and cannot feel or move his lower extremities.

1. Your partner can release the manual stabilization of the patient's head as soon as _____.
   A. the patient is secured to the spine board
   B. he knows that the patient is coherent and will stay still
   C. you complete the trauma assessment
   D. the cervical collar is in place

2. The _____ should be the last part of this patient's body to be secured to the spine board.
   A. legs   **B.** head
   C. torso   **D.** feet

3. What is the most reliable sign of spinal injury in the conscious male patient?

    A. Priapism

    B. Extremity paralysis

    C. Loss of bowel or bladder control

    D. Tenderness along the spine

You are dispatched to the mall for an unconscious person. Upon your arrival, you find a 40- to 45-year-old female who is unresponsive and bleeding from a large laceration to her left temporal region. Witnesses tell you that the patient apparently mistook the *down* escalator for the *up* escalator and fell as soon as she stepped on to it. She had then struck her head on the edge of one of the metal steps and had to be pulled, unconscious, from the escalator. The patient's blood pressure is increasing, her pulse is decreasing, and her pupils are fixed and dilated.

1. How would you secure this patient's airway?

    A. Utilize an endotracheal tube.

    B. Insert an NPA into her right nostril.

    C. Perform the head-tilt, chin-lift maneuver.

    D. Insert an oropharyngeal airway without hyperextending her neck.

2. This patient is suffering from a(n) _____ brain injury.

    A. occipital   **B.** critical

    C. portal-type   **D.** nonlethal

3. Why, in some EMS systems, would you be directed to hyperventilate this patient with supplemental oxygen?

    A. It will reduce the chances of hypoperfusion resulting from a stroke.

    B. It will greatly increase the oxygenation of the blood, compensating for any loss of circulation in the damaged brain tissues.

    C. It can help reduce brain-tissue swelling by lowering carbon dioxide levels and raising oxygen levels.

    D. Large, rapid doses of oxygen have been shown to "kick start" the central nervous system following a trauma to the brain and may prevent further damage.

CASE STUDIES

| CASE STUDY 1 | HE FELL OFF THE ROOF AND WON'T WAKE UP |

You are dispatched to a construction site for a person who has fallen. Upon your arrival, you are directed over to the side of a home that is under construction where you see an approximately 25-year-old male lying on the ground apparently unresponsive. Another construction worker is holding a bloody towel to the man's head and trying to get the patient to talk. Another worker tells you that the man was on the roof when he lost his footing and fell off. You estimate the height to be about 9 feet and see that the man appears to have struck his head on a five-gallon paint can that was sitting on the ground. Your initial assessment finds the man breathing adequately and with a pulse that is strong and regular. The bleeding from the head appears to be controlled.

1. What will be your priorities as you begin to treat this patient? What type of an assessment will you want to perform on this person and why?

2. What device will you use to immobilize and transport this man out to the street to the ambulance?

Your rapid trauma assessment reveals only a deformed right forearm but no other obvious injuries. The patient is beginning to regain consciousness as you place the cervical collar around his neck.

1. As he regains consciousness, how is this man likely to respond to what is happening to him?

2. Once he is secured to the backboard, what will become one of your major concerns about the treatment for this man? How will you manage that concern?

CASE STUDY 2 SOMEBODY CALL 911!

You are driving home from a continuing-education session and come across a motor-vehicle collision. It appears to be a one-vehicle collision in which a car has struck a pole.

1. Why is this event called a "motor-vehicle collision" as opposed to a "motor-vehicle accident?"

2. What hazards might you suspect at the scene of a collision of this type?

You approach the patient as two bystanders are trying to get her out of the vehicle. You advise them that you are an EMT and that the patient is all right where she is. You get access to the patient and introduce yourself. She appears conscious, alert, and oriented. Her skin is warm and dry. She tells you that her neck hurts a bit. As you maintain stabilization, you look for damage in the windshield and steering wheel and see none. You continue to calm the patient and restrict her spine movements. You verify that several bystanders have called 911 on their cell phones.

1. What other things can you look for in and around the car that will help you determine the potential seriousness of the injuries?

2. While you are maintaining stabilization, what can you ask the patient to continue your assessment?

The ambulance arrives and you know the crew members. They ask you to continue stabilization while they continue the assessment and emergency care you began.

1. What information should you tell them about the patient and what you have done thus far?

2. The ambulance crew asks whether you have any idea which device should be used to get the patient out of the car. What do you tell them?

Active Exploration

One of the most important skills you can learn as an EMT-B will be the ability to properly assess and evaluate the MOI. This is important for many reasons including being able to anticipate and predict specific injuries, including possible injury to the spine.

It is important to realize that a significant head injury is likely to result in a cervical-spine injury and to understand that many mechanisms that do not directly affect the spine can cause injury to the vertebrae and the spinal cord.

Once you have determined that there is a chance the patient might have a neck or back injury, your job is to follow through with this suspicion and deliver the most appropriate emergency care based on the MOI and not on whether the patient has pain.

The following activities are designed to help you develop your skills specific to the assessment of and emergency care for patients with known and suspected head, neck, and back injuries.

Activity 1: Roll 'em Over

The reality of the field environment is that you will find patients in any one of a number of possible positions following their injuries. It will be your job to carefully coordinate getting the patient into a position whereby he can be properly secured to a long backboard or similar device. This activity is designed to develop your skills pertaining to the coordinated roll of a patient from the prone position to the supine position.

You will need three of your fellow classmates to assist with this activity. You will all rotate through the different roles in order to experience all aspects of the activity.

1. Have one person lie facedown on the floor to simulate a patient with a suspected spinal injury.
2. Take turns taking the lead role and coordinating each person and what their respective tasks should be. It is *not* necessary for the person in charge to always be at the head of the patient. It is, however, important to always defer to the person at the head when calling out the timing for each move.

3. As the leader, be as specific as you can as you instruct the others on what to do. Assume that your assistants are bystanders with no EMS experience and that you must give them explicit instructions.

4. Take turns managing the "patient" in various positions and rolling him from prone to supine.

What factors will influence which way you will want to roll the patient? What is the best position for each of the helpers? What special considerations must be made for the person in control of the head? Is it best to roll the patient over in just one move, or are two moves more efficient?

You can take this activity one step further by bringing in a long backboard and rolling the patient directly onto the board. How does this make the situation easier or more difficult? What will you do when the person ends up "off center" on the board? What is the best way to get him centered without compromising the integrity of the spine?

Activity 2: One Size Fits All

One of the most difficult things to do is guessing the appropriate size cervical collar for the patient. There are many techniques for doing this, but none is better than experience. This next exercise will help you learn which size collar is the most appropriate to use by just visually inspecting the patient and his body type.

1. Gather an assortment of cervical collars from your lab or department.
2. Take these collars and practice guessing the appropriate size and placing the collars on various people.
3. Purposely choose people of varying size and shape.
4. Practice placing the collars while the "patients" are in the standing position. Then have them lie down, and once again practice placing the collar.

Most manufacturers have labeled their collars with specific names for the various sizes. These can be very misleading since the names are quite subjective.

If your department or school uses just one brand of collar, get to know that brand and how the sizes tend to run. Many collars tend to run larger than their name implies, so do not go by just the name. Practice placing the collars on different sized patients so you will get firsthand experience with what types of patients they actually fit.

There are many factors that influence whether a collar will fit properly or not. There is truly no such thing as a "one size fits all" collar, despite what some of the collar manufacturers would want you to believe.

RETRO REVIEW

1. You arrive at a factory and find that a 43-year-old machinist has a deep laceration running from the base of his ring finger, across his palm and ending about 1 inch proximal to the wrist. He has lost approximately 500 cc of blood but has stopped the hemorrhaging with direct pressure. The

patient's appearance is good and he is calm and coherent. You should
_____.

    A. apply direct pressure and raise the extremity

    B. treat for shock

    C. request an ALS intercept

    D. maintain pressure on the brachial artery

2. Agency names, unit numbers, dates, times, call numbers, and crew members' names are all considered _____.

    A. HIPAA elements   **B.** optional information

    C. template elements   **D.** run data

3. If you notice that your hands are becoming red and itchy after each call, you should suspect a(n) _____.

    A. latex allergy   **B.** hazardous material exposure

    C. excessive use of hand soap   **D.** infectious rash

THINKING AND LINKING

CHAPTER TOPIC	HOW IT RELATES TO YOU AND OTHER COURSE AREAS
Skull injuries	Be prepared for profuse bleeding with any sort of head or face injury that has had enough force to damage the skull. This means BSI precautions and shock management (covered previously in Chapters 2 and 26). Also make sure that your respiratory and suction equipment is handy (including airway adjuncts, O_2, and a BVM) because some skull injuries can force blood and debris into the patient's nose, mouth, and throat or cause a depressed level of consciousness (preventing the patient from maintaining a patent airway or breathing adequately).
Spinal immobilization	Regardless of the call that you are responding to (vehicle collision, syncope, diving incident, seizure, fall, gunshot, and so on), there is always the potential for spinal injury. When checking the ambulance at the start of your shift, ensure that you are carrying an adequate supply of spinal-immobilization equipment (this will be covered more in Chapter 33). Also, until you evaluate (or reevaluate) any possible MOI, do not hesitate to begin treatment by manually stabilizing the patient's head and neck.
Extrication	During extrications (examined in depth in Chapter 34), you will most likely be providing patient emergency care inside of the vehicle. For this reason, you should always carry heavy, turnout-type protective clothing and a good rescue helmet in your ambulance. This will help protect you from the heat, flying glass, and sharp edges common during extrications. Remember, when responding to a collision where the patient is still seated in the vehicle, you will need to bring *both* a long spine board and a vest-type extrication device to the scene.

30

Putting It All Together for the Trauma Patient

CHAPTER SUMMARY

You are familiar with mechanisms of injury and how important they are in determining the emergency care provided for the trauma patient. You have even learned how to assess and treat many trauma injuries and their associated complications—but things on the street may not always be as clear and focused. You must anticipate trauma patients with conditions complicated by medical factors (and vice versa), and patients with two or more (separate) serious injuries—known as "multiple-trauma" patients.

In multiple-trauma situations, your focus should be on the immediate threats to the patient's life (i.e. ABCs, severe bleeding, and so on). Your taking the extra time at the scene to "properly" package the patient may, in certain situations, cause more harm than good.

When managing the multiple-trauma patient, teamwork, timing, and transportation are key to the patient's survival. *Teamwork* means that everybody at the scene knows his job and how it fits into the bigger picture. *Timing* reminds EMS personnel that the patient must be moved to a definitive care facility as quickly as possible. *Transportation* is initiated by first determining which receiving facility would be most appropriate for the patient.

In preparation for the multiple-trauma call, you should continue to practice techniques and assessments, and each member of the crew should have preassigned responsibilities. This will make things go much smoother at the scene with a real patient. Always try to review individual roles en route to the scene. Once you are on the scene, complete your assessment as normal and ensure that the patient's ABCs are stable—if not, intervene as per your training.

With multiple-trauma patients, an unusual situation arises. Is taking the time to properly treat each injury going to cost the patient precious time—and perhaps his life? You need to consider that. Sometimes it may be more beneficial to simply "splint" the patient to a long spine board and transport (while maintaining the patient's airway, breathing, and circulation, of course). Also, be aware of scene safety—remember that certain types of trauma (gunshot wounds, stab wounds, and so on) can indicate danger or a potential instability at the rescue scene.

It is important to be able to adapt to each situation. If you are performing a rapid trauma assessment, for example, and part of the patient's body is not accessible—move on, and worry about that part after extrication.

When treating multiple-trauma patients, guard against your natural urge to treat or "fix" every problem that you identify. You will serve your patient much better by managing the life-threats and letting the receiving facility worry about the injuries that you did not have time for.

PATHOPHYSIOLOGY PEARLS

In 1966, the publication of "*Accidental Death and Disability: The Neglected Disease of Modern Society*" started the whirlwind that is now the Emergency Medical Services. Whether you are just starting in EMS or a veteran, your efforts help make a difference in the lives of the patients you assist.

Trauma is the leading cause of death in persons 1 to 44 years of age. It results in approximately 45 percent of the deaths in persons 1 to 14 years old and 62 percent of the deaths in persons 15 to 24 years old. In the United States, there are approximately 100,000 trauma-related deaths annually.[1]

Our bodies rely on constant perfusion to deliver oxygen and nutrients to the tissues and remove carbon dioxide and other waste products. Any interruption in this perfusion (known as hypoperfusion, or shock) can have a dramatic impact. This hypoperfusion may result from internal or external bleeding (hemorrhagic); dehydration, severe burns, or severe vomiting or diarrhea (hypovolemic); microorganisms in the bloodstream (septic); severe allergic reaction (anaphylactic); cardiac compromise, severe angina, or myocardial infarction (cardiogenic); spinal-cord trauma (neurogenic); and extreme emotional upset or tragedy (psychogenic). It is every EMT's goal to rapidly assess, treat, and transport trauma patients. But even with the best of emergency care, some tissues may be damaged beyond recovery and ultimately succumb to end-organ failure.

According to the American Burn Association, there are over 1,000,000 reported burns annually. Of those reported burns, 45,000 burn patients are hospitalized. About half are admitted to specialized burn centers and the rest are admitted to other hospitals. There are an estimated 700,000 emergency-department visits annually. The average total body surface area of those admitted to burn centers is approximately 14 percent TBSA. About 6 percent of those admitted to a burn center do not survive to discharge, mostly victims of inhalation burns. Burn injuries also make the patient more susceptible to infection.[2]

1 *National Institute of General Medical Sciences, National Institutes of Health*. Trauma, Burn, Shock, and Injury: Facts and Figures. *www.nigms.nih.gov/news/facts/traumaburnfactsfigures.html*
2 *American Burn Association*. Burn Incidence and Treatment in the US: 2000 Fact Sheet. *www.ameriburn.org/pub/BurnIncidenceFactSheet.htm*

We have come a long way in reducing death and disability and, through continued improvement in providing quality emergency medical care, we will continue to reduce this "neglected disease of modern society."

REVIEW QUESTIONS

SHORT ANSWER

1. What is a universal splint?

2. Why is it so important to move trauma patients to a definitive-care facility quickly?

MULTIPLE CHOICE

1. The best way to prepare for multiple-trauma calls is to _____.
   - **A.** practice
   - **B.** inspect the ambulance
   - **C.** restock all supplies
   - **D.** utilize relaxation techniques

2. When treating a multiple-trauma patient, your overall goal should be to _____.
   - **A.** transport immediately
   - **B.** properly immobilize the patient
   - **C.** treat all obvious injuries
   - **D.** treat immediate life-threats

3. Your patient has *multiple-trauma injuries* if he _____.
   - **A.** suffered a crushing blow to the organs in his abdomen
   - **B.** received a concussion during a generalized tonic-clonic seizure
   - **C.** presents with a deformed thigh and paradoxical chest movement
   - **D.** was involved in a head-on vehicle collision

SCENARIO QUESTIONS

You are called to the golf course on the west side of town for an unresponsive man. As you arrive, you are waved over to one of the fairways. You immediately notice several deep, swerving gouges in the grass leading to an overturned golf cart and a man sprawled on the ground. The unresponsive patient is approximately 50 to 55 years old. One of the witnesses tells you that the man just "lost control" of the cart and zigzagged crazily around the fairway before finally flipping the small vehicle over. Another golfer tells you that "Charlie" is a diabetic. The patient is unresponsive, has an obviously deformed left humerus, and loud, snoring respirations.

1. This patient's audible respirations indicate _____.
   - **A.** that he has most likely been drinking
   - **B.** that he suffered a neck injury in the crash
   - **C.** that he has a partially occluded airway
   - **D.** that he is in a postictal state

2. You should have a high index of suspicion that this patient is suffering from (a) _____.
   A. diabetic emergency, cardiac arrest, or spinal injury
   B. multiple traumas, internal injuries, and/or psychogenic shock
   C. heat stroke, spinal injury, or epilepsy
   D. stroke, spinal injury, and/or diabetic emergency

3. How should you treat the patient's humerus injury?
   A. Wrap it with an elastic bandage.
   B. Place the injured arm to the side of his body as you are securing the patient to the backboard.
   C. Apply a rigid splint and wrap it snugly.
   D. Utilize a traction splint.

You and an ALS unit arrive simultaneously at the scene of an ATV crash. A 28-year-old man and his 4-year-old son were thrown into a barbed-wire fence after hitting a partially buried stump. The four-wheeled vehicle had then rolled and landed on the man's legs, crushing both of them and burning one severely. The paramedic tells you and your partner to treat the adult while he treats the unresponsive child. Your patient (who is responsive only to painful stimulus) has deep and profusely bleeding lacerations to his face, neck (laterally), and shoulders; gurgling respirations; abrasions to both hands and arms; open crush injuries on both legs; and a full-thickness burn to his left leg, distal to the knee.

1. What should either you or your partner *immediately* do upon seeing this patient's injuries?
   A. Suction the patient's airway.
   B. Maintain manual stabilization of the patient's head and neck.
   C. Seal the patient's open neck wounds with gloved hands.
   D. Tell the ALS crew that they need to treat this patient first.

2. After completing all life-saving interventions, you should _____.
   A. transport the patient to a definitive-care facility
   B. bandage all open wounds and splint the lower extremities
   C. size and apply a cervical collar
   D. complete a rapid trauma assessment

3. This patient is an ideal candidate for a _____.
   A. pelvic wrap   B. universal splint
   C. Double-Sager® splint   D. PASG

C A S E   S T U D I E S

CASE STUDY 1   THROWN FROM THE VEHICLE

You have responded to a multiple-vehicle collision and are treating a patient who was ejected from one of the vehicles. Your patient is an approximately 20-year-old female who is responsive only to painful stimulus and appears to have stable ABCs.

1. **What additional information will you want to try and gather regarding the MOI for this patient?**

2. On the basis of the MOI that you know so far, what is the most appropriate assessment path for this patient?

Your patient was the front-seat passenger of the vehicle and appears not to have been wearing a seat belt. There was significant intrusion of the passenger compartment from the opposite side and no air bags were deployed. Your baseline vitals on this patient are as follows: blood pressure 106/76; pulse 96, weak and regular; respirations 18, unlabored and of good tidal volume. She has an open wound to her lower right leg with deformity and an open wound to the right side of her head.

1. Is there anything significant about this patient's baseline vital signs?

2. How will you prioritize this patient's injuries for transport?

CASE STUDY 2   "OK. THIS IS GOING TO BE A BIT TOUGH TO BELIEVE, BUT..."

Your ambulance is called for an "impaled object" at 4296 Manor Avenue, apartment 406. When you ask for additional information en route, the dispatcher advises you that a police officer is on the scene and that it is safe. Details will be given to you upon arrival.

You arrive to find the police officer talking with a man in his 20s. The man is sitting on the couch, looking uncomfortable, and apparently naked from the waist down except for a towel covering his genitals. "I'm going to let *you* tell the EMTs about this one, OK?" the police officer says to the man.

"I have a battery, a D cell, stuck in my rectum."

1. How would you perform an initial assessment for this patient?

2. What personal feelings did you have when you read the beginning of the case? If you had them on a real call, how would you deal with them?

"I suppose I could try to tell you that I accidentally sat or fell on it. But that wouldn't be true. I had a couple of drinks and did something stupid," he explains. "If you could just take it out, I can get this over with." He is alert and oriented and complains of minor cramping rectally. He lifts the towel to show you that the battery cannot be seen. The man is young, healthy, has no other complaints, and vitals you consider within normal limits.

1. Can you remove the battery from his rectum?

2. What other emergency care can you provide?

Active Exploration

Managing a trauma patient with multiple injuries can be quite challenging for any EMT-B. What you must develop is an understanding of how to quickly prioritize the patient's injuries and treat the most serious injuries first. You can only properly accomplish this with good training, experience, and a methodical approach to the assessment of the patient.

The following exercises will help you develop both your approach to assessing the patient and your ability to recognize significant mechanisms versus nonsignificant mechanisms of injury.

Activity 1: Which Way Do I Go—Trauma?

You will see presented below a series of short vignettes of trauma patients. These are not full case studies but more basic first impressions of various patients. Your job will be to quickly decide the most appropriate assessment path for each patient. You will remember from Chapter 10, "Assessment of the Trauma Patient," that there are essentially two possible assessment paths you can take for any trauma patient, the rapid trauma assessment and the focused trauma assessment. If necessary, please review these two paths in Chapter 10 of your text before proceeding with this activity.

1. A 36-year-old male who was ejected from a vehicle as it rolled several times. He is unresponsive.

2. A 44-year-old female whose legs are pinned between two vehicles. She is responsive and screaming in pain.

3. A 19-year-old male whose right hand and forearm were caught in an industrial auger and badly deformed.

4. A 6-year-old female who was struck while riding her bicycle. She is responsive and complaining of pain in her pelvic region.

5. A 22-year-old male who fell from a roof onto concrete while cleaning gutters. He is responsive and wants to get back to work.

Activity 2: Which Way to the Nearest Trauma Center?

For many trauma patients, the difference between life and death is rapid transport to a receiving trauma center and immediate surgical intervention. Unfortunately, not all areas of the country are served by such a trauma center.

   This activity will have you investigate what sorts of trauma services are available in your area. Conduct your own research and find the answers to the following questions:

1. What is the difference between a level I, II, III, IV, and V trauma center?

2. What is the nearest trauma center to where you live?

3. Where is the nearest level I and level II trauma center?

RETRO REVIEW

1. If you are not sure whether a patient's breathing is inadequate enough to require artificial ventilations, you should _____.
   A. provide artificial ventilations
   B. recheck the respiratory rate for a full minute
   C. ask your partner to assess the patient's breathing
   D. seek advice from medical direction

2. Fractures and _____ are the most common musculoskeletal ankle injuries.
   A. strains
   B. dislocations
   C. torn ligaments
   D. cartilage separations

3. You respond to an 11-year-old male who crashed an ATV into the side of a shed. The patient suffered a large open wound spanning from his anterior pelvis down to his knee and although you are able to stop the bleeding, the loss is significant. Moments later the patient goes into cardiac arrest. What should you do?
   A. Apply a PASG and transport.
   B. Begin CPR and transport immediately.
   C. Transport the patient to the nearest trauma center.
   D. Apply the AED and prepare to transport.

THINKING AND LINKING

CHAPTER TOPIC	HOW IT RELATES TO YOU AND OTHER COURSE AREAS
Multiple-trauma patients	Your initial suspicions about a patient's potential for multiple injuries will come from analyzing the MOI (Chapter 7). A patient who has fallen down a flight of stairs or has been ejected from a vehicle during a rollover collision (Chapter 7) is, obviously, more likely to suffer multiple injuries than a track athlete who tripped over a hurdle. Also, a patient who has suffered multiple injuries has a higher likelihood of head and spine injuries (Chapter 29). Do not forget the ABCs (Chapter 8) when facing a patient with numerous injuries—your focus will be to keep the person alive.
The three "Ts"	As an EMT-B, you are going to be an integral part of the EMS system (Chapter 1). Your dedication to your agency's Quality Improvement system (Chapters 1 and 14) will help you develop better teamwork, quicker response and treatment times, and safer transports.
Scene safety	Remember that the same MOIs that cause multiple injuries can also make the scene dangerous for you and other responders (Chapter 7). Vehicle-collision scenes (Chapter 34) and terrorist incidents (Chapter 36) are two examples.

31

Infants and Children

CHAPTER SUMMARY

When assessing and treating pediatric patients, you will follow the same concepts as when treating an adult patient. Infants and children have developmental characteristics as well as some anatomical differences that you will have to keep in mind throughout your assessment and treatment procedures. These special considerations will vary among the age groups.

Basic anatomical differences include:

- Head—proportionately larger until age four, more susceptible to injury
- Airway—smaller structures, trachea less rigid, more easily obstructed by disease, foreign, bodies, or position.
- Chest and abdomen—less-developed structures, less protection for internal organs
- Body surface area—larger in proportion to the body mass, more prone to heat loss
- Blood volume—significantly less than for an adult

The child's age will determine whether you gather information from the patient or from a parent or caregiver. In either case, a pediatric patient will take comfort from you communicating with an adult he is familiar with. Remember to approach the child at eye level, be honest, and smile. Your physical exam in young children will start at their toes and work up to the torso and then the head. As in any patient, life-threats need to be managed immediately. When a child is in need of emergency care, the parents or caregivers can show a variety of emotions. You will need to gain the confidence of the parents/caregiver as well as of the patient.

Your assessment strategy for children is very important because they can deteriorate very quickly. They must be reassessed again and again. One method is to use the pediatric-assessment triangle. With this method, the patient's appearance, breathing, and circulation are assessed as you enter the doorway and then continually and more thoroughly once you make contact with the patient. The sequence of assessing the pediatric patient is the same as for an adult patient.

- Scene size-up
- Initial assessment—watch the child's reaction and observe his appearance as you approach him
- Assess mental status
- Assess airway
- Assess breathing
- Assess circulation

A child who presents with any of the following is in need of immediate care and transport:

- Poor general impression
- Unresponsive
- Problems with his airway
- Respiratory distress or inadequate breathing or respiratory arrest
- Signs of shock
- Uncontrolled bleeding

Once you have made a transport decision, you will continue with a focused history and physical exam. This can be accomplished at the scene or en route, depending on the patient's condition. A young patient should be examined on a parent's lap if there are no injuries contraindicating that the child should be moved. The approach you take for the physical exam will vary slightly depending on the patient's age. Remember that pediatric patients can deteriorate quickly, so reassess them often.

There are some special concerns when treating pediatric patients:

- Maintaining an open airway—do not hyperextend or permit flexion; the patient must be in a neutral position
- Oropharyngeal airway insertion—do not rotate the airway as you do for adults
- Artificial ventilations—use appropriate size masks and use only enough volume to make the chest rise

Common causes of shock in infants and children are:

- Diarrhea and/or vomiting leading to dehydration
- Infection
- Trauma
- Blood loss

Children compensate for shock differently than adults do. Once they start developing signs and symptoms, their condition worsens rapidly. Any patient who has the potential for going into shock should be treated with high-flow oxygen, kept warm, and transported as quickly as possible.

Signs of shock in the pediatric patient include:

- Rapid pulse rate
- Rapid respiratory rate

- Pale, cool, clammy skin
- Weak or absent peripheral pulses
- Delayed capillary refill
- Decreased urinary output
- Altered mental status

Respiratory distress is very serious in children. Cardiac arrest in pediatric patients is not typically caused by a malfunctioning heart but by respiratory failure or trauma. It is important to recognize early signs of respiratory distress and provide care before it leads to respiratory failure and/or arrest. You must determine whether the respiratory distress is caused by an obstruction or by disease because the care is different. Signs of respiratory distress include:

- Retractions of accessory muscles
- Nasal flaring
- Abdominal-muscle use
- Stridor
- Wheezing
- Grunting
- Respiratory rate over 60
- Cyanosis
- Decreased muscle tone
- Capillary refill greater than 2 seconds
- Altered mental status
- Decreased heart rate (late sign)

Treatment includes high-flow oxygen, assisted or artificial ventilations if needed, and rapid transport. The patient must continually be reassessed for airway, breathing, and circulation.

Other medical emergencies that are common in pediatric patients are:

- Fever
- Diarrhea and vomiting
- Seizures
- Poisoning
- Altered mental status from a variety of conditions

Sudden infant death syndrome (SIDS) is the sudden death of an otherwise healthy baby in its first year of life. This usually occurs while the child is sleeping. The cause of these deaths is undetermined. Treat the baby as you would any other baby in cardiac arrest and give the parents as much emotional support as possible.

Trauma is the leading cause of death in children. Treating their injuries is basically the same as for adults; however, their anatomical differences create different injury patterns.

- Head—larger in proportion to their bodies, more susceptible to injury
- Chest—structures less developed, less protection for internal organs
- Abdomen—muscles not as strong, less protection for internal organs

Burns are common in children. Remember that their BSA is larger in proportion to their body mass; therefore, maintaining body heat is more challenging. Be cautious using moist dressings on a pediatric burn patient.

Child abuse takes several forms including:

- Psychological
- Neglect
- Physical
- Sexual

Signs of physical abuse include the following:

- Bruising with specific shapes, slap marks, burn marks from cigarettes
- Injuries in various stages of healing
- Broken bones
- Head injuries
- Abdominal injuries
- Bite marks
- Bulging fontanelles indicating possible shaken infant syndrome

Be suspicious of abuse if you notice:

- Repeated calls for same child or children in a family
- Past injuries
- Poorly healing wounds or improperly healed fractures
- Past or recent burns
- Multiple types of injuries to both front and back of the body
- Child fearful of describing how the injury occurred

Also observe the adults involved for inappropriate behavior regarding the emergency.

Signs of sexual abuse include:

- Burns or wounds to the genitalia
- Any unexplained genital injury
- Seminal fluid on the body or clothes of the patient

In cases of suspected sexual abuse, it is important that you preserve as much of the evidence as possible. You must report any suspicions of physical or sexual abuse to the medical staff.

You will encounter children who have special medical needs. Many children with health issues can live at home with the assistance of medical technology. The parents of these children tend to be very well educated regarding their child's condition, needs, and supportive equipment. Common devices you may encounter in an emergency are:

- Tracheostomy tube
- Home ventilators
- Central intravenous lines
- Gastrostomy tubes
- Gastric feeding tubes
- Shunts

Pediatric calls can be the most stressful events that EMTs are involved with. Proper training and frequent review of your skills will give you confidence to treat your patient during the call. Utilize department counseling or a local Critical Incident Stress Management team after stressful calls.

MED MINUTE

Many of the medications used for the adult patient are also used for the pediatric patient. Refer to the appropriate disease or pathology chapter of your Emergency Care textbook for more on medications that may be used in pediatrics. Fever reducers are drugs that may be utilized for the adult but are most commonly associated with the pediatric patient. Aspirin, although it is an antipyretic agent, is not recommended for use in children. This table gives examples of common drugs. Dozens of medications may be available with similar effects.

CLASS OF MEDICATION	MEDICATION NAME(S)	MECHANISM OF ACTION
Antipyretics (fever reducers)	Ibuprofen (Motrin, Advil, and Pediaprofen) Acetaminophen (Tylenol)	Reduce body temperature by stimulating the hypothalamus (temperature-regulation center of the brain) to cool the core temperature.

PATHOPHYSIOLOGY PEARLS

In the first several years of life, a human being experiences significant physical, mental, and emotional development, changing from a small helpless newborn, dependant upon others for his every need, to a young adult who is independent and able to make complex decisions and provide for his own needs.

From birth to 2 years of age, the body is in a rapid stage of growth. During this time, body weight will quadruple. As the brain grows and the neural pathways become more efficient, the infant's gross motor skills develop. By age two, the infant has an idea of basic concepts. Language skills develop from crying, to one or two words, to short sentences. Basic reactions develop into conscious responses.

From 2 to 6 years of age, the brain continues to grow and fine motor skills develop. The body is stronger and more adultlike in proportion. Large body movements, such as running and jumping, are improved and these school-age children are very active. Gender differences in motor skills become apparent. Mental capabilities continue to develop and they now use representation and symbols to express themselves. In just six short years, vocabulary has developed from one or two words to nearly 14,000 words. Children in this group actively use role-playing to interact with others and develop social skills. At this stage of development, children start developing independence, preparing themselves for the future.

From 7 to 10 years of age, growth slows down. The greater heart and lung capacity lead to greater strength and endurance. Like the Energizer Bunny™, this age group can keep on going and going. Mental capacity increases and children of this age start understanding logical principles and analytical thinking. At this stage in life, the child becomes more involved not only with family but also in a variety of outside activities.

From 10 to 20 years of age, major changes again occur as the child becomes a young adult. Puberty usually begins between 8 and 14 years of age. Normally, within a year of the onset of puberty, physical changes begin and a growth spurt occurs. During this time, there are increases in height, weight, and musculature. Growth proceeds from the extremities to the torso, often resulting in a rapid change in height. Near the end of puberty, menarche begins in girls and ejaculation begins in boys. It is also during this time that teenagers undergo a sense of indestructibility. This is a major factor in the risky lifestyle that often leads to severe injury or worse. Mentally, these teenagers begin to understand difficult concepts and articulate general principles and theories. Emotionally, these teenagers often attempt to test authority in their efforts to experiment with independence.

For a human being, the period in which the development from a helpless newborn to a young adult takes place is both a rewarding and a confusing one for the child and the parents. The development of a human being depends on a combination of both nature (hereditary makeup) and the nurture (support and environment) that is provided.

REVIEW QUESTIONS

SHORT ANSWER

1. Explain the oxygen "blow-by" technique.

2. What is a shunt?

MULTIPLE CHOICE

1. Intracranial pressure caused by trauma or _____ may result in fontanelle bulging.
   A. epiglottitis
   B. viral croup
   C. meningitis
   D. anaphylaxis

2. When dealing with parents who have lost a child to SIDS, it is appropriate to express your sorrow for their loss, but only after _____.
   A. determining that they are not at fault
   B. a physician has informed them of the child's death
   C. you have exhausted all resuscitative efforts
   D. attending a stress debriefing

3. _____ is the number-one cause of death in infants and children in the United States.
   A. Drowning
   B. Leukemia
   C. Trauma
   D. Secondhand smoke

4. When treating a child for sexual assault, never _____.
   A. examine the child's genitalia
   B. discourage the child from urinating or defecating
   C. "control your emotions"
   D. say anything that would make the patient feel responsible for the event

5. When a pediatric patient acts younger than his age while under stress, it is called _____.
   A. regression
   B. episodic progression
   C. conversion
   D. stress reorientation

SCENARIO QUESTIONS

You are dispatched to the county fair for an accident on one of the mechanical rides in the children's carnival area. Apparently, a 5-year-old child was thrown from a spinning ride into the side of a metal drum being used as a garbage can. Upon your arrival, you find the child unresponsive in his mother's arms, breathing normally and with blood still dripping from a laceration that extends from the lateral end of his left eyebrow to just superior to the left ear.

1. To insert an oropharyngeal airway in this patient, you should _____.
   A. use the jaw-thrust maneuver
   B. initially insert it upside down and then rotate it into position
   C. check for a gag reflex with your gloved finger
   D. insert it with the tip pointing downward using a tongue depressor

2. You will want to conduct ongoing assessments of this patient *at least* every _____.
   A. 7 to 10 minutes   B. 15 minutes
   C. 6 to 8 miles   D. 5 minutes

3. This patient should be transported while _____.
   A. secured to a spine board   B. in his mother's arms
   C. in the shock position   D. lying on his right side

You are shopping at the grocery store when a woman in the next aisle begins shouting for someone to help her baby. You look around the corner and see a woman frantically hugging a 4- to 5-month-old screaming infant. You see blood dripping from the child's hair. You identify yourself as an EMT-B and ask whether you can help. "I dropped him," she tells you through her tears. "I was trying to reach something on a shelf and I dropped my baby!" You calmly remind her that it was an accident and assess the child's head. You find a small scalp laceration that is bleeding steadily and a bulging anterior fontanelle. You ask a responding store employee to call for emergency services.

1. _____ poses the greatest initial danger to this child's life.
   A. A spinal injury   B. An airway obstruction
   C. Shock   D. A fractured skull

2. The bulging anterior fontanelle is most likely caused by _____.
   A. increased intracranial pressure   B. an impact hematoma
   C. traumatic hypertension   D. the child's crying

3. This patient's scalp wound should be considered _____.
   A. life threatening   B. superficial
   C. radiating   D. secondary

You respond to a residence for a 4-year-old girl who was accidentally run over by her mother's car as she played in the driveway of the home. You arrive to find the girl's mother hysterical while the father holds the crying child. On the basis of your observations of the driveway and the environment around the child, you know that she has lost a good deal of blood from several lacerations. She has a patent airway, her respiratory rate is 28 and her blood pressure is 90 over 64 with a capillary refill time of about 2 seconds.

1. This patient's blood pressure _____.

   A. indicates decompensated shock

   B. is normal

   C. is warning you of the child's impending death

   D. is too low

2. The best way to calm this child's mother is to _____.

   A. lead her a short distance away and explain that she is not to blame and that everything that can be done will be done for the child

   B. ask her to help calm the child

   C. have the father walk her away from the scene while you continue treating the patient

   D. tell her in a direct, authoritative tone to calm down

3. This child's liver and _____ are especially susceptible to trauma due to their larger size and lack of developed protection in the abdomen.

   A. stomach   **B.** pancreas

   C. kidneys   **D.** spleen

C A S E   S T U D I E S

CASE STUDY 1	SHE WAS CHOKING—BUT SHE'S FINE NOW

You are dispatched to a residence for a child choking. Upon your arrival, you are met out in front of the house by a parent who is apologizing for having called you. He states that his 18-month-old is now fine but was choking on a coin just a few minutes ago. His wife performed abdominal thrusts and managed to dislodge the object and now the baby girl is breathing just fine. He is very apologetic and insists there is no longer a problem.

1. How will you manage this situation?

2. What are your concerns since you know the child had an object forcibly removed from the airway?

The father reluctantly allows you into the house to see for yourself that the child is now fine. Upon entering the house, you find the mother seated on the couch clutching the child in her arms. The child is alert and stares at you as you enter. The mother appears to be sobbing.

   As you approach the child and kneel down to examine her, the father says, "See, she's fine. Now you guys can get on your way and save someone who is really hurt." The child begins to cry as you get closer. You notice several large bruises on the child's back as well as bruises encircling the child's right upper arm. Your gut tells you there is more to this situation than first appears.

1. What factors at this scene concern you and why?

2. Do you have any obligation to report your suspicions and, if so, to whom will you report them?

CASE STUDY 2   MY GRANDSON IS HAVING TROUBLE BREATHING

It is about 8:00 P.M. when you are dispatched to a residence where a child is reportedly having trouble breathing. Many things run through your mind, including nervousness as you realize that respiratory problems in children can be quite severe.

You arrive to find an anxious grandfather who leads you to a 19-month-old child who seems to be having respiratory distress. You find the child sitting up in bed and looking toward you as you arrive. He is in his grandmother's arms and buries his head into her as you approach.

1. What parts of the assessment triangle have you observed thus far and what else do you need to know for the "from-the-doorway" assessment?

2. How does the "from-the-doorway" assessment bridge to the initial assessment?

The child continues to avoid eye contact with you and seeks the shelter of his grandmother, which you consider a good sign. You observe the patient as having slight supraclavicular and intercostal retractions. The grandparents tell you that the child has not been himself and has a slight fever that began earlier that day. You note that the child has a hoarse, barking cough. Your partner prepares oxygen for the patient.

1. How will oxygen be administered to the patient?

2. What vital signs will you obtain on this patient?

You find that the patient's pulse is 124, respirations 32, and capillary refill time is less than 2 seconds. The patient's mental status remains the same as he is hidden in his grandmother's arms.

1. What do these vital signs mean? Are they within normal limits?

Active Exploration

Pediatric patients can be some of the most challenging and rewarding you will encounter as an EMT-B. When bad things happen to children, it is a challenge both physically and emotionally. It is a challenge physically because you are so accustomed to treating adult patients that you tend to forget children require special care and techniques. Pediatric emergencies are emotionally challenging because it is difficult to see such a young person, who is so innocent and vulnerable, in any type of distress, especially when it involves severe trauma.

On average, 10 percent of the typical EMS call volume will involve pediatric patients. For this reason alone, many EMT-Bs do not have the amount of experience they would like to have under their belts when treating a critical child.

The following activities will help you become more familiar with the differences and challenges faced when treating the pediatric patient.

Activity 1: Getting to Know You

One of the reasons many EMTs are uncomfortable around pediatric patients is simply the fact that they do not have much experience treating them. This next activity will help you become more comfortable assessing and interacting with a pediatric patient.

There is a pretty good chance that you have either a pediatric family member or a friend with a small child or infant. Explain to them that you would like some experience assessing a pediatric patient and whether they would allow you to perform a simple detailed physical on their child. Explain in detail to the parent what is involved with the EMT detailed physical exam, and perhaps perform the exam on them so they get a better understanding of it.

Have the parent ask the child whether it is all right to have you examine him and explain carefully what is involved. Demonstrate what you will be doing on the parent so the child can see that it does not hurt.

With both the parent's and child's permission, perform the detailed physical exam starting from the feet and working your way to the head. Move slowly and explain to the child exactly what you are doing and what you might be looking for.

Depending on the age of the child, you may or may not get verbal feedback from him. If possible, attempt the exam with the "patient" in both the supine position and while being held in the parent's arms.

How do these two positions differ in terms of your ability to perform a thorough exam?

Activity 2: Mandatory Reporter

Most states have identified specific individuals who are mandated by law to report evidence of suspected child abuse or neglect. In most, if not all states, EMTs are included in this list.

This activity will have you research the laws in your state that define who must report such cases and to whom they must be reported. Using the Internet and individuals you know who are already working in the EMS field, find answers to the following questions:

1. Identify the laws/statutes or regulations that require EMTs to report suspected cases of child abuse and/or neglect.

2. Make a list of the other specific professions or individuals listed in the law who must report such cases, for example, clergy, teachers, and so on.

3. Ask someone you know who currently works in EMS whether they know the law and whether there is a specific company policy addressing this issue.

4. To whom do they report such cases and by what means, written or verbal?

5. What is the difference between abuse and neglect and how might you identify each?

As horrible as it is, child abuse and neglect is a major problem in our society. Staying informed as to your responsibility should you encounter such a case is very important.

RETRO REVIEW

1. The most common advance directive that an EMT-B will see is a(n) _____.
   A. medical-identification device
   B. emergency-vehicle operation manual
   C. do-not-resuscitate order
   D. regional or local protocol

2. Documenting that a patient with a head injury did not lose consciousness is considered a _____.

    A. subjective statement   **B.** pertinent positive

    C. substantive estimation   **D.** pertinent negative

3. _____ collisions tend to cause up-and-over or down-and-under injury patterns.

    A. Rear-end   **B.** "T-bone"

    C. Head-on   **D.** Rotational-impact

THINKING AND LINKING

CHAPTER TOPIC	HOW IT RELATES TO YOU AND OTHER COURSE AREAS
Treating infants and children	You can help counteract the stress related to treating pediatric patients by maintaining your own healthy lifestyle (Chapter 2), striving to be a more effective communicator—which will help with the patients *and* their parents (Chapter 13)—and practicing, practicing, practicing. Nothing reduces anxiety like being prepared.
Hypothermia	When you are treating infants or small children outside (auto crashes, swimming pools, and so on) or in a cool environment (ice-skating rinks, air-conditioned venues), remember to keep them covered with clothing, blankets, or even coats any time that you do not absolutely need them exposed (Chapter 22).
Abuse	You may respond to pediatric calls involving suspected sexual or physical abuse. It is imperative for the well-being of the child that you maintain your professional demeanor (Chapter 1). After the call, you may want to talk about your feelings to other healthcare professionals individually or in a CISD-type setting (Chapter 2). Remember to use your local reporting procedures for notifying the appropriate agencies about abuse (Chapter 14).

32

Geriatric Patients

CHAPTER SUMMARY

EMS calls involving geriatric patients can be very challenging. Each person's body and mind ages differently, so what may be perfectly normal for one geriatric patient may be the sign of something serious in another. Family and caregivers need to be relied on to confirm whether the behavior or condition is normal for that particular patient. Common causes requiring EMS response for an elderly person include:

- Cardiac problems
- Respiratory problems
- Neurological problems
- Injuries from a fall
- Complaints of general illness

Conditions unrelated to the emergency, such as hearing or sight impairment and dementia, can make communicating with the geriatric patient difficult. It is important to situate yourself in a position that allows the patient to see and hear you.

Assessing the geriatric patient is the same as for any other patient, with a few special considerations:

- Scene size-up—Pay close attention to the general condition of the environment in which they live.
- Assessing mental status—What is the patient's normal baseline mental status?
- Assessing the airway—Opening the airway may be difficult due to arthritis. Are there ill-fitting dentures?
- Assess breathing.
- Assess circulation—An irregular pulse may be normal for a particular patient.

- Assessing priority—Geriatric patients are less likely to show severe symptoms and tend to have "vague" complaints.
- Accurate history may be difficult to obtain unless a well-informed family member or caregiver is present.
- Physical exam—Geriatric patients may have a very high or very low threshold for pain. Changes in the spine can make immobilizing a trauma patient challenging.
- Baseline vitals—A geriatric patient's vitals may be outside the "normal" range but normal for that patient.

An older patient's condition will typically deteriorate slowly, so it is important to reassess often and take note of even subtle changes.

The following are common reasons why the elderly need EMS:

- *Pharmacology*—The patient may be on numerous medications, all prescribed from one doctor or from several. There is the potential for the patient to become accidentally undermedicated, overmedicated, or have medications react negatively together.
- *Shortness of breath*—In addition to asthma, the older population can develop diseases such as emphysema and pulmonary edema. Shortness of breath can also be the chief complaint of a patient having a heart attack.
- *Chest pain*—This can be caused by angina, myocardial infarction, pneumonia, or by an aneurysm.
- *Altered mental status*—Common causes are hypoglycemia, hypoxia, stroke, medications, hypothermia, and generalized infections.
- *Abdominal pain*—This can be caused by an abdominal aortic aneurysm, bowel obstruction, or diverticulitis. Abdominal pain in the elderly should always be considered serious.
- *Complaints of general illness*—Dizziness, weakness, and generally not feeling well are vague complaints that can be signs of serious conditions such as internal bleeding or cardiac problems.
- *Depression and suicide*—Depression is very common in the older population. Report any observations of depression or mention of suicide to the emergency department personnel.
- *Falls*—It is important to determine the reason for the fall as well as to treat any injuries sustained in the fall. Your patient may have broken a hip as a result of the fall, but the reason he fell may be due to an abnormal heart rhythm that made him dizzy.
- *Abuse and neglect*—As with younger patients, the elderly patient who relies on others for care may be a victim of abuse or neglect. This may range from neglecting personal needs and hygiene to physical and financial abuse.

One of the biggest concerns for most elderly patients is their loss of independence because of a serious illness or injury. Listening to your patients' concerns and being supportive can help reassure them.

MED MINUTE

Prescription medications account for an exorbitant number of hospital admissions each year. Geriatric patients are highly susceptible to complications from medications because of the number of medications they can be prescribed, often by multiple physicians who do not always consider drug compatibility.

EXAMPLE 1

Consider a patient who has been put on a calcium channel blocker like Cardizem (diltiazem) by his cardiologist and on Tagamet by his family physician. Although these drugs seem to be completely unrelated, they can work together to have negative effects on the patient. Tagamet has been shown to increase the levels of diltiazem in the blood and as a result, the standard dose of diltiazem may actually be too high for the patient, leading to potentially lethal hypotension.

EXAMPLE 2

A patient has been prescribed lithium by his psychiatrist several years ago and continues to take it for a diagnosis of manic depression. Later, the patient is diagnosed by his cardiologist with congestive heart failure and is placed on Lasix. Again, these medications appear to have no relationship to one another and neither physician may realize that interactions exist or that the patient is on the other medication and the opportunity for cross-reactivity exists. Lasix has been shown to slow the speed of lithium elimination and, as a result, the patient may suffer from high levels of lithium and could eventually become lithium toxic.

EXAMPLE 3

A commonly discussed and potentially lethal drug combination is that of erectile-dysfunction medications (Viagra, Levitra, and so on) with nitroglycerin. Both agents cause vasodilation and, just as the previous examples stated, have little to do with each other. The patient's primary care physician and cardiologist could prescribe these medications, and despite good intentions, the patient may experience a hypotensive emergency and could possibly die.

There are many drugs with the potential for reacting and interacting, so it is important to understand that because of their various healthcare complications and needs, geriatric patients with multiple physicians are at significant risk for medication errors and emergencies.

PATHOPHYSIOLOGY PEARLS

It happens to all of us; each day we get a little older. According to the National Center for Health Statistics, the life expectancy for those born in the year 2000 is 76.9 years. This is up from 73.7 years for those born in 1980.[1] This is an increase of about 4.3 percent in over 20 years. If this trend continues, life expectancy will reach 80 by 2020. Certainly, people age differently. Both genetics and lifestyle play a major role in aging, disease processes, and life expectancy.

It is no secret that as we grow older our bodies and minds change. Physically, the most notable changes are in appearance. Changes in the skin and underlying tissues are visible signs of aging. As we get older, we have a

---

1 *Centers for Disease Control and Prevention, National Center for Health Statistics.* Birth, Infant Mortality, and Live Expectancy, 1980–2000. *U.S. Department of Health and Human Services.* www.cdc.gov/nchs/SSBR/023tab.htm.

decline in the abilities of our sense organs. Hearing, seeing, and temperature-sensing capabilities are not as keen as they were in our younger years. Not necessarily as obvious are the changes in body systems. All the body systems function at less than optimal capacity. These changes make us more susceptible to disease and injury.

As we get older, our abilities to receive, organize, interpret, and retrieve information diminish—sort of like your computer hard drive. The more information you save, the more time it takes to process and retrieve that information. Diseases, circulatory problems, depression, and medications all have the potential to impair mental abilities.

Many people (you may even have noticed yourself doing this as you age) will compensate for their physical and mental decline. They may "read" lips more or ask you to speak up a little. They may use glasses to improve eyesight. They may adjust the room temperature to be more comfortable. There are any number of subtle, and sometimes not so subtle, ways to compensate for a decline in physical and mental capabilities.

During the later years, many emotional changes also occur. Retirement, relocation, and loss of friends or relatives all take their toll. One of the most important components of a quality lifestyle is having a good support network of family and friends. Through such a network, the potential for the geriatric patient to thrive is great.

REVIEW QUESTIONS

SHORT ANSWER

1. What is a "triple A"?

2. Explain the difference between diverticul*itis* and diverticul*osis*.

MULTIPLE CHOICE

1. _____ can increase the effects of certain cardiac medications.
   - **A.** Lemons
   - **B.** Whole milk
   - **C.** Grapefruit juice
   - **D.** Beets

2. *Herpes zoster* is more commonly known as _____.
   - **A.** shingles
   - **B.** chicken pox
   - **C.** cold sores
   - **D.** hives

3. Why can assessing an elderly patient's mental status be very difficult?
   - **A.** Elderly patients tend to be uncooperative around people with whom they are unfamiliar.
   - **B.** An altered mental status can indicate a wide variety of ailments.
   - **C.** Many elderly people are ornery and intentionally become a challenge to assess.
   - **D.** An altered mental status may be part of the patient's baseline condition.

4. Elderly males are the segment of the population most likely to _____.
   - **A.** develop colitis
   - **B.** commit suicide
   - **C.** require intubation
   - **D.** neglect their health

5. An older person having a heart attack may present with _____.
   - **A.** sharp chest pain and tremors
   - **B.** hemiparesis
   - **C.** sudden weakness and *no* chest pain
   - **D.** left arm spasms and aching

SCENARIO QUESTIONS

You arrive at the Shady Glen Care Home after being dispatched for a resident who has fallen. You find the patient, a 93-year-old female, sitting in a wheel chair and yelling incoherently while running the fingers of her right hand over her hip. The LVN (Licensed Vocational Nurse) tells you that the patient suffers from Alzheimer's and is rarely ever oriented. You ask about the fall and are told, "She was shuffling down the hallway and then yelled out and collapsed onto the floor. When we were helping her into the chair, I noticed that she didn't seem able to use her right leg. She's been agitated and rubbing her hip since then." You attempt to speak to the patient, and she answers inappropriately and seems confused.

1. What is most likely to be this patient's immediate problem?
   - **A.** Confusion caused by her Alzheimer's.
   - **B.** A stroke.
   - **C.** A hip or proximal femur fracture.
   - **D.** Transient bradycardia.

2. Should you assume that this patient's altered mental status is related to the fall and subsequent injuries?
   - **A.** Yes, always anticipate the worst.
   - **B.** No, she did not receive a head injury.
   - **C.** Yes, the patient may have suffered a stroke.
   - **D.** No, the LVN explained that it is a chronic condition.

Your unit is dispatched to a residence for an elderly man who is complaining of abdominal discomfort. Upon your arrival, you find the patient (an 84-year-old male) sitting comfortably in a recliner. The patient is responsive, pleasant, and tells you that he had just returned from a walk to the park. You ask about his stomach pain and he tells you that it is "no big deal." While your partner starts to obtain vitals, you ask, "Did the pain start while you were at the park?" He laughs, "The park? I haven't been to the park in ages."

1. Due to _____, serious abdominal problems may cause only slight discomfort in elderly patients.
   - **A.** occluded neural pathways
   - **B.** decreased sensitivity to pain
   - **C.** reduced central circulation
   - **D.** organic necrosis

2. This patient presents as a good example of _____.
   - **A.** confabulation
   - **B.** the "1-percent rule"
   - **C.** neuropathy
   - **D.** transient dementia

CASE STUDIES

You are dispatched to an assisted-living facility for a fall victim. Upon your arrival, you are escorted to the third-floor stairwell where you find an approximately 80-year-old female who was found this morning down and injured. She is cold and shivering and responsive to verbal stimulus. The facility manager states that she found Mrs. Brewer this morning and does not know how long she had been in the stairwell. She was last seen just after dinner the evening before.

Your initial assessment finds Mrs. Brewer's respirations shallow at 12 times per minute. Her pulse is 64, weak and irregular and her blood pressure is 104/62. Her skin is pale and cool, and she is not completely aware of what is happening to her.

1. Will you provide any treatment for Mrs. Brewer during the initial assessment?

2. What assessment path do you feel is most appropriate for Mrs. Brewer?

Your physical assessment reveals pain in her right hip and right shoulder. In the few minutes that she has been on oxygen, she seems to be getting more responsive and is able to communicate better. When you ask her how long she has been lying there, she is not sure because she thinks she may have fallen asleep for a while. She is unable to tell you what day it is. You notice that her right leg is rotated inward and appears shorter than the left.

1. What may be the problem with Mrs. Brewer's right leg or side?

2. How will you treat Mrs. Brewer's hip injury, and how will you get her out of the building?

You are called to a residence for a fall. The patient, who appears to be in his 80s, is sitting in a chair at the kitchen table talking with his son who came in to check on him. The son greets you and tells you he found his father on the living-room floor when he arrived today. After he looked his father over, he did not think he had had a fall after all, but he does believe his father "just isn't right." The patient slowly acknowledges your presence. "He just seems slower to me," his son explains.

1. What is the patient's chief complaint?

2. How would you determine whether the patient fell or not?

You concur that the patient does not seem injured although he is slow to answer your questions. He knows the approximate time of day but not the date. He has asked you twice what you were doing there. The son stops by daily to make sure his father has food and that his father's medications are in the labeled pill container that has seven rows (one for each day of the week) and four columns (morning, afternoon, evening, bedtime). His son acknowledges that his father has been "slipping a bit mentally" but is worse today.

1. What are some potential causes of the patient's worsening mental status today?

2. How would you evaluate the causes you have identified?

You examine the patient's medicine container and find that he has gone across the top row rather than down the left-hand rows. After some quick calculations, his son figures out that his father has more than doubled his antidepressant medication and tripled his water-pill doses.

You transport the patient and contact medical direction regarding the potential overdose. Knowing you have a role in prevention, you discuss the issue of the "fall" and medication problems with the nurse who makes a notation on the chart and will involve the hospital's social worker.

Active Exploration

It is no secret that the number of people over the age of 65 is increasing at an alarming rate. According to the federal government general accounting office, nearly 25 percent of the nation's population will be over the age of 65 by the year 2075. To those who will be working in the field of EMS, this statistic means that the number of calls involving geriatric patients is going to increase.

Much like pediatric patients, the elderly have their own unique set of needs and problems that will challenge even the most experienced EMT-B. The following exercises are designed to help you increase your awareness of the unique needs of the geriatric patient and help you become better at providing emergency care for them.

Activity 1: Feeling for (and like) the Patient

This first exercise will help you gain an appreciation of some of the difficulties geriatric patients must overcome in their daily lives. You will need a few supplies for this activity as well as two of your fellow classmates to help you.

Here is a list of what you will need for this activity:

1. One set of ear plugs
2. One ear-protection head set
3. One pair of latex gloves
4. Ten popsicle sticks or tongue depressors
5. One pair of safety glasses
6. One small jar of Vaseline®
7. One deck of playing cards

You are going to simulate three of the most common disabilities that geriatric patients face every day of their lives.

- Rub a small amount of Vaseline® over the lenses of the safety glasses and ask one of your partners to wear them. This will simulate the poor vision that is common in older patients.
- Have another partner don the latex gloves and place a stick down the inside of each finger. This will simulate the severe arthritis that many elderly patients suffer from.
- The third person will place the ear plugs in his ears and don the protective ear muffs. Many elderly patients are hard of hearing and this will recreate this disability.

Now all of you will engage in a friendly game of "Go Fish," attempting to deal with and overcome the respective disability. While it is not possible to recreate what it is really like to have one of these disabilities, let alone all of them all at once, it can provide the EMT-B with a little more insight into some of the challenges faced by the elderly.

Activity 2: Older and Wiser

As you have already learned from reading Chapter 32 in your Emergency Care textbook, the percentage of elderly Americans is growing rapidly. For this reason, the likelihood that you will encounter more elderly patients grows as well. Like pediatric patients, the elderly have their own set of unique characteristics that the EMT-B must understand and deal with. This next activity will serve as a means of developing a better understanding of the elderly and becoming more comfortable with interfacing with them.

Identify an elderly person who would be willing to participate in a practice detailed history and physical exam. This person should be at least 70 years old and older if possible. You will want to spend approximately 30 to 60 minutes with this person, interacting as if you were an EMT-B who had been called to his home for an injury or illness. Complete the following tasks during your time with your subject:

1. Begin by conducting a thorough medical history of your subject.
2. Discuss the experience of aging with him and ask him the greatest challenges that he faces and how you as an EMT-B might help him overcome those challenges.
3. If possible, conduct a detailed physical exam of the subject and make notes of the major differences that you notice between him and the fellow students you are used to practicing on.
4. Discuss your experience with some of your fellow students who have completed the same activity.

There simply is no substitute for adequate preparation. As an EMT-B, you will eventually encounter a wide variety of patients with differing complaints and of various ages. Getting as much experience as possible before you are faced with the real thing will be of great benefit to both you and your patients.

RETRO REVIEW

1. Pediatric febrile seizures are caused by _____.
   - **A.** head injuries
   - **B.** high fever
   - **C.** anxiety
   - **D.** epilepsy

2. History of the present illness, SAMPLE history, focused physical exam, and _____ are the four parts of a focused history and physical exam for a medical patient.
   - **A.** transportation
   - **B.** vital signs
   - **C.** interventions
   - **D.** detailed physical exam

3. You are caring for a 22-year-old female patient who is in active labor with her first child. The contractions are regular and about 4 minutes apart. During a visual exam of the patient's vaginal area, you notice that the umbilical cord is presenting. What should you do?

   A. Cut and tie the cord, advise the mother to begin pushing, and transport immediately.

   B. Elevate the mother's buttocks, administer oxygen, wrap the exposed cord with saline-soaked gauze, and transport immediately.

   C. Gently push the cord back into the vagina and cover the vaginal opening with a sterile gauze pad. Then, place the mother in the Trendelenburg position and transport immediately.

   D. Elevate the mother's buttocks, administer oxygen, wrap the exposed cord with a sterile towel, insert several gloved fingers into the mother's vagina to keep the baby off the cord, and transport immediately.

THINKING AND LINKING

CHAPTER TOPIC	HOW IT RELATES TO YOU AND OTHER COURSE AREAS
Communication	Older patients can sometimes pose a challenge to effective communication (Chapter 13). You will find that strokes (Chapter 19), medications (Chapter 15), dental problems, mental disorders (Chapter 23) and, at times, plain orneriness will affect your ability to talk to the patient. Above all, be understanding of elderly patients. The last time that your patient saw his spouse alive may have been in the back of an ambulance just like yours—in which case, a good deal of anxiety would be normal (Chapter 2).
Mental status	You will find that an older patient's altered mental status (Chapter 19) will sometimes become apparent through bizarre answers, statements, or incessant repetition. It is important to maintain your demeanor—although your patient may be very confused about the situation, he *will* know if you are not taking him seriously. Remember that some mentally altered elderly patients will refuse emergency care and some may even become combative (review Chapter 3).
Pharmacology	Many of your elderly patients will take quite a few different medications (Chapter 15). Although you do not need to know all of the prescription drugs available, it is a good idea to become familiar with some of the more common ones. This will help when the patient cannot actually tell you his medical history (Chapter 9).

CHAPTER

33

Ambulance Operations

CHAPTER SUMMARY

Once just a basic way to transport sick or injured people to the hospital, modern ambulances are a technologically advanced way to bring the emergency department to the patient. Ambulance services have evolved from the undertaker's hearse to the current, fully equipped medium-duty trucks—and they will continue to evolve as technology and prehospital emergency care advances.

An ambulance that is not fully stocked and prepared for patient emergency care is useless. A recommended equipment and supply list has been compiled by the American College of Surgeons and various ambulance services; find out what your particular agency requires and ensure that the ambulance is stocked appropriately. You will find that most supply lists will include items from several main categories. These are control/comfort/protection supplies, initial/focused-assessment equipment, patient-transfer equipment, airway-maintenance/ventilation/resuscitation equipment, oxygen-therapy/ suction equipment, cardiac-resuscitation equipment, bone-immobilization equipment, wound-care/shock treatment supplies, childbirth supplies, road/extrication safety equipment, and supplies (including equipment and medication) for acute poisonings, snake bites, chemical burns, and diabetic emergencies. Some systems require ambulances to have a locked area stocked with narcotic medications and supplies for the exclusive use of paramedics or physicians.

Having the most technologically advanced and well-stocked ambulance staffed by the highest-trained crew in the region will not help a single patient if the engine will not start. Each ambulance service should have a preventive-maintenance program that includes periodic servicing such as oil changes, tire rotations, and so on. Always check with the crew who is coming off duty to see whether they noticed any problems with the ambulance, and then inspect it carefully before you leave.

300

While the engine is off, you will want to check the body condition (to ensure no damage is hindering vehicle operation), the tires and wheels (looking for damage or wear and tread depth—do not forget the inside set of tires on vehicles with dual rear tires), the windows and mirrors (are they all clean, functional, and unbroken?), the operation of all doors and latches, the coolant level and system hoses (waiting for the engine to cool beforehand), the engine fluid levels (oil, brake, power steering, and so on), the battery (or batteries), the upholstery (for damage and cleanliness), the horn, the siren, the seat belts (retraction and latches), and the fuel level.

Then turn the engine on and inspect the dash-indicator lights (do any stay on—indicating a possible problem?), the gauges (for proper operation), the brake pedal (does it compress correctly?), the parking brake, the steering system, the windshield-wiper system, the lighting system (both emergency and standard vehicle lights), the heating/cooling systems (both driver and patient compartments), the transmission-fluid level, and the communications equipment (including portable radios).

Finally, you will inspect the patient compartment and any exterior cabinets. You will check for damage, cleanliness, proper functioning of equipment, and ensure that all needed supplies are present. Restock any deficiencies and let your supervisor know if something cannot be replaced or if equipment is malfunctioning. You will conclude by thoroughly cleaning the interior (for infection control) and the exterior (for public image).

Every agency will have a checklist to guide you through the entire vehicle- and equipment-check-out process.

Now that the ambulance is fully stocked and operational safely, how does the crew get called into action?

In most areas of the country, a person simply dials 911 on any phone and is connected to an emergency medical dispatcher (EMD)—who will, in turn, dispatch the agency most appropriate for the caller's situation (police, fire, or ambulance). Most EMDs are trained to interrogate callers, assign call priorities, provide prearrival medical instructions, continually update responding crews, and coordinate EMS resources with other public-safety agencies.

EMDs will try to obtain as much information as possible from callers in order to provide the responding crews with enough information to properly prepare for the call. The EMD will ask the caller questions about the exact location of the patient, the callback number, the exact problem, and the patient's age, sex, level of consciousness, and whether the patient is breathing.

If the caller is reporting traffic-crash-related injuries, the EMD will inquire about the number (and types) of vehicles involved, the approximate number of patients, if anyone appears trapped, the exact location of the collision, traffic conditions, downed power lines, fires, and so on.

Many regions require EMS personnel to complete an emergency-vehicle-operations course (EVOC) —which includes classroom and behind-the-wheel sessions. These classes teach that safe ambulance drivers are physically and mentally fit, able to perform under stress, positive thinkers, and tolerant of other drivers. Never drive while under the influence of alcohol or drugs, never drive with a suspended license, always wear required corrective lenses, and be responsible enough to admit when you are too stressed, ill, or fatigued to continue driving.

Every state has driving laws specific to the operators of emergency vehicles, relating to speed, right of way, direction of travel, parking, and so on. These exemptions do not, however, allow you to drive without due regard for the safety of others. Doing so can result in reprimands, citations, lawsuits, and even incarceration.

If you are ever involved in a collision while driving an ambulance, the courts will look at two things: 1) were you operating the emergency vehicle with due regard for the safety of others? and 2) were you responding to a true emergency? Most (if not all) jurisdictions follow the concept that a *true emergency* is a situation in which, based on all available information, you feel that life or limb may be in jeopardy.

Studies indicate that people usually will not see or hear your ambulance until it is 50 to 100 feet from them. Always use sound emergency and defensive driving practices and do not let the lights and siren give you a false sense of security. Ambulances commonly have three types of warning devices: a siren, a horn, and a visual warning system. Sirens are becoming less effective due to overuse (drivers can "tune them out" just like car alarms) and advances in automobile soundproofing and stereo systems. It is very possible that others on the road with you are not even aware of your siren. Studies also show that inexperienced ambulance operators tend to drive unnecessarily faster with the siren on. The siren can be a good warning tool if it is used properly. A good alternative to the siren in traffic is the horn—but only use it in the same situations where you would use the siren.

What do you first notice about an ambulance on its way to an emergency scene? The emergency lights. There are many different configurations, but all of them should make the entire perimeter of the vehicle very obvious from any angle. The best lighting packages will include a variety of differing lights in strategic locations. Never use the vehicle's blinking "hazard lights" or four-way flashers during emergency responses—it will be very confusing to the public. Use lights and sirens for emergencies *only*!

In most situations, it is not necessary to use excessive speed when responding to emergency calls. After all, whose ambulance will arrive at the scene every time: the operator who drives safely and consistently or the one who is constantly jumping from the accelerator to the brake while darting in and out of traffic? If you do not show up (or you require another ambulance to respond to *your* collision)—how much help can you be?

During escorted or multiple-vehicle responses, special care needs to be taken. In fact, many systems do not allow escorts unless the ambulance operator is unfamiliar with the area or patient location and must be assisted by the police. Two of the most common dangers with escorted responses result from assumptions by civilian drivers. If they pull over for one emergency vehicle, it is common for them to pull right back out into the lane once it passes—which is unfortunate if your unit is following the first emergency vehicle. The top danger zone with a multiple- or escorted-vehicle response is the intersection. Sirens can blend and mask the approach of multiple emergency vehicles and once the first vehicle passes, the yielding drivers may go—just in time for *you* to reach the intersection. A recent, comprehensive study shows that the majority of ambulance collisions (many of them fatal) occur on clear days with dry roads—at intersections.

Ambulance response can be affected by numerous factors: day of the week, time of day, weather, road construction, railroads, bridges, tunnels, school zones, and so on. For this reason, you should make yourself very familiar with these areas and times and figure out alternate routes *before* being confronted with a delayed-response situation.

So, you have arrived at a vehicle collision ... now what? As you should expect by now, your first step is to size up the scene and establish danger zones. If you notice fire, escaping fluids, or fumes, park your ambulance at least 100 feet away (upwind and uphill, if possible). You can set up about 50 feet away from the wreckage if there are no fumes, fluids, or fire. If you are the first emergency vehicle on the scene, park in front of the wreckage so approaching traffic can be warned by your lights—just remember that the back end of the ambulance will be vulnerable when unloading equipment or loading a patient. Park safely beyond the wreckage if the scene has already been secured prior to your arrival. Always be very cautious when stopped on or near high-speed roadways, or when the road has hills and curves that may hide your ambulance from approaching vehicles. When backing up the ambulance, you will find that there are many blind spots. It is always a good idea to have a spotter stand to the rear of the vehicle and guide you while backing up. As a final safety note when at the scene, drunk drivers are attracted to red, revolving beacons, so it is better to use the vehicle's blinking amber beacons to identify the presence of your vehicle. Also, make sure you set the parking brake and chock the wheels.

Moving the patient into the ambulance only takes four steps: selecting the appropriate carrying device (which will usually be the wheeled stretcher), packaging the patient for transport, moving the patient to the ambulance, and loading the patient into the ambulance. How you cover the patient will be dictated by the weather—a single sheet or blanket if it is warm, several blankets and a plastic sheet if it is cold and raining. All transported patients must be secured to the patient-carrying device by at least three straps—one at chest level, one at hip or waist level, and the third on the lower extremities.

When transporting the patient to the hospital, you must ensure that the stretcher is secured in the ambulance and that the patient is secured to it in the proper position. Do not forget to continue your ongoing assessments, loosen any of the patient's restrictive clothing, prepare for respiratory/cardiac complications, check bandages/splints, and, perhaps most importantly, reassure the patient.

Pediatric patients can be easily overwhelmed and terrified by crashes, emergency care, and transport with unknown people. Many ambulances carry a soft, sanitized toy to comfort children and you may find that having a female EMT-B or police officer may be helpful in calming a child.

Although two EMT-Bs in the patient compartment are preferable during transport, only one is required by law. En route to the receiving facility, you will have several duties to complete, including notifying the EMD of your departure, continuing emergency care as needed, getting additional patient information, continuing ongoing assessments, obtaining additional vital signs, notifying the receiving facility, and rechecking bandages and splints. Also, remember that simply talking to patients can be soothing to them.

It is your responsibility as the EMT-B in the passenger compartment to direct the ambulance operator. If the swaying of the vehicle is having a negative impact on the patient's condition, you are obligated to tell the driver to slow down and drive more carefully. If the patient's condition becomes critical, it is your responsibility to ask the driver to utilize the emergency lights to reduce the transport time. If the patient develops cardiac arrest, you must tell the driver to stop the vehicle so you can attach the AED and allow the

AED to analyze the rhythm without the potential interference from the movement of the vehicle (always notify the receiving facility if the patient's condition changes).

Although brief, your interaction with the receiving staff is crucial to the continued care of the patient. There may be occasions when the receiving staff is busy with patients who are in a more serious condition than your patient; in this case, remain with your patient and continue to treat him until the hospital can assume care. *Never leave a patient in an emergency department without a proper transfer of care.*

You should assist the receiving staff with your patient, provide a verbal report, indicate any changes in the patient's condition and, after the transfer, complete the prehospital-care report (PCR). You must then make sure that you have transferred all of the patient's personal effects and obtained a release from the hospital.

You will also prepare the ambulance for the next call by cleaning, restocking, and preparing the patient compartment (including remaking the stretcher—which should be neat and professional in appearance.)

If no other calls are pending, you should return to quarters. You should always notify dispatch that you are en route to quarters and whether or not you are available for other calls. You should also take this opportunity to air out the ambulance (if necessary) and to refuel. Once in quarters, you should clean and disinfect the ambulance. Remove linens and properly dispose of them, clean all surfaces and disinfect all nondisposable equipment. Prepare yourself also by washing your hands and changing clothing if necessary. Once you have completed everything, contact dispatch and request to be put back in service.

In some situations, it is better for the patient to be transported by helicopter or fixed-wing aircraft. You should always follow local protocols, but usually air transport is used for several reasons. If traffic conditions or scene location will delay traditional transport of a critical patient, if the appropriate receiving facility for the patient's condition is too far away, or if the patient is a high priority for transport (e.g. in shock, a head injury with altered mental status, and so on), air transport may be requested. You will normally *not* call for air transport for a patient in cardiac arrest unless he is hypothermic.

Air rescue can be requested by police, fire, and EMS command at an incident or by you, as an EMT-B, after consulting with your dispatch center about the situation. In addition to your identifying information, you will need to provide the air rescue dispatcher with the exact location of the incident (including distance to nearby towns or cities and visible landmarks) and the location of the landing zone (LZ).

How do you set up an LZ? A helicopter needs a clear space of approximately 100 feet × 100 feet on ground that does not slope more than about 8°. The area should be free from power lines, antennas, towers, vehicles, people, and so on. Mark the LZ with one flare in an upwind location. During night operations, *never* shine a light into the pilot's eyes—he will be using night-vision equipment that can become "blinded" by white light.

Once you have called for air rescue, set up and properly describe the LZ. How do you approach the helicopter once it is on the ground? Easy: *Never approach a helicopter unless escorted by flight personnel.* Beyond that, *never* walk around the helicopter's tail rotor area and keep all vehicles at least 100 feet (and smoking at least 200 feet) from the aircraft.

PEARLS FROM THE PODIUM

- Cleaning, stocking, and checking your vehicle are not the most exciting parts of EMS but are vitally important.
- Decontamination not only prevents you from coming into contact with diseases transmitted by blood and body fluids, it also protects your coworkers and patients.
- A clean vehicle inspires confidence.
- Operating an emergency vehicle with lights and sirens is a great responsibility.
- Motor-vehicle collisions involving emergency vehicles are a tremendous source of lawsuits and injury to EMS providers.

REVIEW QUESTIONS

SHORT ANSWER

1. When is an ambulance run considered to be *completed*?

2. Define a "true emergency."

MULTIPLE CHOICE

1. A childbirth kit should include all of the following items *except* _____.
   - **A.** sanitary napkins
   - **B.** surgical scissors
   - **C.** constriction bands
   - **D.** large, plastic garbage bags

2. Which fluid level should be checked while the engine is running?
   - **A.** Brake
   - **B.** Transmission
   - **C.** Oil
   - **D.** Power steering

3. A mechanical CPR compressor is commonly called a "_____."
   - **A.** pounder
   - **B.** cardioverter
   - **C.** pile driver
   - **D.** thumper

4. Never approach a running helicopter unless you _____.
   - **A.** are coming from the downhill side
   - **B.** have made eye contact with the pilot
   - **C.** are being escorted by the flight personnel
   - **D.** are transporting a patient

5. If your unit is the first to arrive at a vehicle-collision scene, you should park your ambulance _____.
   - **A.** in front of the wreckage
   - **B.** at least 100 feet from the wreckage
   - **C.** beyond the wreckage
   - **D.** no more than 50 feet from the wreckage

SCENARIO QUESTIONS

It is 1730 on Friday and it has been a very busy shift—every time you clear a call, there is another one waiting. As you notify dispatch that you are back on duty, it becomes obvious that things are not going to slow down any time soon. You are sent to a three-vehicle collision on Highway 37. You know the incident location well; it is on a curved part of the roadway just beyond the crest of a hill, and your unit will be the first emergency vehicle on the scene.

1. Once on the scene, where should you park the ambulance?
    A. Between the oncoming cars and the collision.
    B. Between the oncoming cars and the collision, at the crest of the hill.
    C. Alongside the vehicles in the collision.
    D. Past the crash scene by 100 yards.

2. The emergency scene described above should be considered a high-risk area for rescuers because it is during a heavy-traffic time of day, your presence may be obscured by hills and curves, and _____.
    A. the roadway will be wet, increasing the stopping distance for other vehicles
    B. it will be dusk, reducing driver visibility
    C. there is a greater likelihood of intoxicated drivers
    D. approaching vehicles will be traveling at excessive speeds

3. What can you do to reduce or prevent the forward motion of your parked ambulance in the event that it is struck by another vehicle at this emergency scene?
    A. Set the parking brake and chock the wheels.
    B. Turn the front wheels all of the way to the right and place the transmission in "Neutral."
    C. Run an anchor chain from the frame to a nearby large tree or guard railing.
    D. All of the above.

You are delivering a teenaged patient with a swollen, painful, and deformed forearm to the hospital emergency department. You find that the facility is in chaos after receiving four critical patients from a multiple-vehicle collision. A nurse shouts to you, "It's going to be awhile!" and then she disappears into one of the trauma rooms.

1. What should you do with your patient?
    A. Help him onto a hospital cot, ask him to give the PCR to the next available nurse, and return to duty.
    B. Keep him in the ambulance until the facility can assume care for him.
    C. Transport him to another facility.
    D. Wait with him in the emergency department, ensuring that you are not in the staff's way.

2. When providing the receiving staff with a verbal report on this patient, you should stress _____.
    A. that his painful and swollen extremity is also deformed
    B. your displeasure at being made to wait
    C. any condition changes that you have noticed
    D. that the patient might also have a spinal injury

3. Once a member of the receiving staff has assumed responsibility for the care of this patient, what should you do next?
   A. Ask whether you are free to leave and if told *yes*, return to duty.
   B. Proceed to the emergency department's business office to obtain your release paperwork.
   C. Complete the PCR.
   D. Inventory and transfer the patient's personal effects.

CASE STUDIES

| CASE STUDY 1 | DON'T CRASH ON THE WAY TO THE CRASH |

It is just after shift change, and you are completing your preshift inspection of the ambulance when you are dispatched with lights and sirens to a vehicle crash on the main highway just outside of town. One of the local law-enforcement officers who is at the station completing a report also hears the call and heads to his vehicle. As he gets into his patrol car, he tells you to follow and he will run an escort for you to the scene. Your partner who is in the back of the ambulance decides to stay in the back and complete the inventory on the way to the scene.

1. **What are the dangers inherent in following another emergency vehicle with lights and sirens?**

2. **What are the dangers of leaving your partner in the back of the ambulance during code 3 driving?**

To be on the safe side, you ask your partner to join you in the front and forego the inventory check until later. You also decide to allow the police officer to get several hundred yards ahead of you to avoid any chance of other motorists not seeing you in the convoy.
Once you are on the scene, you see that the police officer has positioned his vehicle in front of the crash scene and has begun laying flares in front of his vehicle.

1. **Since you are the second emergency vehicle on the scene, what is the ideal position for your vehicle?**

2. **What other factors should you consider when determining where to park your ambulance at a typical motor-vehicle collision?**

Just after the start of your shift, your ambulance is called to the scene of a pedestrian knock-down colli-sion. You get to the scene and begin to treat the patient. Due to the mechanism of injury, your partner and you decide to place the patient in a cervical collar and on a long spine board. A police officer vol-unteers to return to the rig and get the collar and strap bag and spine board. Your partner maintains c-spine stabilization and you are getting vitals. The officer returns with the board and says, "I can't find the strap and collar bag."

You sigh. Then, you thank the officer and think that he does not know where it is. You go to the rig and you cannot find it either. It is not in the compartment where it should be. You check in the back of the rig, under the bench seat, and quickly in every cabinet it could fit in. Nothing. Your heart sinks.

1. **What happened?**

2. **How can this be prevented?**

You return to your partner and whisper the bad news. He has a similar reaction to yours. He looks at you for an answer and you shrug your shoulders, "It's not there."

1. **What are your options?**

The patient is packaged on the long backboard and moved to the ambulance. You arrive at the hospital and wheel the patient in. The patient is immobilized, but the hospital staff give you a quizzical look. "It works," you say. "And don't ask...."

1. **Can your ambulance return to service after you leave the hospital?**

While at the station a short time later looking for the missing equipment, a car pulls up to the open bay door. A man gets out with your bag, "Your people were at my house last night when my father fell. They must've forgotten this." You thank him sincerely for returning your property and plan to talk to the EMTs from last night's crew when you see them again.

Active Exploration

As a wise EMT once said, "If something has the capacity to both earn you a living and kill you, it deserves some respect." This could not be truer when speaking about the ambulances and fire apparatus that many of you will someday operate. As you have seen throughout your training, the majority of learning to become an EMT-B centers on patient emergency care, as it should. However, there are many other aspects of becoming a good EMT that deserve some attention. Holding an ambulance-driver's certificate does not give you the right to drive in an unsafe manner or demand the right of way from other drivers. Because driving with lights and sirens on is so dangerous, it is essential that you understand the risks associated with code 3 driving and learn how both you and your partner can work together to minimize those risks.

Being prepared for the wide variety of calls you might receive is also very important from an equipment perspective. It is the responsibility of every EMT-B to thoroughly check out his vehicle and equipment prior to each shift and between patients. Developing a standardized routine for doing so will help ensure that everything will be in working order when needed. The following activities will help you become familiar with what it takes to be prepared for an emergency from a nonpatient emergency-care perspective.

Activity 1: Inventory Time

There is no better way to know what is carried on an ambulance or rescue vehicle than to perform a detailed inventory for yourself. This next activity involves doing just that. Since you are taking this EMT class, there is a pretty good chance you will have access to an ambulance at some time during your training. Be prepared for this opportunity ahead of time and plan on doing a detailed inventory when you get the opportunity.

Using a pad of lined paper and a clip board, ask for permission to perform your own inventory on the ambulance. Once you have permission, go through all of the interior compartments and list everything that you find. Then do the same for all exterior compartments.

If you are unsure as to what an item is or what it is supposed to be used for, take the opportunity to ask the on-duty crew. There is no national standard for ambulance inventories, so you can expect to see some differences between agencies.

Activity 2: What's in the Box?

This activity will piggyback right off the previous one and help you understand what the minimum requirements are for the equipment inventory of an ambulance in your area or region.

Most states have minimum-equipment requirements for ambulances. These requirements can vary from region to region within a state or may be standard across an entire state. Your job is to find out who or what agency regulates this requirement and what the actual minimum-inventory requirements are for an ambulance.

Compare the minimum-equipment inventory required by law with the inventory that you obtained from the working ambulance. Was there a big difference between the two lists? Do you feel the minimum-required list is adequate for an emergency ambulance?

| RETRO REVIEW

1. Head injuries, brain infections, and _____ can all mimic a stroke.
   A. vitreousitis
   B. hypoglycemia
   C. bradycardia
   D. hypothyroidism

2. If a patient refuses to sign a care-refusal form, you should _____.
   A. have a law-enforcement officer order the patient to sign it
   B. have a member of the patient's family sign it
   C. have witnesses sign statements attesting to the refusal
   D. just write "refused" on the patient-signature line and sign your name under it

3. CPR that is performed by an untrained layperson with verbal directions from a dispatcher is _____.
   A. about as effective as the CPR performed by a layperson who has been trained
   B. much less effective than the CPR performed by a layperson who has been trained
   C. more effective than the CPR performed by a layperson who has been trained
   D. ineffective and not covered by Good Samaritan laws

THINKING AND LINKING

CHAPTER TOPIC	HOW IT RELATES TO YOU AND OTHER COURSE AREAS
Patient-transfer equipment	Although different EMS systems will require you to have different types of patient-carrying devices, all ambulances will have some type of wheeled stretcher. It is very important to follow all of the patient-lifting and moving guidelines found in Chapter 5—doing so will help save both you and your patient from (further) injury.
Oxygen equipment	You will sometimes need to check the onboard oxygen system in two places: at the tank (Chapter 6) and in the patient compartment. The tank regulator has a main shut-off valve, and some ambulances have an additional shut-off valve in the patient compartment. Only ensuring that one of the valves is open can leave you assuming that your patient is receiving oxygen. This can, obviously, lead to respiratory emergencies (Chapter 16) and potential lawsuits (Chapter 3). If you are using a portable O_2 tank on the wheeled stretcher, make sure that it is properly secured. You may be dismayed at how easily the tanks can roll or slide off during patient movement—causing a very real explosive and/or projectile hazard.
Safe ambulance operation	As you begin to drive ambulances, you will find that other drivers on the road will become distracted by your presence—even when you are not responding to an emergency. Staying very aware of the traffic around you and driving defensively are essential. Also, remember that your driving ability is closely related to mental status and physical conditioning—it will be your responsibility as an EMT-B to maintain both (Chapters 1 and 2).

34

Gaining Access and Rescue Operations

CHAPTER SUMMARY

For every dangerous, unusual, or "one of a kind" situation that a person may get himself into (whether by accident or lack of common sense) there is a group of men and women dedicated and trained to get him out. The role of the EMT-B in rescue operations is an important one—perhaps one of the *most* important. As rescue teams dangle from helicopters, saw through steel wreckage, slide across ice, and navigate tons of rubble, it is the EMT-B who focuses 100 percent on the health and well-being of the patient. To the EMT-B, just reaching the patient and extricating him is not the goal... having the patient survive his injuries and go home to his family is.

Extrication is the process of rescuing people from wreckage, buildings, tunnels, and so on, and the vehicle component has several phases: preparation, size-up, hazard management, vehicle stabilization, patient access, initial assessment and rapid trauma exam, disentanglement, immobilization and removal from the vehicle, providing detailed exams, ongoing assessments, treatment, and transport to the most appropriate facility.

During extrications, patient advocacy and general scene safety must be your highest priorities. Even though you may never actually perform an extrication (fire-department rescue squads handle the majority of those duties), you need to be familiar with the process so you can reassure and prepare the patient before each upcoming step.

Rescue operations have come a long way over the years, culminating in teams that are equipped with the latest extrication tools and trained for almost every type of situation. Although this type of training is beyond the scope of an EMT-Basic course, it is important to be familiar with the protective gear, tools, and processes of vehicle extrication.

Upon your arrival at the scene of a vehicle collision, you must first evaluate for hazards and determine exactly what sort of assistance you may need (other ambulances, fire crews, rescue, police, and so on), the total number of patients, and their priority and mechanisms of injury. Call for additional ambulances first, as you can cancel them if the need decreases. You should quickly determine the extent of the patient's entrapment and the best way to save him. Keep in mind that seriously injured patients have a maximum of one "golden hour" between injury and surgery before their chances of survival begin to decline.

Low-priority patients can afford to wait for rescue squads to free them, whereas high-priority patients may need to be pulled from the wreckage by any means necessary in order to initiate life-saving emergency care. Do not neglect spinal immobilization, even with high-priority patients. Assess whether the vehicle involved is equipped with air bags, in order to determine whether you should consider any complications (such as airborne sodium hydroxide, undeployed air bags, or hidden dash and steering wheel damage).

In rural areas of the United States, ambulance crews can be responsible for their own vehicle rescues. Even in areas where rescue squads are available, ambulance crews may very well be the first on the scene. In these cases, hazard management by the ambulance crews can save time and lives. What types of hazards are normally found at collision scenes? They range from nuisances like broken glass, inclement weather, and slick roads to serious threats like spilled fuel and fires. Traffic also poses a threat, as many drivers are so enamored with the emergency scene that they may not see EMT-Bs until it is too late.

You are no good to patients or fellow rescuers if you are injured or dead. For this reason, you need to maintain attention to safety at all collision scenes—including wearing proper safety gear during rescue operations. Injuries to EMT-Bs at collision sites are commonly caused by careless attitudes toward personal safety, lack of skill in tool use, and physical problems that impede strenuous effort. Unsafe acts or omissions (e.g. failure to select proper tools, failure to recognize unsafe surroundings, lifting heavy objects improperly, and so on) can also cause injuries.

Unlike the past, today's EMS professionals have a wide selection of personal protective equipment (PPE) to choose from. These include lightweight protective helmets with integrated eye protection and protective clothing that is comfortable yet resists flame, fluids, and common chemicals. Highly visible safety vests and reflective helmets should also be worn while working in traffic at night—to reduce the chances of the EMT-B being struck by a vehicle. A good rule of thumb regarding the types of PPE to use at rescue scenes is to match the level of protection being used by those around you.

EMT-Bs involved in rescue operations should carry and use the following types of protective equipment: headgear (no baseball caps or "bump caps"—but a good, solid rescue helmet that is brightly colored and accented with reflective EMS decals), eye protection (either safety goggles with soft vinyl frames or safety glasses with large lenses and side shields), hand protection (disposable latex or vinyl gloves worn under firefighter's gloves), and body protection (a turnout coat and pants or at least a good quality, fire-resistant jumpsuit). You should also consider wearing high-top, steel-toe work shoes.

It is your responsibility to make sure that patients do not receive further injuries during the extrication process. It is not that difficult; just exercise care and shield the patient with appropriate materials. Wool blankets, aluminized rescue blankets, and vinyl tarps can protect the patient from the environment, while spine boards (short and long), heavy blankets, helmets, goggles, and hearing protection can protect the patient from the tools and flying debris of the rescue operations.

Nothing backs up traffic like a collision—no matter how minor. Even if the wrecked vehicles are not blocking any lanes, "rubberneckers" (people who slow down to stare at emergency scenes) will bog down traffic—and even cause further collisions. When you are on the scene in traffic, you should try to assist in directing traffic past the scene. When used properly, flares are very effective at warning drivers about dangerous conditions ahead. Do not throw flares from moving vehicles, avoid combustibles when lighting and placing flares, and do not use flares to direct traffic—they can cause severe burns.

You will occasionally encounter electrical hazards at emergency scenes such as downed power lines, broken utility poles, or damaged pad-mounted transformers. Do not enter these scenes yourself, and prevent anyone else from entering them until a crew from the power company can mitigate the danger.

You will also occasionally encounter vehicles that are on fire—never just assume that "someone else" has contacted the fire department. Although fighting fires is a job best left to those who are extensively trained for it, there are some steps that you can take while waiting for the fire truck to arrive. A 15- or 20-pound-class A:B:C dry-chemical fire extinguisher can extinguish almost anything burning on a vehicle (fuel, upholstery, and so on), except some flammable metals. Always don protective gear before attempting to extinguish a fire.

Vehicle fires will either be in the engine compartment, the passenger compartment, the trunk, or beneath the vehicle (and possibly fed by leaking gasoline). If the fire is in the engine compartment and the hood is open, stand by one of the windshield support posts and direct short, sweeping bursts of the extinguisher into the engine compartment. Use only enough chemical to extinguish the fire and be aware that the blowing powder can be an irritant to airways and open wounds. If the hood is open slightly (just to the locking hood latch) direct the extinguisher's spray into any available engine compartment opening. If the hood is closed completely, *do not* open it or attempt to extinguish the fire. The vehicle's firewall should give you enough time to perform emergency moves on all passengers.

If the fire is in the passenger compartment, apply the extinguisher blast directly to the burning material and try to keep the excess powder to a minimum for the sake of your patients. A fire in the trunk should be left for the fire department—just perform emergency moves on the patients. A fire underneath the vehicle presents a unique situation. If your extinguisher does not put the fire out—as is possible in large fuel-spill fires—you must just stand by and wait for the fire department's arrival, leaving the passengers in the vehicle. Pools of gasoline under a vehicle can be ignited by the car's own catalytic converter, which can reach temperatures of more than 1200°F. The catalytic converter is usually located under the car in the vicinity of the passenger seat.

A:B:C extinguishers can also be used to combat truck fires (depending on the size and level of involvement), which can spread quickly to the body and cargo of the truck. Truck tires are particularly dangerous in a fire as they can explode. Never approach a truck wheel directly when the truck is on fire; stay at a 45° angle from it.

Your decision to begin rescue operations with pooled gasoline under the vehicle will be directed by your own perception of the danger. Be alert for *every* possible ignition source—including your own ambulance's catalytic converter. You may even need to disable the involved vehicle's electrical system to prevent sparks—and sometimes to disable undeployed air bags. What is the best way to do that? Go to the source. You should disconnect the ground ("–") cable from the battery. Disconnecting the positive ("+") cable will also disable the electrical system but may cause sparks during disconnection. Do not cut through the cables unless absolutely necessary—you may need to reconnect the electrical system at some point during the rescue process.

So traffic is controlled, fires are out, and electrical systems have been disconnected—what is stopping you from entering the vehicle to begin patient emergency care? How stable is the vehicle? Can it roll, tip, fall, or slide from where it is currently resting—and what danger does that put you, the patient, and other rescuers in? Before patient emergency care and rescue operations can begin in earnest, you must stabilize the vehicle.

The appropriate vehicle-stabilization procedure depends on what position the vehicle is found in. Did it come to rest on its wheels? Roof? Side? Is the trunk end up in the air? The EMT-Basic course will not train you specifically to stabilize vehicles but understanding what must be done will assist you in your overall understanding of crash scenes and procedures.

If you need to perform an extrication and the vehicle involved is on its wheels, you should set the parking brake and flatten the tires by pulling out the valve stems. Vehicles resting on one side are potentially the most dangerous, as they are unstable and can tip in either direction. Do not allow bystanders to try and tip the vehicle back onto the wheels—you can imagine the additional trauma this may cause to the occupants. Instead, use ropes, jacks, and/or cribbing to increase the number of support contacts that the vehicle has with the ground. A vehicle resting on its roof can be in several positions: trunk and hood off the ground, trunk touching the ground, hood touching the ground, or, with a support collapse, both hood and trunk touching the ground (which is the most stable position that a vehicle can be in).

The most effective support method for all of these "roof presentations" (except for the total collapse, which needs no stabilization) is to crib the voids using 4 × 4 pieces of wood. Never kneel while placing cribbing—stay on both feet and squat down. This way you can quickly move in the event that the vehicle begins to move.

In 1966, the National Highway Safety Act required EMS systems to improve the ability of rescue personnel to extricate trapped patients in a timely manner. The changes made a huge difference in the ability of EMS to provide life-saving emergency care—that is, until the mid-1980s, when extrication times began to creep back up to unacceptable levels. The cause? Ironically, improved vehicle construction was slowing rescue crews down. Initially, the answer seemed to be an increase in training—teaching the rescuers specific techniques to access specific vehicles. This method quickly became too cumbersome.

Out of this challenge came a three-step disentanglement method that proved effective with every vehicle. To begin with, there are two forms of access to a patient: simple and complex. As the name implies, simple access means opening doors, rolling down windows, and so on. Complex access requires tools and training. To begin the process, an access hole is created as far from the patient as possible—through a rear side window, for example. You, as an EMT-B, will then climb into the vehicle and immediately begin assessing the patient, completing the rapid trauma exam, and manually stabilizing the cervical spine. Do not neglect the patient's emotional needs, either. Provide reassurance, explanations, and comfort.

The three steps of vehicle disentanglement are: (1) remove the doors, (2) remove the roof, and (3) displace the front end. Removing the doors and roof allows rescuers a tremendous amount of access to the patient and assists with ventilation. Displacing the front end removes the dash assembly, the steering wheel and column, and the pedals, thus freeing the area around the patient for medical access. If the vehicle has air bags, make sure you disconnect the car's battery, do not put yourself directly in front of the air bag, and do not cut, drill, or heat the air bag assemblies. If the metal of the vehicle is cut or broken, make sure you cover all sharp or dangerous edges.

Use common sense when carrying out this three-step extrication procedure. It may not be necessary to perform all three steps—what if a patient can be adequately accessed just by removing one door? If the sole occupant/patient has ended up in the backseat, would a front-end displacement be required?

As an EMT-B, your hands-on involvement in extrications will depend on your particular community's EMS system. But familiarity with the process will greatly assist you in providing calm and effective patient emergency care in the midst of a rescue operation.

PEARLS FROM THE PODIUM

- Size up the scene carefully to be sure you know the number of patients and the extent of entanglement. This will allow you to call for the appropriate resources early.
- Safety is the primary concern for rescuers during rescue operations.
- Wear protective clothing appropriate for the operation. Be alert for hazards from broken glass, sharp metal, fire, air bag deployment, and the rescue equipment itself.
- Work with fire personnel to get the patient out in the safest and quickest way possible.

REVIEW QUESTIONS

SHORT ANSWER

1. Why should you never attempt to direct traffic by holding a flare?

2. What types of PPE should the EMT-B use during rescue operations?

MULTIPLE CHOICE

1. All of the following are direct threats to safety except _____.
   A. downed power lines   B. spilled fuel
   C. deployed air bags   D. oncoming traffic

2. If it is necessary to disconnect a vehicle's electrical system, you should _____.
   A. remove the key from the ignition
   B. disconnect the positive (red) cable from the battery
   C. unplug the multicolored wiring harness that is commonly found at the rear of the engine compartment
   D. remove the ground cable from the battery

3. Why is your input, as an EMT-B, important in every step of the extrication process?
   A. Because you will most likely be the highest-trained individual present.
   B. Because you could be held civilly liable for any damages suffered by the patient during the rescue.
   C. Because it is your job to keep the patient safe and to prevent further injuries.
   D. Because you will be directing the activities of the rescue squad.

4. _____ bumpers can cause serious injuries to EMS personnel who stand in front of them.
   A. Detached   B. Headed
   C. Reflexive   D. Loaded

5. There are two types of glass used in automobile construction, tempered and _____.
   A. rated   B. laminated
   C. scored   D. tinted

SCENARIO QUESTIONS

You are the first unit to arrive at the scene of a two-car collision and the fire department is on the way. As you approach the wreckage, you observe gasoline pouring onto the ground from one of the vehicles, creating a pool under both. One of the drivers is standing safely on the side of the road, but the other driver is sitting in his vehicle and seems oblivious to everything around him.

1. The gasoline can easily be ignited by either of the vehicles' _____.
   A. catalytic converters   B. spark plugs
   C. wiring harness   D. electrical systems

2. If the pool of gasoline has been ignited, you can attempt to use a 15- or 20-pound _____ extinguisher on the fire.
   A. class A liquid   B. A:B:C dry-chemical
   C. compressed-water   D. DryFoam®

3. If you are unable to extinguish the fire, what can you do to assist the now-trapped motorist?

    A. Attempt to gain access to the vehicle in order to perform an emergency move.

    B. Use your ambulance to push the vehicle off the fire.

    C. Enlist the help of several bystanders to try and roll the car to safety.

    D. Wait for the fire department to arrive and prepare to treat him if he survives.

You arrive at a vehicle rollover crash on a rural highway. You find the car resting on its roof and the driver lying on the ceiling of the vehicle. She is responsive and complaining of severe right-arm pain, and you observe blood dripping steadily from a head wound. She also tells you that her legs "feel weird" and that she cannot move.

1. What should you do?

    A. Pull the patient out of the vehicle by her shoulders, taking care not to twist or turn her spine.

    B. Slide into the vehicle and manually immobilize the patient's head and neck.

    C. Instruct the patient not to move while awaiting the rescue squad.

    D. Reach into the vehicle just far enough to hold the patient's head and neck steady.

2. The most important thing that you can do for this patient while waiting for the rescue squad to arrive is to provide _____.

    A. reassurance   **B.** high-concentration oxygen

    C. water   **D.** blankets

3. What is the best way for the rescue squad to stabilize this vehicle?

    A. Tie ropes from the door jambs to nearby trees or solid structures.

    B. Place two step chocks upside down under the trunk.

    C. Place hydraulic jacks at all four support posts.

    D. Build a box crib with 4 $\times$ 4s under the car.

It has been an unusually quiet, rainy night and you and your partner have just run out of things to talk about when you are dispatched to a semi-truck vs. auto collision. You arrive at a dark stretch of road and see a small sports car crushed beneath a jackknifed big rig. "This isn't going to be pretty," your partner says as he sets the ambulance's parking brake. You step out of the ambulance and turn on your flashlight. You see that the driver's side door of the semi-truck is open and an individual is motionless on the wet pavement below. You start to approach the individual and as you get about 10 feet from him you notice an odd tingling in your legs and lower abdomen.

1. You are experiencing a phenomenon known as _____.

    A. the sixth sense   **B.** an adrenaline rush

    C. ground gradient   **D.** neural reception

2. What immediate action should you take?

    A. Very cautiously continue approaching the motionless individual.

    B. Turn around and hop on one foot to a safe place.

    C. Stay where you are and contact law enforcement.

    D. Drop to the ground and spread your arms and legs.

CASE STUDIES

You are dispatched to a multiple-vehicle collision several miles east of town. You arrive at the scene at the same time as the fire-department rescue squad from the neighboring town. Apparently, things are busy in the area and there are no other resources available to respond. There are several walking wounded on the scene when you arrive and what appears to be two people trapped in one of the vehicles. All the windows are up and intact when you approach the vehicle. One of the patients is moving about while the other one is slumped over and bleeding from the head. One of the firefighters is laying flares while the other is getting the extrication tools out of the truck. You must enter the car to perform an initial assessment on the unresponsive patient.

1. What will be your best method for entry into the vehicle?

2. You have decided to gain entry by breaking one of the windows. Which window will you break and why?

You ask one of the firefighters to break the rear window on the passenger side since that is the side of the car in which the less responsive patient is located. Once all the glass has been cleared away, you reach in and push the button to unlock the door but it does not work. The doors are jammed shut and will not open. You decide to climb into the vehicle to assist the patients inside.

1. What can you do to minimize the chances of getting cut with broken glass as you enter the vehicle?

2. You assess the front-seat passenger and find she is not breathing. She does have a weak slow pulse. What extrication method do you think is most appropriate for this patient?

Your ambulance is dispatched to a motor-vehicle collision at a busy intersection in your town. You can tell by your dispatcher's hurried voice and the phones ringing in the background that it could be a bad one.

    You and your partner arrive at the scene and find a small station wagon on its side in the middle of the intersection. The other vehicle is up ahead on the side of the road with its flashers on. Your partner walks carefully to that vehicle to check the occupant. You see someone moving inside the station wagon.

1. What are the hazards here?

2. Can you begin treating the patient in the station wagon?

3. What additional resources do you need here?

You see a mother trying to get to her child in the back seat. You speak to the mother through the windshield to calm her. The child in the back seat is screaming wildly. You think you would be too if you were in a crash as dramatic as this. You are able to calm the mother and restrict her movement until the car can be secured. You keep a safe distance but see that the child continues crying and appears to be secure in her car seat.

The fire department arrives and stabilizes the vehicle. The windshield is quickly removed, giving you access to the vehicle.

1. What should you be wearing as you enter the stabilized vehicle through the windshield?

2. Who decides what techniques will be used in gaining access to the vehicle?

Active Exploration

As you have discovered so far in your training, there are many hazards awaiting the unsuspecting EMT-B. You must protect yourself from the patient's bodily fluids; you must use great caution when driving the ambulance to and from the emergency scene. You must also use caution when called upon to participate in a rescue operation. You must know your own limitations and take special precautions to ensure your safety and the safety of the patient as well as other rescuers. Depending on where you work and the resources available to you at the scene of an emergency, you may simply stand by and watch as more highly specialized teams extricate the patient from the torn wreckage. In other instances, you may be the only extra pair of hands available and may need to assist directly in the removal of the patient from the wreckage. Whichever the case, it is important you understand and practice good safety techniques when working around a crash scene.

The following activities will help you increase your awareness of the hazards surrounding rescue operations and help you become a more valuable asset to the EMS team.

Activity 1: Get Me Outta Here!

This first activity will give you a greater appreciation for how difficult it can be to remove patients from damaged vehicles when extrication equipment is limited. For this activity, you will need a vehicle and at least two or three of your classmates.

1. Begin by choosing the smallest person in the group and have them lie unconscious on the front seat of the vehicle.

2. The rest of you must carefully remove the unconscious "patient" from the vehicle and to a safe location.

3. You have no extrication equipment for the first few rounds of this activity and must use your rescuers to carefully remove the patient from the car.

4. Take turns being the leader and directing the other rescuers to do what you need. Be clear and concise with your directions each step of the way.

For the second round, have the "patient" slump down with his legs caught under the dash of the car. Your third round may involve the removal of a "patient" from the rear of the car with no rear doors.

Plan each challenge carefully and take turns being leader, patient, and rescuers. This is as much an exercise in communication as it is in learning to move a patient. Remember to use good body mechanics with every move.

If you have some equipment available with you, you may want to try using a long backboard or vest-type extrication device as well.

Activity 2: What's on Your Truck?

Just because you will soon be an EMT-B does not mean that you are expected to have all the answers. The best EMTs do however know what resources are available to them and how best to access those resources.

This next activity involves finding out what local resources you might have for gaining access to entrapped patients, whether in a building or a vehicle. Identify someone you know who works in the local EMS system and ask them the following questions:

1. What resources are available in your area to handle a major vehicle extrication? Is there more than one resource?

2. What resources are commonly utilized to stabilize a vehicle during an extrication?

3. Is there a resource trained in confined-space rescue? Where is it located?

4. Is there a resource specifically trained for high-angle or cliff rescue? Where is it located?

5. Is there a resource specifically trained for trench rescue? Where is it located?

6. Is there a resource specifically trained for swift-water rescue? Where is it located?

As we have stated many times, knowing what resources are available and how best to access those resources is very important for the well-being of both the EMT-B and the patient.

RETRO REVIEW

1. How should you reassess the posterior body of a patient who has been secured to a long spine board?

    A. Carefully logroll the patient with the help of several other rescuers.

    B. Tilt the spine board at an angle and visually inspect the posterior of the patient's body.

    C. Reassess as much of the patient's back as you can touch without moving the patient.

    D. There is no need to reassess the patient's posterior body once secured to a spine board.

2. A common side effect of nitroglycerin is _____.

    A. chest pain   **B.** hypotension

    C. blood clotting   **D.** dementia

3. You are dispatched to a rollover collision on the freeway during rush hour. Due to the severity of the vehicle damage, the rescue crew has estimated that it will take approximately 20 minutes to free your patient from the wreckage. Your patient has two crushed and trapped extremities, a profusely bleeding forehead laceration, and abdominal tenderness. Regarding the transportation of this patient, you should _____.

    A. request a police escort

    B. suspect internal injuries

    C. call for air rescue

    D. recheck vital signs every 7 to 10 minutes

THINKING AND LINKING

CHAPTER TOPIC	HOW IT RELATES TO YOU AND OTHER COURSE AREAS
Working in traffic	There is always the possibility that one of your fellow rescuers at the scene of a vehicle collision may be struck by a passing motorist. You will then need to calmly notify dispatch of the new situation (Chapter 13) and prioritize the scene using a triage system (covered in Chapter 35).
	Dont forget your own safety (Chapter 7) and understand that such an event may necessitate a critical-incident stress debriefing (CISD) (Chapter 2).
Vehicle fires	In addition to the trauma injuries associated with a vehicle collision (Chapter 7), you should also be prepared to treat respiratory emergencies (Chapters 6 and 16) and burns (Chapter 27) in the event of a vehicle fire.
	Also, remember to park your ambulance a safe distance from any fire or potentially flammable event (Chapter 33)—the oxygen that you carry can quickly make the situation much worse (review Chapter 6 for oxygen-safety information).
Unstable vehicles	You may be required to treat crush injuries and amputations (Chapters 27 and 28) for both patients and First Responders resulting from vehicles that have not been properly stabilized.

35

Special Operations

CHAPTER SUMMARY

Imagine being the first crew on the scene of an airline crash, a passenger train derailment, or a rollover bus crash. You know how to assess, treat, package, and transport a single patient … but what about 10 patients? 25? 100+? Where do you even begin? *Special operations*, which encompasses both multiple-casualty incidents and hazardous-materials incidents (which are sometimes in the same event), is an area of the EMS that you, as an EMT-B, need to be familiar with.

Hazardous materials (also simply called *hazmats*) are, according to the U.S. Department of Transportation, "Any substance or material in a form which poses an unreasonable risk to health, safety, and property when transported in commerce." Hazmats are everywhere and you will be responding to incidents involving them. As a matter of fact, many hazardous-materials incidents begin as routine EMS calls. It will be up to you to recognize a hazmat, initiate the appropriate response, and know your role in that response.

What is that role? As an EMT-B, you will be highly trained in emergency care but will still be a layperson when it comes to hazardous materials. Special training is required to understand hazmats and to make the scene safe following a spill or accident. Your initial role in a hazmat incident will likely be to report it and then stay back at a safe distance and let the experts take care of the situation.

The Environmental Protection Agency (EPA) and the Occupational Safety and Health Administration (OSHA) are the two federal agencies responsible for developing hazmat guidelines—for both training and response. According to OSHA, "training is required for all employees who participate, or who are expected to participate, in emergency response to hazardous substance accidents." There are four levels of training: **First Responder Awareness** (incident recognition and reporting), **First Responder Operations** (protection of persons, property, and environment *outside* of the incident), **Hazardous Materials Technician** (plugging, patching, and stopping escape of hazmat), and **Hazardous Materials Specialist** (advanced knowledge and skills to command activities at the site).

Most EMT-Bs are trained just to the Awareness level, but it will be your quick recognition and effective communication that will lay the foundation for the entire incident. Where are hazmat incidents likely to occur? Logically, these will most likely be where hazardous materials are used, produced, or transported—factories, laboratories, agricultural areas, highways, and railways. As part of a community's EMS system, you should be familiar with the types and locations of the hazardous materials in your area. What do they make in that factory by the railroad tracks? What are the by-products of that chemical plant on Highway 9? You should also spend time with local police and fire agencies developing preincident plans for known hazmats.

When you initially arrive at the scene of a potential hazmat incident, *do not* rush in and take action. Never assume that the scene is safe—your assumption could cost you dearly. Always evaluate the scene from a safe distance. Once a hazmat is recognized, only individuals trained to the Technician level or above should enter the scene. You must consider all patients leaving a hazmat scene contaminated until proven otherwise.

You may be the first to identify that a hazardous-materials incident exists. If you are called to the scene for more than one medical patient—think hazmat! Your first priority at the scene of a hazmat incident is your safety, the safety of your crew, and the safety of the public. You will need to determine a *danger zone* and a *safe zone* (which should be on the same level as, but upwind of, the danger zone). Try to keep people out of the danger zone and convince those already in it to move to a decontamination area. You should stay in the safe zone at all times.

For some hazmat incidents, you will need to mobilize fire departments, other ambulance crews, rescue teams, law-enforcement personnel, and local and/or state hazardous-materials experts. Luckily, you can usually do all of this with one call to your agency's dispatch center. It will be up to you to implement your area's Incident Management System and to stay in command until relieved by someone higher in the chain of command.

In order to prevent the situation from becoming worse, you should set up perimeters, direct people to safe areas, and evacuate if necessary. *Do not* risk personal safety by making rescue attempts. You should also redefine your previous danger and safe zones into a hot zone, warm zone, decontamination corridor, and cold zone. Stay in the cold zone.

You should also attempt to determine exactly what hazard is involved in the incident—it is difficult to assess the potential dangers otherwise. Since it is obviously not safe to enter the warm or hot zone in order to determine the hazmat, you must do it from a distance. Use binoculars to locate signs, labels, or placards (utilizing the National Fire Protection Association [NFPA] or US DOT identification systems). Invoices, bills of lading, and shipping manifests (if they can safely be obtained) will show the exact materials involved. Just be aware that recent studies indicate that placards, labels, and shipping papers can be wrong much of the time—so never act hastily on the assumption of hazmat identification.

How else can you obtain information about the possible materials involved in an incident? Check the material safety data sheets (MSDS), interview individuals who have been in the hot zone, consult your unit's copy of the *Emergency Response Guidebook* (ERG), contact CHEMTREC or CHEM-TEL, and do not forget about regional poison-control centers. When contacting any of the above services, be prepared to provide information, such as your name; the location and type of the incident; any placards, identification numbers, or labels; the shipping company and type of vehicle(s) involved; local conditions (weather, schools, hospitals, and so on); and any injuries or exposures. If there is no way to identify the materials involved, the hazmat experts will be able to identify them once they are on the scene.

Once the hazmat scene is up and running, EMS will have two responsibilities: monitoring and rehabilitating hazmat team members and treating the injured. How do I rehabilitate team members? The health and well-being of each hazmat worker is paramount in maintaining the integrity of the entire operation. In order to enter the hot zone, these individuals must put on chemical-protective suits and breathing apparatus. This apparatus causes both physical and thermal stress on the rescuer, requiring the need for evaluation before, during, and after emergency operations (including vital signs, temperatures, and so on). This should be done in a special area called the *rehab sector*—which should be located in the cold zone, protected from the weather, large enough for multiple crews, easily accessible to EMS, and situated to allow the crews easy access back to the emergency operations. The rehab sector should also be used for prehydration, hydration, and in extended operations, nourishment of crews.

Hazmat or terrorist incidents involve civilians and/or First Responders. It is essential to set up an effective decontamination process to *clean* individuals leaving the hot zone and to protect the EMS crews who will be treating them in the *treatment sector* of the cold zone. It is important to remember that patients who have been "field decontaminated" will not be completely free from all contaminants. For this reason, EMTs in the treatment sector should utilize appropriate personal protective equipment and clothing to prevent secondary contamination. If patients are to be transported, cover the patient area of the ambulance with plastic to collect the runoff from the decontamination process. Also, consider any equipment used on these patients to be disposable—stethoscopes, spine boards, blood pressure cuffs may all need to be disposed of.

At a hazmat scene, you will encounter four types of patients: uninjured and not contaminated, injured and not contaminated, uninjured and contaminated, and injured and contaminated (who you will, occasionally, be required to treat). To begin with, you must determine the substance that the patient was exposed to and look up the appropriate precautions and first-aid in the Emergency Response Guidebook. Use PPE that affords splash protection, manage the patient's ABCs, remove his clothing, and rinse with large amounts of water (especially the patient's dense body hair, navel, armpits, ear canals, crotch, fingernails, and so on). Use tepid water if available (to prevent hypothermia), avoid rinsing contaminants into open wounds, and try to contain the runoff. Following treatment of the patient, decontaminate yourself—which may include disposing of your clothing.

The term *decontamination* has been used numerous times, but what exactly does it entail? Decontamination takes two main forms: gross and secondary. Gross decontamination is the removal or neutralization of **most** of the contaminant but not all. Secondary decontamination removes **most** of the *residual* contaminants—it is much more thorough than the gross decontamination. Decontamination processes normally utilize emulsification (surfactant, soap, and so on), chemical reaction (neutralization), disinfection (for biological contaminants), dilution, absorption, removal (vacuuming, and so on), and disposal (removing contaminated object[s] from patient). Always utilize proper PPE when running a decontamination line and prioritize patients on the basis of the triage system.

Finally, you will need to decontaminate those wearing PPE and those who are not. Individuals wearing PPE should have their protective suits rinsed, scrubbed from the head down, and rinsed again before removal. Patients not wearing PPE should be instructed, via a public address system, to remove all clothing, jewelry, watches, and so on. Dry and water-reactive contaminates should then be brushed off, vesicants should be blotted off, and then the patients should undergo a 2- to 5-minute water rinse—utilizing a low-pressure system to avoid aggravation of soft-tissue injuries and creation of an aerosol out of contaminants. Washing and rinsing should begin with the head and face and move down from there. Provide these patients with a covering as soon as possible, both for modesty and for protection from the elements.

A multiple-casualty incident (MCI)—sometimes called a multiple-casualty situation (MCS)—is an incident that places a great demand on EMS equipment and personnel. While the most common MCI is an automobile collision with three or more patients, each EMS jurisdiction defines an MCI a little differently. The key definition, however, is that the *event itself* challenges or hampers the EMS systems' ability to respond. Once you are working as an EMT-B, you may regularly encounter MCIs with three to 15 patients—but large-scale casualties are very rare and will likely be a "once in a career" event. The common thread in all MCI plans, though, is that they should be as effective with three patients as with 300.

The main difference between the management of small- and large-scale MCIs is that the latter unfolds over longer periods of time and requires greater dependence on outside agencies. All EMT-Bs should be familiar with their local disaster plan—the predefined instructions that designate how each agency should respond to particular types of disasters. Good disaster plans should address events likely to occur in the region, be well publicized, be realistic, and be rehearsed.

Since every large-scale incident needs a planning structure and organizational hierarchy, most areas of the country utilize the Incident Management System (IMS)—also called the Incident Command System (ICS) in some regions. The two most commonly used functions of the IMS are for "command" and "operations." Command, which is an essential part of any emergency-response plan, consists of an individual (initially, the highest ranking person to arrive at the scene) who is responsible for management of the incident. This individual will stay in command until replaced or until the incident has concluded. Since it has been shown that one person cannot effectively manage more than six individuals in an emergency environment, the incident commander will begin appointing sector managers as the incident grows in complexity. Command has two methods: singular and unified. Singular command means that only one agency controls the resources for an incident, whereas unified command means that several agencies work independently but cooperatively.

Once the incident command is established, two phases of action begin: scene size-up/triage and organization/delegation. While awaiting backup, the crew(s) initially on the scene will complete the triage process and prepare for reinforcements. Once further personnel arrive, the incident commander may pass command to a higher ranking responder or remain in command. In a unified response, the command from each service would come together and assume command corporately. The command post (whether singular or unified) is normally set up at the edge of the scene—within sight of the events but far enough to accommodate planning and communications. Some systems designate the command post by placing two traffic cones on top of the vehicle being used.

The initial scene size-up is a sweep to determine what needs to be done. First, put on the appropriate identification and then move through the incident (or observe from a distance during hazmats) and determine everything—from the number of patients (including the so-called "walking wounded") to the types and extent of resources needed to manage the scene. Then pick up the radio, take a deep breath, and *calmly* report the scene condition and resources needed. When giving the initial report, you should speak clearly and in short sentences so that the gravity of the situation will be understood by the dispatch center and other resources. You should give yourself a unique command name (e.g. "First Street Command" or "Rockville Quarry Command") to distinguish yourself and your incident from other units using the same frequency. You must also give responding units information on what equipment should be brought, how to access the scene, what to do upon their arrival, and whether you are activating the regional disaster plan.

Once backup begins arriving, use as much face-to-face communication as possible—it cuts down on radio traffic and can be more effective. The communication flow at the scene should follow the flow of the incident's organizational chart.

Getting organized early and aggressively is very important, as is thinking and ordering *big*! If you have a planned structure for the incident, you will be able to direct resources as they arrive and reduce the chances of "freelancing," or rescuers showing up and working their own agenda. Many systems have illustrated the important points of their incident-action plans on "tactical worksheets" for use in the field—if yours is one of these systems, use the worksheet!

The area that you, as an EMT-B, will spend most of your time in during an MCI is called the EMS sector. This sector can be broken down into smaller, more specific sectors, on the basis of incident need. As you bring your ambulance to the scene, you will be directed to a particular sector officer who will give you instructions. Complete your task and report back to that officer.

Triage ("to sort") is the process of sorting multiple patients into one of four categories: treatable life-threatening illnesses/injuries, treatable but not life-threatening illnesses/injuries, "walking wounded," and the dead or fatally injured. The purpose of triage is to provide emergency care based on the severity of need, without neglecting five patients to work on one.

You can start the triage process by directing anyone who can walk to move to a particular location—this "weeds out" those who do not need immediate emergency care. With those who remain, you need to rapidly assess each one, stopping only long enough to open airways or stop severe bleeding. Once you have triaged the entire group, then go back and begin providing more extensive emergency care—beginning with the top-priority patients and working your way to the walking wounded. Once no other patient requires immediate emergency care to prevent death or disability, you may begin assisting fatally injured patients.

The most commonly used triage system is called START—*Simple Triage and Rapid Treatment*. You begin by, once again, separating the "walking wounded" from the group. Assess the remaining patients for RPM (Respiration, Pulse, and Mental status) and tag them as follows: Immediate (red) have altered mental status and/or no radial pulse and/or respirations greater than 30 per minute. Delayed (yellow) are alert and/or have a radial pulse and/or respirations less than 30 per minute. Minor (green) are typically the walking wounded and have good respirations, perfusion, and mental status. Deceased (black) have no respirations after airway is opened or have no pulse or respirations. You would then complete the cycle by retriaging the minor (green) patients—just because they could walk earlier does not mean that they are not critically wounded.

Although different areas use slightly different triage systems, it is very important that regions have a standardized triage program. Many MCIs are multiagency incidents and it is imperative that everyone be "on the same page." Also—as you are triaging—you must physically label each patient with a *triage tag*. These tags (of which there are different styles) alert other rescuers as to which treatment group each patient belongs to. In well-organized incidents, these categorized patients will even be moved to separate triage sectors for treatment. In some large MCIs, triage tags may be the only form of prehospital documentation—so always notate vitals, treatments, and so on, on your patient's tag.

The final EMS sectors at the MCI scene are for *staging* and *transportation*. As ambulances have been arriving to assist with the incident, they have been directed to wait in the *staging sector*. Once the first few patients have been prepared for transport, the ambulances will be called to the *transportation sector* to load and proceed to the appropriate medical facility. The transportation officer will coordinate with all of the local hospitals so that no facility will become overwhelmed with patients, or receive patients that they were not expecting. Once the ambulance has transferred the patient to the hospital, they will most likely be ordered to return to the staging sector to await further instructions.

Medical facilities should be notified of large-scale MCIs as soon as possible. This will allow them to call in extra personnel and prepare their emergency departments. During major MCIs, the transportation officer (or his assistant) should be the only person contacting the hospitals. This is also one instance where you will *not* need to provide a radio report to the receiving facility—that, again, will be the transportation officer's job, although his report may be as short as, "You're getting an 'immediate' patient with severe bleeding."

PEARLS FROM THE PODIUM

- Triage (roughly) means "to sort."
- The early stages of a multipatient incident are the most critical. Call for adequate help early, institute the ICS, and triage patients.
- The response and procedures used in MCIs varies depending on the number of patients.
- An MCI is defined as an incident that exceeds the resources of an EMS system. This may include an MVC with three patients and major incidents with more than 100 patients.
- If air medical evacuation is available in your area, know how and when to contact them. Know their procedures for setting up an LZ.

REVIEW QUESTIONS

SHORT ANSWER

1. Explain the difference between singular and unified command in a mass-casualty incident.

2. Where are hazardous-materials incidents likely to occur?

MULTIPLE CHOICE

1. The common philosophy among incident-command experts is that each leader can effectively manage only up to _____ people.
   A. eight   B. three
   C. six   D. ten

2. The four levels of training for hazardous-materials-response participants are First Responder Awareness, _____, Hazardous Materials Technician, and Hazardous Materials Specialist.
   A. First Responder Technician
   B. Hazardous Materials Responder
   C. Hazardous Materials Commander
   D. First Responder Operations

3. In large-scale-emergency incidents, the _____ is responsible for coordinating rest rooms, meals, and crew rotations for rescue personnel.
   A. incident commander   B. staging officer
   C. communications coordinator   D. treatment officer

4. Utilization of a _____ system following a tour-bus crash gives the largest number of patients the greatest chance for survival.
   A. CISD   B. hazmat
   C. triage   D. MSDS

5. During large-scale MCIs, incident sector officers are usually identified by _____.
   A. brightly colored vests
   B. color-coded flags erected above each area
   C. clearly labeled helmets
   D. lapel pins

SCENARIO QUESTIONS

You and your partner are relaxing at a coffee shop when you hear a loud screeching sound in the distance. The floor begins vibrating, lightly at first and then violently. You try to keep your coffee from spilling as the little coffee shop is shaken by wave after wave of thundering jolts, accompanied by the ceaseless sound of crashing metal. Your partner yells, "Is this an earthquake?" You fear that it is *not*. Then, the noise and motion stop abruptly, to be replaced by silence. You step out the front door and your fear is confirmed. About half a mile up the railroad tracks, there is a smoking maze of twisted wreckage. Row after row of railroad cars are bent and scattered on both sides of the track—some on their sides, some upside down, and some no longer recognizable. As you watch, the first human shape lurches from one of the passenger cars and falls into the dirt beside the tracks.

1. After notifying dispatch of the incident, you should _____.
   A. proceed to the scene and begin triaging patients
   B. set up incident sectors and lay out the appropriately colored equipment
   C. use your unit's binoculars and initially survey the scene from where you are
   D. park near the crash scene and set up a command post

2. The first patient whom you approach after beginning the START triage process is alert, has a radial pulse, and is breathing at a rate of 24 per minute. He has several angulated extremity fractures and complains of numbness in his legs. You would place a _____ tag on this patient.
   A. red   B. yellow
   C. green   D. black

3. What is the best way to begin the triage process for this scene?
   A. Use your unit's PA system and direct all individuals who can walk to leave the train.
   B. Put on your turnouts, take a stack of triage tags, and start searching through the train car nearest you.
   C. Designate your partner as the triage officer, help set out treatment tarps, and await the other rescuers.
   D. Assist the walking wounded to move into the designated staging area.

You and your new partner arrive at the scene of an early-morning auto collision and find three cars involved. Through your scene size-up, you locate seven people: two are standing on opposite sides of the road talking on cellular phones, three are unresponsive (one in each vehicle), another is entangled under a dashboard and yelling for help, and the last one is lying on the pavement, staring blankly and moving her mouth as if trying to speak.

1. In this MCI, you will assume the position of _____.
   A. triage commander   B. operations manager
   C. incident commander   D. treatment officer

2. What is the most appropriate initial radio broadcast to dispatch?
   A. "Dispatch, this is Unit 75 on Thompson Road about 2 miles south of Porter. We are currently on scene with that three-car MVA and I've got two standing individuals, one in each car that seems unresponsive, an entangled male adult and another unresponsive female. We need assistance ASAP."
   B. "Dispatch, this is Unit 75. We are on scene with a three-car MVA. I've got one severely entrapped "delayed" patient and four additional "immediate" patients. Dispatch a rescue squad and five paramedic ambulances. I will now be called Thompson Road Command, and I need police for traffic control."

    C. "Dispatch, this is Unit 75 out with that three-car MVA on Thompson Road. I've got five patients total and one is going to need extrication. Send me one fire unit, four paramedic ambulances, and some traffic control."

    D. "Dispatch, this is Thompson Road EMS Command. I need a rescue squad for an entrapped "delayed" patient and five paramedic ambulances. Please also get police out here for traffic control."

3. This incident will have a _____ command structure.

    A. singular   **B.** parallel

    C. unified   **D.** generational

You are called to a local factory for a worker who complained of feeling ill, before collapsing next to the assembly line. You know from previous community-EMS training that the factory uses and produces a wide variety of chemicals in its manufacturing processes. As you pull the ambulance around to the rear of the building, you see numerous large trucks, trailers, and holding tanks—each with placards displaying different content codes on them. You cannot see anybody walking around outside and no one seems to be waiting to greet you.

1. What should you do?

    A. Contact dispatch and request a hazmat specialist.

    B. Take your equipment and cautiously walk into the building.

    C. Move the ambulance to a safe location and survey the scene with binoculars.

    D. Have dispatch contact the factory and ask somebody to meet you outside.

2. If this were a hazardous-materials incident, you would park your ambulance _____.

    A. 1,000 feet downwind

    B. uphill, upwind, and by a line of trees

    C. upwind and on the same level as the factory

    D. 600 to 800 yards away, facing the opposite direction

3. If you needed to identify the contents of the various vehicles and holding tanks, you would _____.

    A. look up your CHEMTREC binder

    B. consult the current ERG

    C. access your ambulance's CHEM-TEL database

    D. check for the vehicles' shipping manifest

CASE STUDIES

CASE STUDY 1	IT'S A GAS

You are dispatched to a train derailment about 20 miles north of town. Since you were already on that side of town when the call came in, you anticipate a 10-minute response time. You are advised that several agencies will be responding to the incident as there is the possibility of multiple casualties.

    A mile or so from the scene, you can see dark black smoke billowing into the sky from the vicinity of the scene. As you approach the scene, you can see a double-tanker truck that has been broadsided by a freight train. The cab of the truck is engulfed in flames, and several of the tanker cars on the train have derailed and tipped onto their sides.

1. What consideration will you make before positioning your vehicle at the scene?

2. What information will you want to report to dispatch regarding the incident?

You position your vehicle in a safe location from the incident. A passing motorist has stopped and is observing the scene through a pair of binoculars. You ask to use the binoculars and focus in on the tanker truck. The placard that is visible on the rear tank is 1202. You can see one of the placards on the rail cars and it reads 2438.

1. What is the chemical for 1202 and what is the threat to the rescuers?

2. What is the chemical for 2438 and what is the threat to the rescuers?

| CASE STUDY 2 | A CAR JUST CRASHED INTO MY BUILDING |

You are called to the scene of a one-vehicle collision (van vs. building). Your partner and you arrive first on the scene. The van hit the corner of a dentist's office and took out several feet of brick and 2 × 6s. The van came to rest in an adjacent parking lot. Six people are walking around the van, and you see at least four more sitting inside. The driver is one of these and he is slumped over the wheel.

1. What would you do for the scene size-up?

2. How many patients do you have?

3. What initial assistance and equipment should you call for?

You assume EMS command, and your partner begins to triage patients. You check inside the building from a stable surface and find that the dentist and hygienist were knocked out of their chairs inside the building and are injured slightly ("minor"). The patient with the unfinished root canal is unhappy but unhurt. Your partner reports back that he has seven patients outside. Two are "immediate," two are "delayed," and three are "minor." He suspects that the driver of the van had a seizure. You tell him that there are two patients inside the building.

The additional units that you called arrive as well as a few off-duty personnel who heard the call. You begin to direct them to appropriate areas and tasks. One off-duty person is assigned as transportation officer and another as treatment officer. You direct the placement (staging) of arriving ambulances to prevent a snarl at the scene. A fire-department incident command is set up. You discuss your concerns for the building's structural problems and issues with stabilization of the van with fire command. The fire department begins work.

1. **What does the treatment officer do?**

2. **What does the transportation officer do?**

Active Exploration

If your career as an EMT-B lasts long enough, it is only a matter of time before you find yourself knee deep in an MCI. Keep in mind that the term "multicasualty" can involve as few as three patients and as many as 3,000. The definition of an MCI is not tied directly to a specific number of patients but rather to the ability of the specific EMS system to respond to the incident appropriately. Most systems define an MCI as any event involving multiple casualties (patients) whereby the ability to effectively respond is challenged or hampered by the event itself. For this reason, it is likely that large metropolitan EMS systems can manage incidents involving many patients without actually declaring an MCI. On the other hand, a small rural EMS system may need to declare an MCI and request additional resources with an incident involving only three or four patients. Bottom line, it just depends on the size of the system, the experience of the individuals involved, and the resources available.

The same principles apply when responding to a suspected or confirmed hazmat incident. If you work in EMS long enough, there is a good chance you will become involved in such an event. More than most incidents, the hazmat incident has the potential for causing harm to the responding rescuers if they are not alert, aware, and prepared for such a response. The following activities will help prepare you for these types of events.

Activity 1: Are We Prepared?

Most communities across the nation have prepared for and have a plan of action in the event of a major disaster or incident with the potential for causing multiple casualties. Whether you realize it or not, these plans are in place and many communities have large stockpiles of medical supplies for just such an event. As a member of the EMS team, you will be called upon to assist in your community and be a part of the overall response plan. This first activity will have you investigate and discover what is being done to prepare for such an event in your community.

1. Contact your local EMS agency or fire department and arrange to speak to someone who can offer information on the disaster plan in your area.

2. Find out what plan, if any, is in place for your community. Who is responsible for the plan and how is it kept up to date?

3. What part, if any, do local EMTs play in the plan? How will they contact or communicate with those trained and ready to assist with the medical needs of such an event?

4. Are there large stores of medical supplies that will be accessible in such an event?

5. Should all EMTs notify the EMS agency of their training and be put on a list for possible callout in such an event?

As an EMT-B, you possess the knowledge and skills to lend vital help in the event of a large disaster. Knowing whether there is a local plan and understanding the scope of that plan and the resources available to you are essential to ensure an appropriate response.

Activity 2: Methyl Ethyl Bad Stuff

This next activity will better prepare you in the event of a suspected or known hazardous-materials spill. Becoming familiar with and knowing how to use the Emergency Response Guidebook (ERG) is an important skill for any EMT-B. It is the goal of the DOT to provide a free copy for each emergency-response vehicle in the United States.

As you go about your daily routine, begin to pay attention to the various placards around you. Take a moment to write the numbers down as you see them. Also, make note of where you saw them, such as on a tanker truck or on the side of a building.

Once you have accumulated several of these placard numbers, take some time to locate an ERG and look up the specific numbers in the guidebook. Copies of the guidebook can be found at all emergency-response agencies as well as on-line at the following address:

http://hazmat.dot.gov/gydebook.htm

While free copies are made available to all emergency-response agencies, personal copies can be purchased for $20.00 through the Online Government Printing Office at:
http://bookstore.gpo.gov/index.html

It is one thing to know the book exists and another to feel comfortable using the book to identify potential threats at the scene of an emergency. By completing this activity, you will become more familiar with the use of the book and the types of materials that exist in and around your community.

1. Which of the following would not be considered part of the on-scene assessment and emergency care of a trauma patient?

   A. The ABCs with spinal precautions.

   B. Loading the patient into the ambulance.

   C. A detailed physical exam.

   D. Immobilization.

2. If, during an extrication, you need to displace the vehicle's steering wheel and find that the air bag has not yet deployed, you should do all of the following, except _____.

   A. disconnect the battery terminals, starting with the negative one

   B. avoid cutting or heating the steering wheel hub

   C. ensure that no objects are placed in front of the air bag

   D. remove the positive battery cable first

3. You are dispatched to a local ice arena for a leg injury. Upon your arrival, you find the patient, a 16-year-old male, writhing in pain on the ice and clutching a nearly amputated foot. According to witnesses, the patient had been skating very fast and fell and crashed into the arena wall. You examine the foot and find that it is only attached to the leg by about 1/4 inch of skin. You should _____.

   A. complete the amputation, stop any bleeding, and package the foot according to local protocols

   B. apply a bulky pressure dressing to the stump, wrap the attached foot with a sterile dressing, and treat for shock as you transport immediately

   C. use sterile gauze pads to stop bleeding from the leg, bandage ice packs onto the foot, and reassure the patient as you transport

   D. replace the foot back onto the stump, bandage it in place, and treat the patient for possible shock and hypothermia as you transport

THINKING AND LINKING

CHAPTER TOPIC	HOW IT RELATES TO YOU AND OTHER COURSE AREAS
Hazmat incidents	Hazmat incidents will test your overall skills more than any other type of call except, perhaps, for terrorist incidents (covered in Chapter 36). These skills include sizing up potentially mysterious scenes (Chapter 7) and communicating clearly with dispatch (Chapter 13) to treating multiple patients with a wide range of medical symptoms (Chapter 25) and trauma injuries such as chemical burns (Chapter 27).
Decontamination	Even with the best of efforts, there is always a chance that you will transport some hazardous residue along with your patient. That is why it is imperative that you use all appropriate PPE (Chapter 2) and clean your ambulance and equipment completely after each patient (Chapter 33).
Multiple-casualty incidents	You never know when you may find yourself as the initial incident commander for an MCI. Your professional demeanor (Chapter 1) and communication skills (Chapter 13)—on the radio/phone to dispatch or in person to patients and other rescuers—will be tremendously important in coordinating chaotic events.

36

Terrorism and EMS

CHAPTER SUMMARY

"A violent act dangerous to human life, in violation of the criminal laws of the United States or any segment to intimidate or coerce a government, the civilian population or any segment thereof, in furtherance of political or social objectives." That is how the U.S. Justice Department defines terrorism. As a future EMT-B, what is the key phrase in that statement? "A violent act dangerous to human life." Regardless of political aims or social objectives, terrorism is a threat to human life—which, by default, will soon put you into this particular struggle. What do people do when there is an explosion? An unexplained mass illness? Or when airliners are flown into buildings? They call for emergency services—and soon you will be responding to that call. That is why you need a basic knowledge of terrorism and terrorist methods.

According to the FBI, there are two types of terrorism: domestic and international. Domestic terrorists focus their attacks on the government and/or citizens of a nation, without foreign direction. There are domestic terrorist groups who define themselves by their beliefs in environmentalism, religion, racism, and extreme politics—just to name a few. International terrorists are, as their name indicates, directed or influenced by governments or organizations beyond the borders of the targeted nation. There is a current trend toward international terrorism motivated by religion or ideology.

In addition to firearms, terrorists may use technological hazards such as Chemical, Biological, Radiological, Nuclear, or Explosive (CBRNE) agents—often called weapons of mass destruction (WMD).

The most important concept that you must understand when dealing with a terrorist attack is that *first responders are often the principal targets*. Terrorists have a history of utilizing delayed secondary devices specifically to injure law-enforcement and EMS personnel. Never assume that the scene is safe until it is cleared by the appropriate agency. You must also be aware that the emergency scene created by a terrorist attack will also be a crime scene—and that it must be treated as such.

It is important, though, to not let these additional factors distract you from following your agency's established procedures. Regardless of the cause of the MCI, responders must still set up the incident-command system and follow protocol. Failure to do so will cause confusion and unnecessary complications.

So how does a responding EMT-B recognize a terrorist attack that may not be obvious? The mnemonic OTTO was developed to remind you of what to be alert for when responding to any MCI or hazmat incident. It stands for Occupancy or location, Type of event, Timing of event, and On-scene warning signs. Are you responding to a possible symbolic or historic site, public building or assembly area, controversial business or infrastructure facility? Has there been an explosion or incendiary device? How about firearms? Are you on your way to a nontraumatic MCI? The answers to these questions might point to a terrorist act. What about timing? Is the incident happening on a day of significance? Since the government siege on the Branch Davidian compound in Waco, Texas and the bombing of the Murrah Federal building in Oklahoma City were both on April 19, that date has been identified as a potential "attack day" by antigovernment extremists. On-scene warning signs can include unexplained patterns of illness or death; eye and mucous-membrane irritation; unusual clouds, plumes, or even spray devices; or lab equipment in odd locations. Also, be suspicious of containers that appear out of place at unusual incidents—they may be secondary devices.

Before you can protect yourself at terrorist-attack scenes, you must understand what you may be exposed to. Use the acronym TRACEM-P to help remember. Thermal harm can be caused by extreme heat or extreme cold. Radiological harm comes from nuclear fuel, waste, or bombs. Asphyxiation results from exposure to gases that are heavier than air, such as argon and carbon dioxide. Chemical harm is produced by toxic or corrosive materials. Etiological harm is initiated by exposure to bacteria and viruses. Mechanical harm can be the result of firearms or the shrapnel from a bomb. Psychological harm can result from any violent or traumatic event—and is perhaps the most potent weapon wielded by terrorists.

Your protection, as you respond to a potential terrorist attack, is based on reducing or minimizing exposure through the concepts of *time, distance,* and *shielding*. Minimizing the *time* you spend at the scene will prevent prolonged exposure to danger and will reduce your disruption of the crime scene. Maximize your *distance* from the hazard—or projected hazard—area. *Shielding* can refer to an array of defenses, from the literal—such as sheltering behind a building—to the figurative—like getting vaccinated against a contagious disease.

Chemical incidents can include many classes of hazardous materials (including industrial- and military-type agents)—inhaled, absorbed, ingested, or injected. Chemical-incident patients may be subject to a variety of harms: thermal, asphyxiation, mechanical, psychological, and (obviously) chemical.

Biological incidents will be initiated by inhaled or ingested bacteria, viruses, or toxins and may either be focused in a small group or widespread and epidemic. Bacteria are single-celled organisms that grow in a variety of environments and are divided into two categories: those that grow in the human body and those that grow outside of the human body but produce toxins that can affect the human body. Viruses are the smallest known entities capable of reproduction—they flourish *inside* of human cells, causing those cells to produce more viruses. Toxins are poisons produced by living organisms.

How is an *exposure* calculated? It is simply the dose or concentration multiplied by time. Chemical doses are measured in milligrams per kilogram of body weight and biological doses in fractions of micrograms per kilogram of body weight. Agent concentration is measured in parts per million. So, by reducing the dose, concentration, or time, you reduce the exposure. Infectious-dose data are standardized—and are based on a 70-kg or 150-pound male in good health. Patient variations from that baseline will cause variations in the results of exposure.

Biological agents can be introduced into the body in four main ways (with some being much rarer than others): absorption, injection, inhalation, and ingestion. Although absorption is uncommon, ingestion can occur easily—such as through eating or drinking prior to undergoing decontamination. Injection (whether accidental or intentional) is another highly likely route of introduction. Inhalation, however, poses the largest threat to humans in terms of biological-agent exposure.

We have mentioned it extensively, but what exactly *is* contamination? It is contact with a material (liquid, solid, or aerosol) that is present where it does not belong (hard or soft surfaces, skin, hair, or clothing) and that is harmful to humans, animals, and/or the environment. So, is an exposure a contamination and vice versa? Not really. Exposure indicates entrance *into* the body, whereas contaminants cling *to* the body or clothing. Biological agents can cause the following harms: chemical, etiological, mechanical, and psychological.

If biological agents are suspected, work to limit exposure and contamination. Proper PPE can be an effective barrier against exposure—with adequate equipment protecting the wearer's skin, face, hands, feet, body, head, and respiratory system.

According to intelligence sources, it is highly unlikely that terrorists will be able to obtain and detonate a nuclear device. It is possible, however, that they will spread (or disperse) dangerous radioactive materials with either conventional explosives (referred to as a "dirty bomb") or by sabotaging or attacking a nuclear power facility. The challenge in identifying a nuclear/radiological incident is that symptoms can be delayed for hours or days. Nuclear/radiological incidents can cause harm in the following ways: thermal, radiological, mechanical, chemical, and psychological.

The only real protections in a nuclear/radiological incident are time, distance, and shielding. Assume that every explosive incident has disseminated either radiological, biological, or chemical materials; this will assure an appropriate response until such time as the cause can be determined.

Explosive attacks (currently terrorism's most common weapon) can be delivered using a wide variety of methods (from pipe bombs to vehicle bombs) and directed at any number of targets (buildings, crowds, rescue workers, and so on). Explosives can be designed to disperse chemical, biological, or radiological materials and be built to detonate in a variety of ways—pressure, light, movement, radio transmissions, and so on. Also, due to the proliferation of suicide bombers, keep in mind that the perpetrator(s) may be among the patients at the scene—and search all patients for weapons prior to transport. (Note that in everyday situations a search for weapons would be performed by police. In situations such as these, you may uncover a device during your patient assessment.) *Untrained personnel should never attempt to neutralize an unexploded device.* Explosive incidents can cause thermal, asphyxiation, radiological, chemical, etiological, mechanical, and psychological harm.

The most common means for dissemination of CBRNE materials (especially biological, chemical, or nuclear/radiological elements) is by enabling them to enter the respiratory tract, which is also the most effective way of creating mass casualties. The deeper into the lungs the material is "placed," the longer the exposure and the more severe the reaction.

Other means of dissemination depend upon the agent used. For instance, some biological agents cannot survive the acidic environment of the stomach, thereby negating their use as an ingested weapon. Some agents, however, such as anthrax, can survive ingestion—and that possibility raises fears of the terrorist contamination of our water supplies. Normal dilution, filtration, and chlorination processes, however, reduce the chance of that happening.

Dermal (or percutaneous) exposure can be very effective for blister agents (vesicants) but less effective for biological agents. Healthy, unbroken skin provides an excellent barrier. Some biological, and many viral, agents can be disseminated very effectively through person-to-person contact. If the agent has an extended incubation period, it is possible to infect large segments of the population before anything is ever detected. This is the concern with such illnesses as smallpox and hemorrhagic fever.

Chemical agents cover the whole range of physical properties: they may be in a solid, liquid, or gaseous form; they may be soluble or insoluble in water; they may have a strong odor or none at all. A chemical's volatility is important because it will determine whether there is rapid evaporation (causing respiratory danger) or delayed evaporation (causing extended exposure). Chemical agents are classified in several ways: choking agents, vesicating agents (chemically change exposed skin), cyanide agents (prevent cellular utilization of oxygen), nerve agents (prevent the nervous system from functioning properly), and riot-control agents (tear producing).

Biological agents are microorganisms (bacteria and viruses) or toxins that can cause disease processes. Any biological agent can be weaponized and disseminated; some are just not very effective. Biological agents that are used as weapons will most likely be infective, virulent, toxic, stable, and lethal. As a weapon, biological agents have a benefit over their chemical counterparts in that they are easily produced and can replicate over time—increasing the effectiveness of the attack as time passes.

Some of the more common biological agents that can be weaponized are anthrax (which can cause open sores and, in respiratory form, death), cholera (a diarrheal disease that may cause death from dehydration or electrolyte imbalance), plague (which can result in severe respiratory distress and death), Q fever (which causes diaphoresis, malaise, and fatigue but has a low fatality rate), and tularemia (which causes fever, headache, and weight loss, and has a 5- to 10-percent mortality rate).

Toxins, which are chemical compounds created by living organisms, can and have been utilized effectively as weapons—but they will not reproduce or spread beyond the target area. Some of the more dangerous toxins available to terrorists are botulinum (one of the deadliest agents known), ricin (which causes severe necrosis), staphylococcal enterotoxin B (more incapacitating than it is fatal), and trichothecene myotoxins (which cause vomiting, hypotension, shock, and death—usually within 12 hours).

Viruses are the simplest microorganisms but perhaps the most insidious. A virus will attach to a cell and override that host's own DNA/RNA—causing the cell to assist the virus in replicating itself. Due to severe logistical issues, the weaponized use of viruses—although possible—is highly unlikely. Viruses that *may* be encountered include smallpox (a highly contagious disease that causes flu-like symptoms and a blistery rash and is fatal in 30 percent of unvaccinated cases), encephalitis (which causes swelling of the brain and all associated neurologic results, and is incapacitating but rarely fatal), and viral hemorrhagic fevers such as ebola and dengue fever (viruses that alter the clotting characteristics of blood, as well as capillary permeability, causing systemic hemorrhaging and liquefaction of solid organs, and leading to death in up to 90 percent of cases).

If a terrorist organization were to use nuclear or radiological technology as a weapon, it would likely take one of four forms: a military nuclear device (*very* unlikely), an improvised nuclear device (possible but probably not without the intelligence community first becoming aware of it), a radiological dispersal device (or a "dirty bomb"—which would be the most probable of all radiological weapons), or sabotage of an existing nuclear facility (again, *possible*, but very unlikely due to security and redundant safety features). The three body systems that are most affected by radiation exposure are the musculoskeletal (blood production in the bone marrow), gastrointestinal, and central nervous.

Incendiary devices are much more probable as weapons of terrorism than nuclear or radiological devices. These devices, such as Molotov cocktails and propane bombs, can cause thermal injuries, blast injuries, and death. Follow local protocols when treating burns and soft-tissue or musculoskeletal injuries.

As an EMS responder to a potential terrorist action, it is very important that you understand how to apply tactical considerations to isolate the site, contact the appropriate authorities, identify possible agents used, and protect assets. Your priorities should be, in order of importance, protection of life, stabilization of the incident, and protection of property.

First, realize that responding to a terrorist action will be unlike any other call that you will receive. It will most likely be on a large scale, have unknown secondary hazards, and involve masses of panicked (and potentially injured) civilians—while the terrorists may still be in the area just waiting for you to arrive. In addition to all of that, it will be the largest crime scene that you may ever encounter.

You will first need to perform a scene size-up and begin establishing outer and inner operational perimeters to isolate the scene—which, initially, may be a challenge due to crowds of potentially contaminated people fleeing the scene, debris, rubble, and lack of personnel. As soon as law enforcement is available, you should turn over the perimeter responsibility to them.

This leads us to the subject of initial notification. It will *not* be your job, as an EMT-B, to notify law enforcement, local, state, and federal agencies, and so on regarding a terrorist incident—but you need to provide your dispatch center with a calm, clear picture of what has occurred and what response is needed, much like a hazmat incident. Your dispatch center will then make all of the appropriate notifications.

You need to be observant for indicators of specific chemical, biological, or radiological agents. Be suspicious of your surroundings. Should that stainless-steel box be there? Is there any reason for lab equipment to be lying in the alley? Why does that tanker truck not have a placard on the cargo? Consult your Emergency Response Guidebook or contact the CHEMTREC or CHEM-TEL hotlines for assistance with identifying or responding to substances. Also, pay close attention to illness patterns among patients whom you are treating. Are there particular signs or symptoms that many of them are displaying?

Once the scene is isolated, the proper notifications have been made, and the dangerous materials present (if any) have been identified, what next? The last, yet equally important, step in the response to a terrorist incident is to ensure the protection of assets. What exactly does that mean? The military calls it "force protection." You must partner with law enforcement, security, and, potentially, even the National Guard to ensure the safety of EMS resources. Personnel, transport vehicles, and supplies will all be critically important in the aftermath of a terrorist event. Perimeter control, traffic control, and scene-access control are all effective ways to protect EMS operations.

Your responsibilities, with respect to asset protection, will be to look for any initial security threats, contact dispatch and request protection, establish staging and triage sectors in safe zones, advise EMS command about security concerns, and report any suspicious individuals or activities.

PEARLS FROM THE PODIUM

- Terrorism can come in many forms, including domestic or international, and use many methods including CBRNE (chemical, biological, radiological, nuclear, or explosive).
- Terrorism may seem quite distant to you, or quite likely, depending on where you practice EMS—but every EMS provider could respond to a terrorist incident.
- Occupancy, type, timing, and on-scene warning signs (OTTO) is one method to use for clues to a terrorist attack.
- Time, distance, and shielding are the factors you should consider when protecting yourself from a terrorist incident.

REVIEW QUESTIONS

SHORT ANSWER

1. What is the difference between a *strategy* and a *tactic*?

2. Why do government facilities operate with a higher state of security awareness on April 19?

MULTIPLE CHOICE

1. *Hazmats* are a subcategory of a much broader field known as _____.
   - **A.** biological hazards
   - **B.** technological hazards
   - **C.** ideological hazards
   - **D.** primary hazards

2. What do the letters in the mnemonic OTTO stand for?
   - **A.** **O**rganization, **T**actics, **T**iming, and **O**pportunity.
   - **B.** **O**ccurrence, **T**ransfer, **T**ransportation, and **O**rientation.
   - **C.** **O**ccupancy, **T**ype, **T**iming, and **O**n-scene.
   - **D.** **O**rder, **T**ransition, **T**echnicality, and **O**bstruction.

3. If a bacterial or viral agent has been "weaponized," then it most likely has been altered into a(n) _____ form.
   - **A.** respirable
   - **B.** injectable
   - **C.** thermal
   - **D.** ingestible

4. Terrorists have a history of using secondary devices to target _____.
   - **A.** civilians
   - **B.** military personnel
   - **C.** buildings
   - **D.** emergency responders

5. The three types of events that should raise your awareness of possible terrorist involvement are explosions, incidents involving _____, and nontrauma MCIs.
   - **A.** large vehicles
   - **B.** firearms
   - **C.** public figures
   - **D.** utility lines

SCENARIO QUESTIONS

It has been a relatively light-call day and you are just about done reading a new novel. Dispatch breaks the silence and tells you to head toward the county courthouse to assist a unit already at the scene for a "few" medical patients. As you pull up in the ambulance, you see absolute pandemonium! There are people everywhere—75 to 100 at least—all in various stages of collapse. You see some people vomiting, some motionless in the street, a bailiff is convulsing on the sidewalk, and you see a fellow EMT-B dragging himself through the glass double doors of the courthouse.

1. How should you handle this situation?
   - **A.** Immediately contact dispatch for more assistance and begin triaging patients.
   - **B.** Run over to the EMT-B and question him about the situation.
   - **C.** Contact dispatch, calmly explain your assessment of the scene, and set up an incident-command post while waiting for backup.
   - **D.** Move your ambulance a good distance away while relaying the entire situation to dispatch, and set up an incident-command post.

2. The first ambulance crew on the scene apparently did not _____.
  A. evaluate the OTTO signs
  B. initiate the START program
  C. maintain contact with the CBRNE agents
  D. establish a TRACEM-P post

3. You should suspect that the courthouse was attacked with a _____.
  A. radiological device   B. vector contaminant
  C. chemical weapon   D. gastrointestinal vesicant

You are dispatched to the mall following some sort of explosion. You were not that far away and arrive at the same time as the fire department. Shoppers are pouring from the entrance to the mall and scattering in the parking lot. You stop a young woman who is bleeding from a scalp wound. "What happened in there?" you ask. The girl says through her tears, "That guy … he walked right into the crowd and … and he just blew up." She then pulls away from you and runs off.

1. Due to the potential for response targeting, you should _____.
  A. contact the IED hotline
  B. only treat patients in the exclusion zone
  C. allow law enforcement to clear the scene
  D. immediately install isolation barriers

2. This situation is an example of a(n) _____.
  A. incendiary event   B. tertiary device
  C. suicide bombing   D. zoonotic incident

3. Before transporting patients from this scene, you should _____.
  A. obtain REM readings
  B. seek clearance from the triage officer
  C. perform a gross decontamination
  D. search them for weapons

It is surreal that the building is now gone. You had just passed it on the way to lunch and now you are approaching the scene after dispatch told you that the Museum of Commerce and Industry was destroyed by a "truck bomb." As you approach the designated staging area, the staging officer tells you to just park and wait. You pull in next to six other ambulances and wait, watching as dark smoke billows into the sky from the rubble that once was a structural masterpiece.

1. Any time there is an explosion, you should anticipate _____.
  A. the introduction of thermal–pH conditioning
  B. a virulent fallout
  C. the dispersion of radiological materials
  D. weaponized ebola

2. You should have a high index of suspicion for _____.
  A. possible criminal involvement
  B. asbestos smoke around the scene
  C. illnesses caused by thermal residue
  D. secondary devices

3. The general purpose of a terrorist attack is to inflict _____ harm.

    A. etiological   **B.** psychological

    C. architectural   **D.** physiological

CASE STUDIES

CASE STUDY 1	THERE HAS BEEN AN EXPLOSION AT THE STADIUM

It is 1715, and you are working the ambulance in a large metropolitan area when you receive a dispatch to respond to a local sporting arena for a possible explosion. There is a major play-off game being held between two national teams and you know of several of your colleagues who are working medical support at the game. Dispatch advises there are multiple injuries and that there are multiple resources responding to the incident. As you approach the arena, you can see smoke coming from one section of the north side.

1. What characteristics of this scene cause you to suspect a possible terrorist event?

2. Given what you know so far, what types of injuries can you expect to see?

As you approach the scene, you are advised by dispatch to contact incident command on tactical channel 3. You can see hundreds of people rushing out of the exits on the north side and spilling out into the parking lot. You make radio contact with incident command and are advised to stage your vehicle in the east parking lot and begin setting up a triage and treatment area to help manage the injuries.

1. What factors must be considered when establishing command, treatment, and triage areas for such an event?

2. Aside from the threat of contamination from a primary attack, what other threats must the EMT-B keep in mind when responding to suspected acts of terrorism?

You are called by the police to a family-planning clinic on the outskirts of town. The clinic has been the site of several protests over the past few months. You arrive and meet a police captain outside the building. He tells you that a receptionist opened a letter that contained a threatening note with an unknown white powder. The suspicion is that it may be anthrax.

1. Is this a terrorist act?

2. What type of harm is this event (using the TRACEM-P categories)?

The employees of the clinic have been briefed what to do for events such as this. The area was isolated and only two employees were potentially exposed after the letter was opened. The employees were reportedly in good health before the incident and have no complaints now. A hazardous-material team and the FBI have been contacted.

1. Should you have contact with these patients now? If not, when?

The hazmat team arrives and decontaminates the patients and appropriately collects any contaminated waste. They turn their attention to the office as the patients are brought to you at the ambulance.

1. What BSI precautions are required at this point?

2. Can these patients be transported to the hospital?

Active Exploration

To get an understanding of just how much the topic of terrorism has hit the EMS community, you can look at how many EMS textbooks now have a chapter or appendix dealing with the subject. Just three years ago, very few Paramedic, EMT, or First Responder textbooks even touched on the topic. Now you will have difficulty finding a textbook that does not.

Among the EMS community in the east, terrorism has been seen, felt, heard, smelled, and touched. For those who responded to the incidents of September 11, 2001, terrorism could not be more real or more frightening. For those of us who witnessed the events on the television, the experience was horrific and surreal, to say the least, but we did not experience it firsthand as so many of our colleagues did. Our experience was filtered by the media and the very distance we happened to be from ground zero. No matter where we were or how we experienced it, the affects of that attack were real, and they made an everlasting impact on EMS and the way EMS is viewed by our country and the government.

The following activities will help you develop your understanding of the potential of terrorist acts and how they might affect the community we live in.

Activity 1: Choose Your Weapon—Biological

While the threat of a terrorist attack is real, it is still quite rare when compared to the number of other EMS calls EMTs see each day in this country. For that reason, the information available to EMTs and First Responders in their textbooks is minimal. The next two activities will have you conduct an in-depth exploration of at least two WMD of your choice. For the first activity, we want you to refer to Chapter 36 of your Emergency Care textbook and select one "biological" weapon to learn more about. In doing so, we want you to find out as much about the agent as you can and answer the following questions:

1. Have there been any recent (past five years) incidents involving the agent you selected?

2. What was the method of dispersal of the agent?

3. What was the outcome in terms of casualties and injuries?

4. What are the signs and symptoms of exposure—early and late?

5. What can the typical EMT do to treat someone exposed to the agent?

6. How does an EMT protect himself from becoming exposed?

Activity 2: Choose Your Weapon—Chemical

For the first activity, we want you to refer to Chapter 36 of your Emergency Care textbook and select one "chemical" weapon to learn more about. In doing so, we want you to find out as much about the agent as you can and answer the following questions:

1. Have there been any recent (past five years) incidents involving the agent you selected?

2. What was the method of dispersal for the agent?

3. What was the outcome in terms of casualties and injuries?

4. What are the signs and symptoms of exposure—early and late?

5. What can the typical EMT do to treat someone exposed to the agent?

6. How does an EMT protect himself from becoming exposed?

┃ RETRO REVIEW

1. When treating a high-school football player with a suspected spinal injury, you should leave his helmet in place, unless _____.
   A. the patient is in cardiac arrest
   B. the helmet fits snugly and does not allow for head movement
   C. removing it might cause further injury
   D. the patient is appropriately responsive

2. Which of the following would be included in a verbal patient report but not necessarily in a radio report?

   A. The patient's chief complaint.   **B.** The patient's medical history.

   C. The patient's ongoing vital signs.   **D.** The patient's mental status.

3. The definition of poison is _____.

   A. any toxin capable of destroying living cells

   B. a substance that causes instant or eventual death

   C. any manufactured or organic chemical that can be absorbed, inhaled, injected, or ingested

   D. any substance that can harm the body

THINKING AND LINKING

CHAPTER TOPIC	HOW IT RELATES TO YOU AND OTHER COURSE AREAS
Targeting First Responders	When responding to a potential terrorist incident, *do not* forget that the use of secondary devices to injure or kill rescuers is a common terrorist tactic. You should have a high index of suspicion for the area surrounding the scene and exercise appropriate caution before approaching it (covered generally in Chapter 2 and specifically in Chapter 35).
On-scene warning signs	Fight the urge to develop "tunnel vision" at potential terrorist incidents. During your scene size-up (Chapter 7), you should try to keep a broad focus and make note of anything suspicious (people, containers, vehicles, and so on). Your top priority after recognizing an unsafe element at the scene is to take action to protect yourself and others (Chapter 2).
	Remember that the scene size-up process should continue as long as you are at the scene.
Explosions	Explosions do have the potential of spreading biological, chemical, or radiological materials, but you should also anticipate such "normal" injuries as burns and both blunt and penetrating trauma (Chapter 27).
	Keep in mind that a patient who was near enough to be injured by an explosion (or the accompanying shock wave) is likely to have head or spinal injuries also (Chapter 29).

37

Advanced Airway Management

CHAPTER SUMMARY

Airway management is the most critical component of treating any patient. Without a patent airway, your patient will die regardless of all other interventions performed.

The major structures of the airway are:

- Nasopharynx—area that air passes through when inhaled by the nose
- Oropharynx—area that air passes through when inhaled by the mouth
- Hypopharynx—area just superior to the opening of the trachea and the esophagus
- Trachea—windpipe
- Epiglottis—leaf-shaped structure that acts as a cover to the opening of the trachea
- Vallecula—the "valley" created where the tongue and epiglottis meet
- Larynx—voice box
- Vocal cords—contained in the larynx
- Cricoid cartilage—the cartilage ring at the inferior portion of the larynx
- Mainstem bronchi (right and left)—the trachea splits into two separate airways, one for each lung
- Carina—where the trachea splits into two mainstem bronchi
- Alveoli—where oxygen and carbon dioxide are exchanged in the lungs

It is important to understand the issues that can cause the respiratory system to fail to the level that requires an advanced airway. The body requires that certain functions be intact in order for a patient to breathe adequately. These include:

- A functioning respiratory control center in the brain, located in the brainstem
- A patent airway

- An intact chest wall
- The ability for oxygen and carbon dioxide to be exchanged in the alveoli

Injuries or illnesses that affect any one of these areas can cause respiratory problems. Your assessment of the adequacy of a patient's breathing will be crucial in determining whether basic or advanced airway management is needed. Inadequate breathing presents with the following findings:

- Rate—outside the normal range
- Rhythm—irregular pattern
- Quality—abnormal breath sounds, chest expansion, or breathing effort
- Shallow or deep
- Cyanosis
- Cool, clammy skin
- Agonal respirations

Pediatric respiratory anatomy and physiology differ from those of adults. Children also exhibit different signs and symptoms of respiratory failure. Anatomy and physiological differences include:

- All structures are smaller and more easily obstructed
- Tongue is proportionately larger
- Trachea is softer and more flexible, can be pinched off if the head is extended too far while opening the airway
- Narrowest area of the airway is at the circoid cartilage
- Chest wall is softer, diaphragm more heavily depended on for breathing

In addition to exhibiting the same signs and symptoms for inadequate breathing as adults, pediatric patients may present with the following additional signs and symptoms:

- Slower than normal heart rate
- Weak or absent peripheral pulses
- Retractions
- Nasal flaring
- Seesaw breathing

Keep in mind that respiratory failure in children and infants is the number one cause of cardiac arrest.

The first step in managing an airway is to perform oropharyngeal suctioning to remove any fluids from the oropharynx.

Endotracheal intubation is the placement of a tube through the mouth and vocal cords into the trachea to secure the airway. This is accomplished by using a laryngoscope with an appropriate size blade to visualize the vocal cords for correct placement. The advantages of endotracheal intubation include:

- Complete control of the airway
- Minimization of aspiration
- Better oxygen delivery to the lungs
- Allows for deeper suctioning of the airway

Complications can include:

- Slowing of the heart rate
- Soft-tissue trauma and broken teeth
- Hypoxia
- Vomiting
- Right mainstem intubation
- Esophageal intubation
- Accidental extubation

Equipment needed for intubation includes appropriate BSI precautions, a laryngoscope, an endotracheal tube of appropriate size, a stylet, a 10-cc syringe, something to secure the tube with, water-based lubricant, and a suction device.

Indications for performing endotracheal intubation include the following:

- Inability to ventilate the apneic patient
- Need to protect the airway of a patient without a gag reflex or cough
- Need to protect the airway of a patient unresponsive to any painful stimuli
- Cardiac arrest

Below is a basic list of steps for intubating a patient. You must practice these skills on a regular basis throughout your career.

1. Utilize BSI and prepare all equipment
2. Visualize the glottic opening and vocal cords with a laryngoscope
3. Use Sellick's maneuver if necessary
4. Insert the endotracheal tube so that the cuff is just past the vocal cords
5. Inflate the distal cuff
6. Ensure correct tube placement and correct if needed
7. Secure the tube in place, marking depth of placement
8. Perform ongoing assessments

An attempt to intubate should not last longer than 30 seconds. Ventilate the patient for 1 minute before making a second attempt.

Indications for intubating a child are similar to those for an adult. The child's anatomical differences can make visualizing the vocal cords more difficult. Cuffed tubes are not utilized on children less than 8 years of age, so it is very important to select the correct tube size. Remember that children are more sensitive to hypoxia than adults, so children must be monitored carefully during intubation attempts. The procedure is similar to the one for adults with the following important differences:

1. Rate of ventilation must be appropriate for the child's age
2. Heart rate must be monitored closely
3. Head should be in "sniffing position," not hyperextended
4. Little force is needed
5. Epiglottis is less rigid than in an adult; may obstruct view of glottic opening
6. Hold onto the tube until it is well secured—pediatric tubes are easily dislodged
7. Be sure you observe bilateral chest rise and fall during ventilation
8. Heart rate should increase after correct placement of the endotracheal tube

In addition to the placement of an endotracheal tube, an EMT-B may also be permitted by local protocol to place a nasogastric (NG) tube in an infant or child. This is a tube that is inserted through the nose and into the stomach to alleviate gastric distention of the stomach and proximal bowel area during ventilations. Indications for use of the NG tube include:

- Inability to effectively ventilate the patient due to distention of the stomach
- Unresponsive patient with gastric distention

Major facial trauma or head trauma is a contraindication to the use of the NG tube.

To insert the NG tube, prepare all equipment needed. Oxygenate the patient well before proceeding. Measure the tube from the nose, around the ear to below the xiphoid process. Lubricate the end of the tube and pass it downward along the nasal floor. Confirm that the tube is in the stomach by aspirating stomach contents. Secure the tube in place.

Individual local protocols may also allow the EMT-B to perform orotracheal suctioning, commonly performed through an endotracheal tube. Indications for performing orotracheal suctioning include:

- Obvious secretions in the airway
- Poor compliance with BVM ventilations

Complications include:

- Cardiac dysrhythmias
- Hypoxia
- Coughing
- Damage to the lining of the airway

Other advanced airway devices that may be available for EMT-Bs to utilize, depending on local EMS system protocol, include a multilumen airway (Combitube), a laryngeal-mask airway (LMA), and automatic transport ventilators (ATVs).

PEARLS FROM THE PODIUM

- The ability to use advanced airway techniques is a great responsibility.
- It is important to practice your skills during initial training and at regular intervals afterward—especially if you do not frequently practice advanced airway insertion.
- Be sure you know your protocols and the indications for using advanced airways.
- Suction is critical. It is not uncommon for patients to vomit during the insertion or withdrawal of advanced airways. Have suction ready.
- Be sure that you confirm placement of your advanced airway when it is inserted and monitor the airway position throughout your treatment of the patient.

REVIEW QUESTIONS

SHORT ANSWER

1. What is the most common use of the NG tube in regard to advanced airway management?

2. Why are breath sounds not the only indicator of proper endotracheal tube placement in pediatric patients?

MULTIPLE CHOICE

1. The endotracheal tube can be used to direct oxygen, medication, or a _____ directly into the trachea.
   - **A.** stylet
   - **B.** saline flush
   - **C.** suction catheter
   - **D.** laryngoscope

2. Deep suctioning a patient for more than 15 seconds can cause all of the following except _____.
   - **A.** bronchospasm
   - **B.** gastric distention
   - **C.** hypoxia
   - **D.** cardiac dysrhythmia

3. A straight laryngoscope blade lifts the epiglottis and a curved blade fits into the _____.
   - **A.** vallecula
   - **B.** larynx
   - **C.** carina
   - **D.** oropharynx

4. The most serious complication of orotracheal intubation is _____.
   - **A.** bradycardia
   - **B.** right mainstem intubation
   - **C.** accidental extubation
   - **D.** esophageal intubation

5. An EMT-B should only make _____ attempt(s) to intubate a patient.
   - **A.** three
   - **B.** two
   - **C.** four
   - **D.** one

SCENARIO QUESTIONS

You arrive at a local park on Saturday afternoon. You immediately see a group of people waving frantically and shouting for you. The original call was for an individual who was having trouble breathing. As you approach, the group separates, exposing a young woman who is lying on the ground fighting to breathe. There is tremendous swelling in her hands and face. "Are you allergic to anything?" you ask her. The patient shakes her head weakly. "Did you get stung or bitten by anything today?" The patient has become unresponsive and one of the bystanders says, "Yes. She got stung by a bee about twenty minutes ago."

1. The most appropriate airway technique you can perform for this patient right now is to _____.
   - **A.** insert an NPA
   - **B.** intubate orally
   - **C.** perform a tracheotomy
   - **D.** insert an NG tube

2. If you notice gurgling sounds during the epigastric auscultation of this patient, you have _____.

   A. pushed the tube too far past the carina

   B. neglected to inflate the cuff properly

   C. placed the tube correctly

   D. performed an esophageal intubation

3. If you are having difficulty visualizing the glottic opening, you should ask your partner to apply _____.

   A. a new laryngoscope blade   B. ice packs to reduce swelling

   C. cricoid pressure   D. the Smithson maneuver

The rescue squad has quickly finished extricating a 53-year-old male patient who became unresponsive during the disentanglement procedure. The patient's pulse is quickening and his respirations have stopped. The patient is rapidly becoming cyanotic.

1. As soon as you have access to this patient, you should ensure an open airway and immediately _____.

   A. insert an endotracheal tube

   B. begin rescue breathing

   C. suction the hypopharynx

   D. administer high-concentration oxygen

2. Besides a return to normal color, how else might you be able to tell that your artificial ventilations are sufficient for this patient?

   A. The patient's capillary refill time will decrease.

   B. There will be equal bilateral breath sounds.

   C. The patient will begin to cough.

   D. The patient's pulse will slow.

3. During this emergency, you would use a _____ mm orotracheal tube on this patient.

   A. 4.5   B. 7.5

   C. 9.0   D. 10.5

CASE STUDIES

CASE STUDY 1   MAN NOT BREATHING

You are dispatched to a homeless shelter for a man not breathing. Upon your arrival, a police officer on the scene directs you to an alley at the back of the shelter. There you see an approximately 30-year-old male patient of average size who is being ventilated with a BVM by a firefighter. The police officer tells you that one of the shelter staff discovered the man about 20 minutes ago and called 911. He is a regular at the shelter and has a known history of drug abuse. You perform a quick initial assessment and find that the man is breathing approximately 4 times per minute and has accepted an OPA from the firefighter. You decide to place an endotracheal tube into this man's airway.

1. What size ET tube will you use for this patient?

2. What steps will you take prior to attempting intubation of this patient?

You have prepared the tube by inserting the stylet and testing the cuff with the syringe. The firefighter has been hyperventilating the patient at a rate of 24 per minute for about 45 seconds when you ask him to stop and move aside so you can place the tube.

1. You have placed the blade of the laryngoscope into the patient's mouth and are still having difficulty visualizing the glottic opening; what will you do?

2. You pass the tube on the first try and quickly inflate the cuff. How will you confirm proper placement of the tube?

| CASE STUDY 2 | I THINK THERE IS SOMETHING WRONG WITH MY WIFE |

Your ambulance is dispatched for a "sick person" at 14 Gwendolyn Circle. The dispatcher is not able to obtain further information. You arrive and cautiously approach. A man meets you at the door and looks a bit worried. "It's my wife," he says. "She doesn't look good."

You arrive in his living room and find his wife slumped over in a chair. You look at her and immediately suspect she is in cardiac arrest. You and your partner carefully move her to the floor where your suspicions are confirmed. Your partner radios for ALS assistance.

1. Why did the husband not know his wife was without a pulse?

2. If CPR had begun, would you reach for the AED or the ET tube first? Why?

Before any decisions are made the patient vomits. She vomits copiously. It is a thick pasty substance that is difficult to suction. You suction with a rigid tip catheter and cannot get it all, so you switch to just the wide suction tubing. You clear the airway although it takes the better part of 15 seconds. The patient vomits again. Copiously.

1. You have already suctioned for 15 seconds and now the thick vomitus returns. What do you do?

2. What may be causing the vomiting?

It is time to intubate and you reach for the equipment. The patient remains pulseless. CPR is continued with hyperoxygenation while you prepare for intubation. CPR is stopped while you attempt to intubate. You see more vomitus and suction while you are trying to view the cords. Even with suctioning, you cannot see anything. You cease your intubation attempt and resume CPR. The patient is oxygenated again. The second attempt is again negative. The woman is large, at least 130 kg, and this complicates your attempts at visualization. BVM ventilations are relatively effective when the patient is not vomiting.

1. Now what do you do for airway control?

Active Exploration

Regardless of whether or not your EMS system allows EMT-Bs to intubate, it is important for every EMT-B who may assist in such a procedure to know and understand what is happening. A wise paramedic once said that a paramedic is only as good as his EMT partner. There is truth in that statement and your goal as an EMT is to become as valuable as you can when assisting more advanced care providers in the field.

As a well-informed EMT-B, you will want to become familiar with your local protocols for advanced airway management as well as with the tools and techniques used to establish an advanced airway. While you may not be placing these airways directly, you will need this knowledge to better assist those who will.

The following activities will help you develop the knowledge and skills necessary to place or assist in the placement of advanced airways.

Activity 1: Toy with the Tools

The road to becoming familiar with the equipment and techniques used in placing advanced airways is simple: get your hands on the equipment. While you cannot practice placing these airways on one another, you can get your hands on the tools used in the process and familiarize yourself with them.

Ask your instructor or perhaps a paramedic friend to show you the tools used in the placement of these airways. You will want to get your hands on an endotracheal tube, a stylet, a syringe, and a laryngoscope at the very least.

1. Practice placing the stylet into the tube and shaping the tube in different ways.
2. Use a syringe to inflate the cuff at the end of the tube to test its integrity.
3. Place several different blades on the laryngoscope handle and test the light on each blade for function.
4. Learn how to change the batteries in the handle of the scope.

Ask a paramedic the difference between the curved and straight blades and their recommended uses.

Activity 2: Dr. Sellick, I Presume

This next activity will help you become familiar with the technique known as "Sellick's Maneuver." This procedure, also known as cricoid pressure, is well known by emergency physicians, nurses, respiratory therapists, and paramedics. It was originally performed to provide indirect pressure on the esophagus during artificial ventilations to minimize aspiration of stomach contents and the flow of air into the stomach. It is also helpful in aiding in the visualization of the glottal opening when placing an advanced airway such as an endotracheal tube.

Ask for the assistance of a fellow student and practice locating the proper location for this maneuver. The procedure is best performed with the use of the thumb and two fingers—the index finger and middle finger. Follow these steps:

1. With your simulated patient lying supine on the floor, place your index finger directly over the cricoid notch to facilitate location.
2. Now place your thumb and middle fingers on either side of the cricoid membrane for stabilization.
3. Using all three fingers, apply downward pressure evenly on the cricoid membrane.
4. Do not apply pressure to your partner. This activity is for positioning practice only.

Just how much pressure to apply is debatable, but in most cases, the paramedic requesting assistance will advise you when enough is enough. It is important to keep in mind that too much pressure can damage the trachea, so caution must be used.

Cricoid pressure is applied when requested during intubation of the unresponsive patient and when ventilating the nonbreathing patient.

RETRO REVIEW

1. Why should a low-pressure water system be used for decontaminating patients following a hazardous-materials incident?
   A. To avoid aggravating soft-tissue injuries.
   B. To prevent the creation of an aerosol out of dry chemicals.
   C. To avoid further contamination due to overspray.
   D. All of the above.

2. You respond to a single-vehicle crash on a country road late one rainy night. Upon your arrival, you see that a pickup truck has overturned and slid into some heavy foliage on the side of the road. As you are getting the gear from the back of the ambulance, your partner, who was approaching the overturned truck, shouts "This sounds really weird, but my legs are tingling!" What should you do?
   A. Tell your partner not to move and immediately contact dispatch.
   B. Walk over to your partner and see whether you notice the same sensation.
   C. Tell your partner to quickly hop on one foot back to the ambulance.
   D. Run over and tackle your partner to the ground.

3. Asking your patient to smile, to put her arms out in front of her for 10 seconds, and to say something like "The grass grows tall on the terrace," are all three elements of _____.
   A. the Apgar Scale
   B. the Cincinnati Stroke Scale
   C. the START Scale
   D. the Rochester CVA Scale

THINKING AND LINKING

CHAPTER TOPIC	HOW IT RELATES TO YOU AND OTHER COURSE AREAS
Orotracheal intubation	Of all the procedures that you, as an EMT-B, will perform, the intubation process is probably going to be the most disturbing to the patient's family. Your effective communication skills (Chapter 13), confident (practiced) technique, and professional appearance (Chapter 1) will go a long way toward reducing the stress and fear that the family is feeling.

Do not forget to have suction equipment ready while attempting intubation (Chapter 6); there is always the chance that you may trigger the patient's gag reflex. |
| Nasogastric tube insertion | A pediatric patient who has been artificially ventilated (Chapters 6 and 31) by a lay rescuer prior to your arrival will commonly have excess air in the stomach and bowel. Many lay rescuers will be too "aggressive" with air pressure and ventilation timing while acting under the stress of the situation (Chapter 2).

Thanking lay rescuers for providing patient emergency care until your arrival and complimenting their abilities are two small actions that not only assist with your agency's public relations, but also show you to be a courteous and professional EMT-B (Chapter 1). |
| Deep suctioning | Medical or trauma patients who have already aspirated substances such as blood and vomitus (Chapter 6) before your arrival may need orotracheal (sometimes called "deep") suctioning.

Always be prepared with orotracheal suctioning equipment when responding to a patient with an altered mental status (Chapter 19), a possible drug or alcohol overdose (Chapter 21), or any "gurgling" respirations. |

THIS WORKSHEET CORRESPONDS TO CHAPTER 27, PAGE 245 OF THIS TEXT

We suggest that you first make several copies of this sheet. Using a pencil, pen, or marker of some kind, shade in specific areas of each of the images and have a fellow student estimate the body surface area (BSA) affected. Compare your results with the images on page 617 of the Emergency Care 10 textbook.

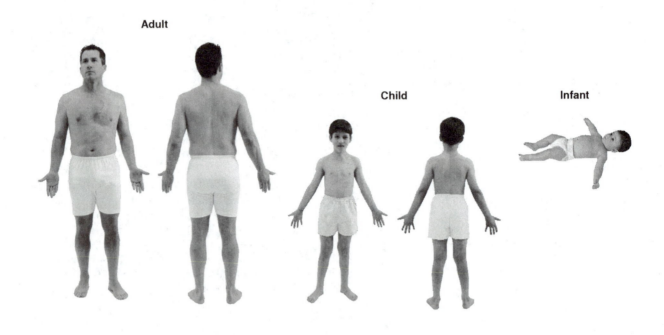

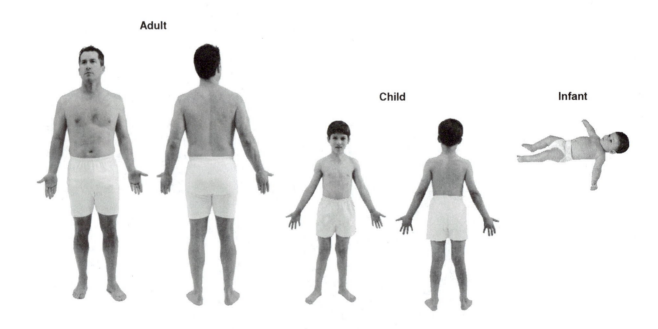

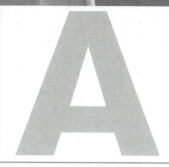

Answers to Chapter Review Questions

ANSWERS TO CHAPTER 1
INTRODUCTION TO EMERGENCY MEDICAL CARE

ANSWERS TO SHORT ANSWER QUESTIONS

1. *Answer:* *The most important role of an EMT-B is to ensure the best possible emergency care for the patient. This includes addressing the patient's needs, bringing up any of his concerns to the hospital staff, and "speaking up" for the patient who might not be able to.*

2. *Answer:* *A telephone-access system for reporting emergencies that is capable of automatically identifying the caller's phone number and location. It assists the dispatcher in sending emergency personnel to the scene even if the caller is confused, becomes unresponsive, or the phone is disconnected.*

ANSWERS TO MULTIPLE-CHOICE QUESTIONS

1. *Answer:* *b.* *Each EMS system has a Medical Director, a physician who is ultimately responsible for medical direction, or oversight of the patient-care aspects of the EMS system.*

2. *Answer:* *a.* *The color of a patient's skin, lips, and/or nail beds can be an important indicator of the patient's condition. An EMT-B with color vision problems may not be able to effectively assess the patient's skin.*

3. *Answer:* *d.* *Without regular continuing education, it will be difficult to maintain, let alone improve, standards of quality.*

4. *Answer:* *c.* *NREMT (National Registry of Emergency Medical Technicians)*

5. *Answer:* d. *Development of the modern Emergency Medical System began during the 1960s.*

ANSWERS TO SCENARIO QUESTIONS

1. *Answer:* c. *A policy or protocol authorizing an EMT-B to perform particular skills in certain situations (e.g. administering glucose to a diabetic patient) is called a standing order.*

2. *Answer:* b. *An enhanced 911 system allows a dispatcher to send emergency personnel to a scene, even if the caller cannot provide his location.*

1. *Answer:* d. *A dead or injured rescuer is of no use to a patient. Your first responsibility is always to keep yourself safe.*

2. *Answer:* a. *In 1966, the U.S. Department of Transportation began developing standards for emergency medical care. Most EMT-Basic courses today are based on models developed by the DOT.*

ANSWERS TO CASE STUDY QUESTIONS

1. mutual aid
2. Emergency Medical Dispatcher or EMD
3. First Responders
4. ALS intercept

Personal safety—Not arriving until the scene is safe, clearing the crowd
Safety of the crew, patient, and bystanders—Clearing the crowd
Patient assessment—Assessing the ABCs, checking for further injuries
Patient emergency care—Dressing the chest wound, applying oxygen
Lifting and moving—Moving the patient to the stretcher, then to the ambulance
Transport—Choosing the trauma center and transporting him there
Transfer of care—Providing a report to the hospital staff
Patient advocacy—Ensuring his mother is called

ANSWERS TO RETRO REVIEW QUESTIONS

No questions or answers for this chapter.

ANSWERS TO CHAPTER 2
THE WELL-BEING OF THE EMT-BASIC

ANSWERS TO SHORT ANSWER QUESTIONS

1. *Answer:* *Eustress is a positive form of stress that helps people work under pressure and respond effectively. Distress occurs when the stress of a situation becomes overwhelming, causing the sufferer to become ineffective.*

2. *Answer:* *An organism that causes harmful effects by way of infection, such as a virus or bacteria.*

ANSWERS TO MULTIPLE-CHOICE QUESTIONS

1. *Answer:* a. *defusing session*
2. *Answer:* c. *Maintain a safe distance from the scene.*

3. *Answer:* c. *heavyweight, tear-resistant gloves. Standard latex or nonlatex gloves are adequate to protect you from exposure to blood or other body fluids.*

4. *Answer:* b. *bargaining*

5. *Answer:* d. *Retreat, Radio, and Reevaluate*

ANSWERS TO SCENARIO QUESTIONS

1 *Answer:* b. *acute stress reaction*

2. *Answer:* b. *setting aside time to do nothing but relax*

3. *Answer:* d. *a normal response to an abnormal situation*

1. *Answer:* c. *Latex or vinyl exam gloves only.*

2. *Answer:* a. *Occupational Safety and Health Administration*

3. *Answer:* c. *Just before examining the patient.*

ANSWERS TO CASE STUDY QUESTIONS

1. Due to the bleeding, it is essential that you wear protective gloves before making contact with this patient. The persistent cough is also very suspicious, and you might want to place a mask on yourself or perhaps on the patient.

2. You will want to get as much medical history as possible on this patient. The cough should be a big concern since this man could have tuberculosis, which can be spread by his coughing.

1. It is probably a good idea to add at least eye protection and probably a face mask as the potential for blood to splatter is present.

2. At this point, the persistent cough is a major concern given the little that is known about this patient. You will need to take extra airborne precautions and upgrade to an N95 mask for you and the patient if possible. You do not want to take any chances if the patient ends up having TB.

A patient holding a pencil looking "angry"—A pencil can be a weapon—and a dangerous one at that. An apparently agitated patient should also cause concern.

A large dog standing just inside the door of a home with a person lying apparently unresponsive inside—Even when patients or family members say, "It's OK—he doesn't bite," be careful. Dogs can sense the stress in their owners and act unpredictably.

A tractor trailer (tanker) overturned on the roadway—Hazardous (explosive, flammable, corrosive) materials and a potentially unstable vehicle top the list of hazards here.

A house from which a 911 call was received but no one answers the door—Sometimes quiet scenes can be an indicator of danger even though the quiet may seem to indicate the opposite. This could mean that a patient became unresponsive after calling, the people inside cannot hear you, or it could be a sign of danger.

A person who is lethargic, with alcohol and marijuana visible—Alcohol and drugs can cause unusual behavior and can be associated with crime and violence. Major warning signs here.

A three-car collision on a four-lane-interstate highway—In addition to the danger from spilled gas, downed power lines, and hazardous materials, traffic may actually pose the most danger to you. Cars will be whizzing by while the drivers try to get a glimpse of the wreckage. They may not see you. This kills many providers each year.

ANSWERS TO RETRO REVIEW QUESTIONS

1. *Answer:* b. *off-line medical direction (Chapter 1)*

2. *Answer:* c. *Obtaining liability insurance. (Chapter 1)*

ANSWERS TO CHAPTER 3
MEDICAL/LEGAL AND ETHICAL ISSUES

ANSWERS TO SHORT ANSWER QUESTIONS

1. *Answer:* Negligence requires that the EMT-B had a duty to act, failed to provide the standard of care and, as a result, caused harm to the patient.

2. *Answer:* A DNR order is completed and signed (usually by the patient and his physician) in advance of any event where resuscitation might be indicated.

ANSWERS TO MULTIPLE-CHOICE QUESTIONS

1. *Answer:* c. The Health Insurance Portability and Accountability Act (HIPAA)
2. *Answer:* c. police officer
3. *Answer:* d. You may provide emergency care based on implied consent.
4. *Answer:* a. duty to act
5. *Answer:* a. consent to treat minors or incompetent adults

ANSWERS TO SCENARIO QUESTIONS

1. *Answer:* c. explain to her that, based on the seriousness of the collision, if she does not accept your help, her condition may worsen
2. *Answer:* a. multiple-casualty incident (MCI)
3. *Answer:* d. No, an unemancipated individual under the age of majority is not allowed to make emergency-care decisions.
1. *Answer:* b. maintain the patient's airway
2. *Answer:* d. No, the DNR released you from your duty to act.
3. *Answer:* c. There is no legal way to ignore a valid DNR.

ANSWERS TO CASE STUDY QUESTIONS

1. This presents a somewhat difficult moral dilemma for the junior member of the team. You must respond as quickly as possible because that is what is right for the patient. Allow your partner to eat his meal while you drive to the scene. You may even be able to conduct an initial assessment on Mr. Jones while your partner finishes his meal. Should there be anything seriously wrong with Mr. Jones, you will both be there in a timely manner to assist him.

2. As an EMT-B working for an agency, you have a legal and ethical duty to respond to all calls for assistance. Failure to do so in a timely manner can result in disciplinary action from your employer and perhaps legal action from the patient or his family.

1. As long as Mr. Jones is competent to make his own decisions and you do not feel his life is in danger, he has the right to refuse transport, and his daughter cannot make him go.

2. You must explain to Mr. Jones what might happen to him medically if he does not go to the hospital and his condition does worsen. You should also have him sign either a "release at scene" or an "against medical advice" form before you leave the scene.

1. Yes. Absolutely. Unquestionably. Honesty is always required. If the hospital administers additional medications without knowing this was given, it can negatively affect patient outcome.

2. You are going to be in some trouble—you violated protocol. But not in as much trouble as you would be if you tried to cover it up.

In the event of an error, your agency will have to take some action. This could range from counseling by the medical director and additional training to more serious actions such as suspension (although this would be rare in an event such as this). Protocols are a serious thing. If you tried to cover up an error, it would not be unusual for you to have your certification suspended or revoked and for you to face disciplinary hearings. The difference: dishonesty. EMS involves trust and integrity. We see people at their worst and when they are vulnerable. EMTs must be honest, trustworthy, and act with integrity at all times.

3. Yes, although how it is done may vary widely. One option would be to document the call as it happened and to make a note at the end of the narrative that states "Upon arrival at the hospital, the patient thanked us for administering the nitro and mentioned that it was his wife's. Dr (doctor's name) was advised immediately upon arrival at the emergency department."

ANSWERS TO RETRO REVIEW QUESTIONS

1. *Answer:* d. *The BSI precautions used are based on preventing exposure to blood and other potentially infectious materials. (Chapter 2)*

Answer: c. *National Highway Traffic Safety Administration (Chapter 1)*

ANSWERS TO CHAPTER 4 THE HUMAN BODY

ANSWERS TO SHORT ANSWER QUESTIONS

1. *Answer:* *Voluntary muscles, or skeletal muscles, support and allow for movement of bones. Involuntary muscles, or smooth muscles, are found in the gastrointestinal system, lungs, blood vessels, and urinary system. The cardiac muscle is only found in the heart.*

2. *Answer:* *The midaxillary line is an imaginary line (extending vertically from the armpit to the ankle) that divides the human body into front and back halves.*

ANSWERS TO MULTIPLE-CHOICE QUESTIONS

1. *Answer:* a. *semi-Fowler's*
2. *Answer:* d. *motor*
3. *Answer:* a. *pulmonary vein*
4. *Answer:* d. *epidermis*
5. *Answer:* b. *manubrium*

ANSWERS TO SCENARIO QUESTIONS

1. *Answer:* c. *Femur, radius, and ulna.*
2. *Answer:* a. *Dorsalis pedis*
1. *Answer:* b. *Trendelenburg*
2. *Answer:* d. *On the anterior side of the hand.*
3. *Answer:* a. *brachial*

ANSWERS TO CASE STUDY QUESTIONS

1. The patient is found lying on his back, which is known as the supine position.
2. This man is complaining of pain and has deformity on the anterior side of his right leg just proximal to the knee. He also has pain and deformity just proximal to his left ankle.
3. The liver is the organ that takes up most of the space in the upper right quadrant of the abdomen.

1. The patient was found in a prone position. If he were rolled over (as would be necessary for airway care), he would be in a supine position.
2. The tibia and fibula are the bones of the lower leg. This injury is distal to the knee and proximal to the ankle.
3. The bone of the upper arm is the humerus. It is distal to the shoulder and proximal to the elbow.

1. Trendelenberg position.

ANSWERS TO RETRO REVIEW QUESTIONS

1. *Answer:* b. *death and dying (Chapter 2)*
2. *Answer:* d. *four (Chapter 1)*
3. *Answer:* c. *Leaving competent and oriented patients who refuse emergency care (Chapter 3)*

ANSWERS TO CHAPTER 5 LIFTING AND MOVING PATIENTS

ANSWERS TO SHORT ANSWER QUESTIONS

1. *Answer:* *A Reeves stretcher (also called a "flexible" stretcher) is made of canvas, or some other flexible material, with carry-handles sewn into each side. It is for use in confined places such as narrow hallways.*
2. *Answer:* *Make sure that as great an area of your fingers and palms as possible is in contact with the object to be lifted or carried. All fingers should be bent at the same angle and hands should, ideally, be kept at least 10 inches apart.*

ANSWERS TO MULTIPLE-CHOICE QUESTIONS

1. *Answer:* d. *urgent*
2. *Answer:* b. *stair chair*
3. *Answer:* c. *In the recovery position*
4. *Answer:* a. *has a suspected spinal injury*
5. *Answer:* d. *keep the weight close to your body*

ANSWERS TO SCENARIO QUESTIONS

1. *Answer:* d. *Grab the patient's shoulders and drag him straight out of the vehicle.*
2. *Answer:* b. *Raise the foot-end of the long spine board 8 to 12 inches.*
1. *Answer:* c. *A Stokes stretcher.*
2. *Answer:* a. *He should be fitted with a cervical collar, secured to a short spine board, and moved to a long spine board.*

1. Assuming that the bathroom is too small for a backboard or flat stretcher, you will need to carefully slide the patient out into the bedroom where you will have more room to work.

2. This will depend on the available room inside the bathroom. Try and get two of you in the bathroom and one person reaching in through the doorway.

1. You can use either a soft, flat stretcher that will be the most comfortable or a long back board or scoop stretcher to move her downstairs.

2. You will need to secure her firmly to one of the devices mentioned above and carefully carry her down the stairs feet first. If available, use two people at each end of the carrying device.

1. In addition to the usual size-up issues (e.g. will ALS be necessary?), you will need additional personnel to lift the patient. You may also need to "remodel" a bit by opening up doorways or removing door frames and windows to get the patient out of the house.

2. Stretchers are usually rated for between 400 and 600 pounds. This depends on the stretcher. Ratings vary widely. Stretchers are an important—but often taken-for-granted—piece of equipment. Stretchers must be maintained and inspected regularly.

1. The patient should not be carried by any fewer than 8 rescuers—possibly more. You may actually consider dragging the patient or using a winch for some parts of the move. The Sked device (www.skedco.com) and the Morrison Medical Jumbo Stretcher (www.morrisonmed.com) are examples of devices used for obese patients.

2. The fire department will be a key resource. Calling for an engine (or two) for additional manpower is a start. You may also want to call a rescue company with more tools, in the event carpentry is needed. A winch may also be helpful depending on the situation. Because of the complaint of worsening respiratory distress, Advanced Life Support (ALS) would also be a good idea.

ANSWERS TO RETRO REVIEW QUESTIONS

1. *Answer:* b. *supine (Chapter 4)*
2. *Answer:* c. *enhanced 911 (Chapter 1)*
3. *Answer:* a. *Enabling (Chapter 2)*

ANSWERS TO CHAPTER 6 AIRWAY MANAGEMENT

ANSWERS TO SHORT ANSWER QUESTIONS

1. *Answer:* *Although Bourden gauge flowmeters are tremendously versatile and will function regardless of the positioning of the oxygen cylinder, it is not designed to compensate for back pressure. As a result, a kinked hose or dirty filter can dramatically affect the accuracy of the gauge.*

2. *Answer:* *Respiratory failure occurs when breathing has deteriorated to the point where oxygen intake is not sufficient to support life. Respiratory arrest means that breathing has completely ceased.*

Answers to Multiple-choice Questions

1. *Answer:* a. *200*
2. *Answer:* c. *16 French*
3. *Answer:* b. *the patient's tongue*
4. *Answer:* c. *cerebrospinal fluid*
5. *Answer:* d. *chest trauma*

Answers to Scenario Questions

1. *Answer:* c. *check his mouth for vomitus. If present, turn the patient to the side and suction his mouth*
2. *Answer:* a. *One breath every 5 seconds.*
3. *Answer:* c. *causes the patient's chest to rise*
1. *Answer:* d. *leave the head and neck in a neutral position*
2. *Answer:* a. *sealing the stoma and attempting ventilation through the mouth*
1. *Answer:* b. *The patient's blood will need a higher saturation of oxygen to compensate for the loss of red blood cells.*
2. *Answer:* c. *21 percent*
3. *Answer:* d. *Nonrebreather mask with 15 lpm*

Answers to Case Study Questions

1. Your first concern is whether he has a clear airway and is breathing. You must kneel beside him and attempt to rouse him. Place your ear next to his nose and mouth to assess his breathing status. Proper BSI is a must with this patient.
2. There is a strong likelihood that you may have to ventilate this patient. You will want a pocket mask at the very least and preferably a BVM. Having portable suction at the ready is also important since it appears that he may have already vomited once.

1. Noisy breathing always means some degree of airway obstruction and gurgling is indicative of upper airway obstruction. Provide oral suction to clear out any fluids in the upper airway.
2. Respirations that are eight and shallow are not adequate for this unresponsive man. You will need to supplement his breaths with some additional manual ventilations. This is best accomplished using a BVM hooked up to supplemental oxygen. You will want to enhance his eight breaths with the BVM and interpose at least four more to bring his rate up to a minimum of 12 per minute.

1. Nonrebreather mask 10 to 15 lpm.
2. Nasal cannula 2 to 4 lpm.
3. Pocket face mask or BVM with oxygen attached to the device at 15 lpm. Oral airway to be inserted if gag reflex is absent. Jaw thrust used to protect the spine. One breath every 5 seconds in support of existing respiratory effort.
4. Nonrebreather mask 10 to 15 lpm.
5. Nonrebreather mask 10 to 15 lpm.
6. Pocket face mask or BVM with oxygen attached to the device at 15 lpm. Oral airway to be inserted if gag reflex is absent. One breath every 5 seconds. Remain alert for vomiting.

1. *Answer:* c. *sitting, a stair chair (Chapter 5)*
2. *Answer:* d. *tibia and fibula (Chapter 4)*
   Answer: b. *proximal (Chapter 4)*

ANSWERS TO CHAPTER 7
SCENE SIZE-UP

ANSWERS TO SHORT ANSWER QUESTIONS

1. *Answer:* *When a projectile, such as a bullet, travels through tissue at a high velocity, the accompanying pressure wave creates a temporary cavity that is much larger than the projectile. This cavitation can cause considerable trauma along the path of the projectile.*
2. *Answer:* *Having an* **index of suspicion** *means that the EMT-B has an awareness of and suspects possible injuries on the basis of the mechanism of injury.*

ANSWERS TO MULTIPLE-CHOICE QUESTIONS

1. *Answer:* c. *readily available*
2. *Answer:* a. *velocity*
3. *Answer:* d. *mechanism of injury*
4. *Answer:* a. *perform a scene size-up*
5. *Answer:* b. *resources*

ANSWERS TO SCENARIO QUESTIONS

1. *Answer:* d. *All of the above.*
2. *Answer:* b. *at least one full span of wire from the pole to which the broken line is attached*
3. *Answer:* a. *100 feet*
1. *Answer:* d. *The shouting that you heard upon your arrival.*
2. *Answer:* c. *Immediately retreat to a safe position and contact dispatch for law enforcement assistance.*

ANSWERS TO CASE STUDY QUESTIONS

1. You might expect to find hazards such as emergency traffic en route to the scene, traffic at the scene, unstable vehicles, fire, explosion, leaking fuel, broken glass, body fluids.
2. Safety for you and your partner is your top priority. Once the scene is safe for you, then consider the safety of the other personnel arriving at the scene, the bystanders, and then the patients.
1. You must take proper BSI precautions and bring extra gloves with you. It is likely that you will be treating multiple patients at a scene like this. Watch for sharp glass and metal as you enter vehicles to treat patients.
2. Certainly having enough ambulances to transport all the patients is essential. You will want law enforcement there to take over traffic control and provide any extrication equipment to deal with trapped patients. You must consider the most appropriate place for the helicopter to land should any of the patients need to be transported.

1. Look at the scene from a distance. Ambulances should have binoculars in the cab that will allow you to obtain information from a safe distance.

2. The fire department would be a good start. In the event of a leak from the tanker or a fire, they are the people to have around.

3. Using your binoculars, you should look for a placard that indicates the presence of hazardous substances. Also be alert for things that might seem obvious or simple but include people running away, vapor clouds, fire, smoke, and other signs of danger.

1. This is gasoline and it is flammable.

2. In the Emergency Response Guidebook. This tells you this information as well as evacuation distances, specific health hazards, and more. Every emergency vehicle should have one.

1. Number of patients, BSI, a closer look at the damage for MOI determination, and any additional resources you may need for multiple or critical patients

ANSWERS TO RETRO REVIEW QUESTIONS

1. *Answer:* c. *abandonment. (Chapter 3)*
2. *Answer:* d. *EMTs should consider evidence preservation while treating the patient. (Chapter 3)*
3. *Answer:* a. *NREMT (Chapter 1)*

ANSWERS TO CHAPTER 8
THE INITIAL ASSESSMENT

ANSWERS TO SHORT ANSWER QUESTIONS

1. *Answer:* *An action taken by an EMT-B to correct any life-threatening or non-life-threatening problem.*
2. *Answer:* *Without a consistent and systematic approach to the initial assessment, it is more likely that you may overlook or neglect a life-threatening problem.*

ANSWERS TO MULTIPLE-CHOICE QUESTIONS

1. *Answer:* b. *24*
2. *Answer:* c. *Capillary refill*
3. *Answer:* a. *appearance*
4. *Answer:* d. *clinical judgment*
5. *Answer:* b. *smelling*

ANSWERS TO SCENARIO QUESTIONS

1. *Answer:* d. *The patient's respiratory rate.*
2. *Answer:* b. *Observed her, spoke to her, and provided painful stimulus.*
1. *Answer:* d. *Performing the jaw-thrust maneuver.*
2. *Answer:* c. *general impression*

ANSWERS TO CASE STUDY QUESTIONS

1. You must tap and shout to establish any type of responsiveness. If the patient is unresponsive, you must kneel as close to him as possible with your ear next to the patient's nose and mouth and assess his airway and breathing. If he is breathing, you must then reach in and assess the carotid pulse.

2. If you were unable to manage the patient's airway or ventilate the patient with the helmet in place, it must be removed. In most cases, if it is a full-face helmet, it must be removed to adequately manage the airway or ventilate the patient.

1. Due to the inadequacy of respirations, it is necessary to roll this patient face up, remove the helmet, and assist his respirations.

2. In this instance, since you have the fire department on the scene, it is probably best to ventilate this patient with a BVM hooked up to supplemental oxygen. You will also want to suction to manage the bleeding in his upper airway.

1. The patient has exhibited some classic postures indicating difficulty in breathing. These include dangling his feet over the edge of the bed and the "tripod position" illustrated by his hands outstretched and resting on his knees. The fact that he is sweaty could indicate that his problem is severe.

2. Your general impression should be that of a serious patient. The initial impression (based on your observations in question #1) should be that of a male patient in respiratory distress, with a potentially serious condition. The general impression (experienced providers call this the "look test") is that of a sick patient who may require rapid emergency care and transport because you suspect his condition could deteriorate even more.

1. The patient's airway is clear, so suction would not be required. Oxygen should be started immediately with a nonrebreather mask. There is no bleeding. Transport decision/priority is discussed in the next question.

2. This patient would receive a high priority for transport. His respiratory distress, rapid pulse, cool and sweaty skin, and position indicate that he is a potentially serious patient.

3. Yes. While transportation should not be delayed, having ALS respond to the scene if they are close or meeting you along the route to the hospital would be beneficial. Medical patients can often benefit from the medications carried by paramedics.

1. The patient now needs to receive assisted ventilations. As discussed in Chapter 6, when the respirations become fast and shallow and when the patient can barely speak and becomes sleepy, the patient must receive ventilations with either a pocket face mask or a BVM. It will seem awkward ventilating a patient you can still talk to—but it will also be lifesaving!

ANSWERS TO RETRO REVIEW QUESTIONS

1. *Answer:* c. *corner of the mouth to the tip of the earlobe (Chapter 6)*
2. *Answer:* d. *The EMT acted within protocols. (Chapter 3)*
3. *Answer:* d. *Stokes basket (Chapter 5)*

ANSWERS TO CHAPTER 9 VITAL SIGNS AND SAMPLE HISTORY

ANSWERS TO SHORT ANSWER QUESTIONS

1. *Answer:* *If you neglect to obtain vital signs and a SAMPLE history, you will be unaware of any important patient conditions or trends. This could cause you to neglect a critical treatment or delay much-needed transport.*

2. *Answer:* A pulse oximeter sends different colors of light into the tissue on the tip of a finger or an earlobe. It then measures the amount of light that returns and calculates the percentage of oxygen in the patient's blood.

ANSWERS TO MULTIPLE-CHOICE QUESTIONS

1. *Answer:* a. an obstruction from the tongue
2. *Answer:* b. Pertinent past history
3. *Answer:* c. hypovolemia
4. *Answer:* b. regularity
5. *Answer:* a. liver abnormalities

ANSWERS TO SCENARIO QUESTIONS

1. *Answer:* b. L
2. *Answer:* c. Ask open-ended questions whenever possible.
1. *Answer:* c. temporary stress
2. *Answer:* a. auscultation

ANSWERS TO CASE STUDY QUESTIONS

1. Considering the age of the patient, these vitals are well within the normal limits.

2. You will want to know whether anyone saw him fall and whether the observer can tell you why he fell or how he may have landed. You will also want to know whether the patient can answer any questions and whether he remembers the event or why he may have fallen.

1. Due to the mechanism of injury, it is likely this man has some internal injuries. The change in his vital signs is consistent with someone going into shock.

2. You will want to take a set of vitals on this patient every 5 minutes due to the fact that he is unstable and getting worse.

1. It is not uncommon at a medical facility to have a bit of confusion at the time of patient transfer. Although you would not normally think it would be the case—it is. The nurse has told you that the patient is having difficulty breathing (which the patient does not agree with), that he has COPD, and that his sats (oxygen saturation) are low at 90 percent.

2. Ask questions of the nurse and the patient. You also have a packet that will likely include the patient's medications, history, and possibly more.

3. Oxygen saturation is the percent of hemoglobin in the blood that is saturated by oxygen. It is one piece of the puzzle. Low oxygen saturations mean one thing: the patient needs oxygen. Always evaluate the patient's respiratory rate and depth, mental status, skin color, and other signs of respiratory problems including use of accessory muscles to determine whether the patient is breathing adequately. Never withhold oxygen from a patient who needs it because his sats are "normal."

The patient continues to deny breathing difficulty although he appears winded. He fires another joke at you. You realize he really just appreciates the company. As you ask him about his problem, he tells you that he was a smoker and has had emphysema for years. He is on oxygen in his room at 2 lpm via cannula and this was turned up to 4 lpm before your arrival. You quickly glance at the fact sheet on the patient's paperwork and see that he has dementia.

4. The history of dementia should throw up a flag. This does not mean that you should not talk to your patient at all—but you may need to verify the information he provides you. The nursing staff may be able to provide information on the reliability of his complaints and statements.

5. OPQRST is an excellent tool to help you remember all the questions you should ask including when the respiratory distress came on, what he was doing when the distress came on, does anything make it worse or better, is there any pain associated with breathing, how bad the distress feels to him, and how long he has had it. Since he seems to be downplaying the distress, some answers may come from the staff at the nursing facility.

   The nurse returns and tells you that he had an albuterol "breathing treatment" about 20 minutes ago and takes numerous medications that are listed on the papers she gave you. He is up to date on his med administration today. He has a pacemaker and has had one prior heart attack. He has high blood pressure and diabetes for which he takes a pill. His last hospitalization was 10 days ago for the same problem.

6. You should have more information on the signs and symptoms as noted in the OPQRST information in question 4. You know nothing about his allergies, but his medications are listed in the paperwork, his past history was outlined relatively well for you. His last oral intake and the events that led up to the call for EMS also require more information to be complete.

ANSWERS TO RETRO REVIEW QUESTIONS

1. *Answer:* d. *acetabulum (Chapter 4)*
2. *Answer:* a. *personal sacrifice (Chapter 3)*
3. *Answer:* b. *Always use appropriate infection control practices. (Chapter 6)*

ANSWERS TO CHAPTER 10 ASSESSMENT OF THE TRAUMA PATIENT

ANSWERS TO SHORT ANSWER QUESTIONS

1. *Answer:* *You should use your sight, touch, smelling, and hearing to complete an effective rapid trauma assessment. The only sense that you will not be using is taste.*
2. *Answer:* *If the mechanism of injury exerts great force on the upper body, if there have been blows to any area above the collar bones, or if there is soft-tissue damage to the head, face, or neck from trauma, it is appropriate to apply a cervical collar. If the patient complains of pain to the neck and or spine (back).*

ANSWERS TO MULTIPLE-CHOICE QUESTIONS

1. *Answer:* d. *normal circulation*
2. *Answer:* c. *Manually stabilizing the patient's head and neck.*
3. *Answer:* a. *Damaged capillaries.*
4. *Answer:* b. *Battle's sign*
5. *Answer:* d. *the patient*

ANSWERS TO SCENARIO QUESTIONS

1. *Answer:* c. *the rapid trauma assessment*
2. *Answer:* b. *rapid trauma assessment*
3. *Answer:* a. *after completing the rapid trauma assessment*

1. *Answer:* a. *internal bleeding*
2. *Answer:* d. *flail*
3. *Answer:* c. *lung collapse*

ANSWERS TO CASE STUDY QUESTIONS

1. Once you have determined the scene is safe, you will want to conduct an initial assessment including her mental status and her ABCs. You must ensure that she has a clear airway and is breathing, then check the status of her pulse.
2. You may need to roll her if you cannot perform an adequate assessment of her ABCs facedown. If you can assess her facedown and find that any one of the ABCs needs attention, then you must roll her to treat the problem.

1. Due to the serious mechanism of injury this patient endured, you must perform a rapid trauma assessment.
2. As long as there are no life-threatening problems with this patient, it will be appropriate to perform a detailed physical exam. This is probably best performed en route to the hospital.

1. This would be considered a nonsignificant mechanism of injury. The significant mechanism of injury would indicate the potential for serious, hidden injury, which is not likely in this case. This does not mean that additional injuries are not possible. Question #2 addresses this point.
2. Yes. When the patient fell, she could have tried to catch herself, injuring her wrist, arm, or shoulder. When she hit the ground, she could have also struck her head. You should also inquire about whether the woman may have felt dizzy, passed out, or had heart palpitations prior to the fall to help rule out medical problems that may have caused the fall.

   The patient states she went to the ground carefully and does not believe she has further injuries. She denies feeling dizzy or passing out. "I just missed the end of this blasted thing!" she says.

   The patient has remained oriented and has not complained of further injuries in the few minutes you have been talking to her.
3. The patient would receive a focused examination of the ankle. If she hurt another extremity in the fall, that would be examined as well. If multiple problems were encountered, a head-to-toe exam would be more appropriate.
4. An altered mental status is a significant sign of injury—and it means that she might not recall or be able to accurately relay the events surrounding her fall to you. A conflict between the patient's recollection of the events and those of friends/bystanders may also indicate a more serious underlying problem. If you have doubts about how serious a patient's injury may be, always err on the side of caution.

ANSWERS TO RETRO REVIEW QUESTIONS

1. *Answer:* c. *cavitation (Chapter 7)*
2. *Answer:* b. *concealment (Chapter 7)*
3. *Answer:* d. *extremity lift (Chapter 5)*

ANSWERS TO CHAPTER 11
ASSESSMENT OF THE MEDICAL PATIENT

ANSWERS TO SHORT ANSWER QUESTIONS

1. *Answer:* Position yourself so that you are on the same level as the child and ask the SAMPLE and OPQRST questions with very simple, easily understood words.

2. *Answer:* Patients with difficulty breathing who have a prescribed inhaler, patients with chest pain who have prescribed nitroglycerin, and patients having allergic reactions who have a prescribed epinephrine auto-injector.

ANSWERS TO MULTIPLE-CHOICE QUESTIONS

1. *Answer:* a. wallet cards
2. *Answer:* c A woman suffering an allergic reaction following a bee sting
3. *Answer:* c. A head-to-toe physical examination is critical for medical patients.
4. *Answer:* d. focused
5. *Answer:* a. Quality

ANSWERS TO SCENARIO QUESTIONS

1. *Answer:* c. Ensuring and maintaining an adequate airway.
2. *Answer:* b. Search for prescription bottles, medical equipment, or medical-identification devices.
1. *Answer:* d. Gather the history of the present illness.
2. *Answer:* c. blood pressure, respirations, capillary refill, pulse, skin, and pupils

ANSWERS TO CASE STUDY QUESTIONS

1. You will want to know which came on first, the pain or the difficulty in breathing. You will also want to know whether she has a history of cardiac or respiratory problems.

2. Because she is conscious and presenting with a "medical" complaint, you should follow the "focused medical assessment."

1. Because her primary complaint is respiratory, you may want to suggest that she sit up to make it easier to breathe. Only do so if she is no longer feeling dizzy.

2. Given the fact that she is experiencing both pain and difficulty in breathing, your best bet will be a nonrebreather mask, at an appropriate flow rate to keep the bag full.

1. This patient seems to be in minimal distress with some sort of respiratory condition. His ability to talk in full sentences and play down his condition does not lead you to think that his condition puts him at immediate risk of being critical or worsening.

2. The husband says he is all right, the wife is concerned. It is not uncommon to have differing opinions between spouses. The question of whether the wife knows her husband plays down symptoms or whether she worries too much is one you might have trouble answering at the scene. It should add to your index of suspicion as you move forward. If you ask the patient whether he is having pain or difficulty breathing and

he says "Not really," you should be aware he may be minimizing his condition and explore it further.

Your initial assessment reveals a patient who is able to speak full sentences and states that he feels like he is breathing "OK—except sometimes I can't stop coughing." His breathing is adequate and his pulse is a bit rapid. His skin is warm and dry. Your pulse oximeter reveals a reading of 96 percent.

3. The pulse oximeter is nice for taking readings before and after giving oxygen. But even if you saw a reading of 100 percent on the device, you would still give oxygen. Most agree that readings of 95 percent or below reflect hypoxia and that readings below 90 percent are indicative of a more severe condition. But remember it is a device—it should never cause you to withhold oxygen from patients.

4. This patient would probably be best with a nasal cannula with oxygen at 2 to 4 lpm. He is not in severe distress. The mask may also get in the way of his coughing and phlegm removal.

5. Rapid transport is probably not necessary. He shows no signs of instability, has an alert mental status, and minimal respiratory distress. If he had more severe distress, inadequate breathing, chest pain, poor skin color, or other more serious indicators, he would be a high priority.

    You begin to take a patient history while your partner takes vital signs. The patient tells you that he worked in a factory for years—long before respiratory protection was common practice and has developed a chronic lung disease. He has good days and bad days. He still does not think this is all that bad. He developed the cough over the past several days. It gets a bit worse when he is active. He has had breakfast and lunch normally. He is allergic to penicillin.

6. Getting more information on signs and symptoms would be appropriate. Ask things like, "Do you have pain?" (especially chest pain) and expand the OPQRST in relation to the respiratory distress (e.g. "Does anything make your breathing worse or better?"). The E (events) in SAMPLE is underestimated in importance. Has anything been different recently? Does something cause the coughing? Just because the patient is sitting in a chair now does not mean he was when this happened.

7. Most patients with respiratory distress find that sitting upright is most comfortable and best for their breathing. Unless spine injuries or inadequate breathing prohibit it, this is the usual transport position as well as the position of comfort.

ANSWERS TO RETRO REVIEW QUESTIONS

1. *Answer:* b. *respiratory-distress (Chapter 6)*
2. *Answer:* a. *8 lpm (Chapter 6)*
3. *Answer:* c. *HIPAA (Chapter 3)*

WORKSHEET FOR FILL-IN-THE-BLANKS ACTIVITY

PATIENT ASSESSMENT—MEDICAL

ANSWER KEY

SCENE SIZE-UP	ACTION/VERBAL RESPONSE
* *Assess scene safety (CRITICAL CRITERIA)*	I am determining whether the scene is safe.
Determine the nature of illness	I am determining the nature of illness.
Determine the number of patients	I am determining the number of patients.
Assess the need for additional help	I am determining the need for additional help.
Take cervical spine precautions as necessary	I am taking/directing appropriate c-spine precautions.

INITIAL ASSESSMENT	ACTION/VERBAL RESPONSE
Verbalize general impression of patient	I observe an approximately ___ -year-old male/ female patient who appears to be in mild/moderate/severe distress (determine one and state it).
Determine responsiveness/level of consciousness	*Eyes open/awake*: "Hello, my name is _____, and I am an EMT; I am going to take care of you. What is your name? How old are you?" I have determined that the patient is awake and alert (if eyes are open but patient seems confused, say so). Eyes Closed: Determine responsiveness using: Alert – Verbal – Painful – Unresponsive.
Determine chief complaint	"What seems to be the problem?"
Identify apparent life-threats	I am identifying and managing apparent life-threats.
* *Assess airway/initiate appropriate airway management (CRITICAL CRITERIA)*	If patient speaks to you: I have determined that the airway is patent. If patient does not speak or is not responsive: I am assessing the airway for patency.
* *Assess breathing/initiate appropriate oxygen therapy (CRITICAL CRITERIA)*	I am assessing breathing for: adequate rate and tidal volume, labored or easy. At this time, I would initiate oxygen therapy, if appropriate (specify the device and appropriate flow rate).
* *Assess circulation (CRITICAL CRITERIA)*	I am assessing for presence of a pulse at the carotid artery (unresponsive patient) or radial artery (responsive patient) and assessing approximate rate, strength, and regularity.
* *Assess and control severe bleeding (CRITICAL CRITERIA)*	I am assessing for and controlling severe bleeding.
Assess skin signs	I am assessing the skin for color, temperature, and moisture.
State priority of patient for transport	At this time I have determined that the patient is *low* or *high* priority (select one).

DETERMINE APPROPRIATE ASSESSMENT PATH	FOCUSED HISTORY-PHYSICAL or RAPID MEDICAL ASSESSMENT
Perform focused history and physical examination or, if indicated, complete rapid medical assessment.	I am focusing my history and examination on the body part or body system relating to the chief complaint. In the case of an altered mental status, I may defer this until en route to the hospital and move directly to a rapid medical assessment.
Signs and Symptoms (assess history of present illness)	
"**O**" – Onset	When did it start? What was the patient doing?
"**P**" – Provocation	Does anything make it better or worse?
"**Q**" – Quality	What does it feel like? (i.e. tight, sharp, dull, and so on)
"**R**" – Region/radiation	Where is it? Does it move or go anywhere?
"**S**" – Severity	How bad is it, on a 1–10 scale?
"**T**" – Time	How long does it last?
Allergies	Is the patient allergic to foods or medications?
Medications	Does the patient take any medications? (prescribed/nonprescribed including vitamins, herbal remedies, birth control pills, illegal drugs)
Past pertinent history	Has this ever happened before? Was the patient seen by a physician? Diagnosis? Does he have a history of diabetes, high blood pressure, cardiac or breathing problems, or seizures?
Last oral intake	What and when did the patient last eat?
Event leading to present illness (rule out trauma)	What happened today that led the patient or someone to call 911?
Vital Signs	I will now obtain *baseline vital signs*: Blood pressure: by auscultation Respirations: rate, depth, and quality Pulse: rate, regularity, and quality
Interventions	I will perform or delegate the following interventions.
Transport (reevaluates the transport decision)	At this point I feel the patient is *emergent and should be transported immediately* or *nonemergent and does not require immediate transport* (select one).

Detailed Physical Exam

Head	I am examining the head for symmetry, scars.
Face	I am examining the face for equality of facial muscles.
Eyes	I am examining the eyes for size, equality, reactivity to light, color, pink and moist conjunctiva.
Ears	I am examining the ears for drainage (color).
Nose	I am examining the nose for flaring, drainage (color), singed nostrils, and foreign bodies.
Mouth	I am examining the mouth for loose/broken teeth, foreign bodies, blood or mucus, pink and moist soft tissue.
Neck	I am examining the neck for stoma, jugular vein distention, tracheal deviation, medical alert necklace, scars, and accessory-muscle use.
Chest	I am examining for equal chest rise, lung sounds, subcutaneous emphysema, retractions, and scars.
Abdomen	I am examining the abdomen for distention, scars, rigidity, referred pain, guarding, and pulsating mass.
Pelvis	I am examining the pelvis for incontinence of urine, pregnancy (crowning, bloody show, broken a water).
Legs	I am examining the legs for distal circulation sensation motor function, scars, track marks, medical alert jewelry, equal pulses bilaterally, pedal edema, capillary refill.
Arms	I am examining the arms for distal CSM, scars, track marks, medical alert bracelet, and equal pulses bilaterally, capillary refill.
Back	I am examining the back for scars, sacral edema.

ONGOING ASSESSMENT

Repeat initial assessment	I will now repeat my initial assessment of the patient to determine whether there has been any change in his condition.
Obtain secondary vital signs and compare with baseline	I would obtain and record a second set of vital signs and compare with the baseline vitals.
Repeat focused assessment regarding patient complaint or injuries	I would repeat a focused assessment on the patient to determine any other complaints or injuries not found or reported previously.

ANSWERS TO CHAPTER 12 ONGOING ASSESSMENT

ANSWERS TO SHORT ANSWER QUESTIONS

1. *Answer:* Trending is the process of evaluating the changes in a patient's condition over time.

2. *Answer:* The ongoing assessment consists of the following steps: Repeat the initial assessment (to find any life-threatening problems), reassess the vital signs, repeat the focused assessment (as it relates to the patient's specific complaint or injuries), and evaluate any interventions that you performed.

ANSWERS TO MULTIPLE-CHOICE QUESTIONS

1. *Answer:* a. When you are performing lifesaving interventions.
2. *Answer:* c. 5
3. *Answer:* d. flicking the feet

ANSWERS TO SCENARIO QUESTIONS

1. *Answer:* a. Nothing would be assessed in an ongoing fashion.
2. *Answer:* c. None. You should be focused on ventilating the patient and monitoring her pulse.
1. *Answer:* a. press on the back of his hand
2. *Answer:* b. When repeating the initial assessment.

ANSWERS TO CASE STUDY QUESTIONS

1. Your first concern should be his respiratory rate. Someone who is breathing at a rate of 10 and shallow is in need of immediate attention. After that, you will need to be concerned about his ability to manage his own airway during transport.

2. In response to his respiratory status, you will want to put him on 15 lpm by nonrebreather mask and closely monitor signs of perfusion. If at any moment you feel he is still not getting enough oxygen, you will have to begin manual ventilations with a BVM. As far as position is concerned, you will want to place him in the recovery position to help control his airway.

1. You will want to reassess his respiratory status and determine whether he appears to be getting enough oxygen with the mask in place. You will also reassess his ABCs and vital signs.

2. You will need to assist his respirations with a BVM and supplemental oxygen.

   A. Normal vital signs (no illness or injury)
   B. Developing shock (patient bleeding internally)
   C. Head injury (increasing pressure on the brain)
   D. Uninjured patient in a car crash who was very nervous, then calmed down

1. D
   P: 104 R: 24 BP: 138/86 Pupils: equal/react Skin: warm/dry
   P: 88 R: 16 BP: 120/76 Pupils: equal react Skin: warm/dry
   P: 86 R: 16 BP: 122/78 Pupils: equal react Skin: warm/dry

2. A
   P: 76 R: 12 BP: 116/68 Pupils: equal/react Skin: warm/dry
   P: 80 R: 12 BP: 120/72 Pupils: equal/react Skin: warm/dry
   P: 80 R: 14 BP: 120/70 Pupils: equal/react Skin: warm/dry

3. B

  P: 84 R: 16 BP: 124/64 Pupils: equal/react Skin: warm/dry

  P: 92 R: 22 BP: 126/68 Pupils: equal react Skin: cool/dry

  P: 108 R: 24 BP: 120/60 Pupils: equal/react Skin: cool/moist

4. C

  P: 72 R: 14 BP: 140/86 Pupils: equal react Skin: warm/dry

  P: 68 R: 18 BP: 152/88 Pupils: equal/react Skin warm/dry

  P: 56 R: 10 BP: 192/92 Pupils: react/sluggish Skin: cool/dry

ANSWERS TO RETRO REVIEW QUESTIONS

1. *Answer:* c. *flicking his feet (Chapter 11)*
2. *Answer:* b. *orthopedic (Chapter 5)*
3. *Answer:* d. *medical ID devices (Chapter 11)*

ANSWERS TO CHAPTER 13 COMMUNICATIONS

ANSWERS TO SHORT ANSWER QUESTIONS

1. *Answer:* Eye contact shows that you are interested in your patient, attentive, and at ease with what you are doing.

2. *Answer:* When a scene is potentially dangerous, the emergency dispatcher will often have an ambulance wait, or "stage," at a nearby safe location. The ambulance will then stand by until law enforcement has cleared its entry.

ANSWERS TO MULTIPLE-CHOICE QUESTIONS

1. *Answer:* a. *repeater*
2. *Answer:* d. *question the physician*
3. *Answer:* b. *use medical terms*
4. *Answer:* c. *cellular phones*
5. *Answer:* d. *involve the parents as much as possible*

ANSWERS TO SCENARIO QUESTIONS

1. *Answer:* c. *speaking unnaturally.*
2. *Answer:* a. *contact on-line medical direction*
1. *Answer:* d. *That his arm was badly damaged in the machine and could not be recovered. This makes reattachment very unlikely.*
2. *Answer:* b. *"Community General, this is BLS4 en route to your location with a 20-minute ETA. We've got a 17-year-old male patient with a right arm amputation, proximal to the elbow. The arm was caught in a hay baler and couldn't be recovered. The patient has no pertinent medical history and is alert, oriented, and never lost consciousness. His vital signs are: pulse 97; respirations 24 and unlabored; skin is pale, cool, and moist; and blood pressure is 112 over 74. The exam indicates that the right arm trauma is the sole injury and bleeding is controlled. We've placed the patient in the Trendelenburg position with a nonrebreather and 15 liters of O_2 and are keeping him warm. The patient's level of pain has increased from seven to nine but mental status is unchanged and there's been only a slight increase in pulse and respiration. Do you have any orders for us?"*

ANSWERS TO CASE STUDY QUESTIONS

1. You should acknowledge the dispatch by replying with something such as, "Dispatch, this is Ambulance 1, copy dispatch and responding code 3 to Baker and 1st street for a fall victim."

2. Having multiple units responding with lights and sirens to the same scene can be very dangerous. It is possible that you and one of these other vehicles could arrive at an intersection at the same time. You would want to ask dispatch from what location the other units are responding and be extra alert for other code 3 traffic.

1. Dispatch, Ambulance 1 on scene at Baker and 1st street.

2. Whenever possible, you will want to advise dispatch of any additional information that may be helpful to other responding units. It is important that everyone be made aware of potential hazards as early as possible. You will also want to request the utility company to manage the downed power lines.

1. The name and unit number of your ambulance should be given initially. The mental status of the patient has not been given. This is very important in painting the patient picture. Any physical exam findings should be noted in the report. The treatments you gave and any response by the patient to these treatments are also missing.

2. The hospital could hear the radio transmission and they were ready. The patient's complaint, a brief history (although noting heart, blood pressure, and diabetic problems may be appropriate in some areas), vital signs, and an ETA were included.

ANSWERS TO RETRO REVIEW QUESTIONS

1. *Answer:* a. *duty to act (Chapter 3)*
2. *Answer:* c. *sign, symptom (Chapter 9)*
3. *Answer:* d. *white blood cells (Chapter 4)*

ANSWERS TO CHAPTER 14 DOCUMENTATION

ANSWERS TO SHORT ANSWER QUESTIONS

1. *Answer:* *A pertinent negative is an examination finding that is important because it is either absent or negative. A patient who has chest pain should also be asked whether he has shortness of breath. Even if the answer is no, it is something you must know.*

2. *Answer:* *The PCR has many functions. It is the legal record of patient emergency care, it provides information for administrative functions, it is a resource for EMS education and research, and it is a necessary part of every Quality Improvement program.*

ANSWERS TO MULTIPLE-CHOICE QUESTIONS

1. *Answer:* d. *triage tag*
2. *Answer:* c. *Patient seemed confused when trying to recall events leading to the injury.*
3. *Answer:* b. *omission*

ANSWERS TO SCENARIO QUESTIONS

1. *Answer:* b. *Yes. The receiving staff needs to know because the patient may experience complications due to your error.*

2. *Answer:* *d.* *The QI team may be able to improve the new-hire training program.*

1. *Answer:* *c.* *that the patient suffered a stroke*

2. *Answer:* *a.* *Patient's spouse states that patient complained of a severe headache. The patient has weakness on his right side and answers questions with inappropriate words.*

ANSWERS TO CASE STUDY QUESTIONS

1. You are responding to a call concerning a <u>71-year-old</u> retired mechanic who was up on a <u>6-foot ladder</u> changing a light bulb in his garage when he <u>fell</u> and injured himself. He is <u>responsive when you arrive</u> but according to his wife who heard the fall, he was <u>unconscious</u> on the floor <u>bleeding from the head</u> when she found him. She called 911 immediately and placed a washcloth over the cut on his head and waited for the ambulance to arrive.

2. What was the cause of the fall? Did the patient slip or lose his balance? Does he not remember why he fell, suggesting a possible underlying medical cause for the fall?

1. You must document all emergency care given and all attempts to persuade him to go. You must also document that you informed him of the possible consequences of not receiving further care. You must also carefully document any action or statement on his part that might indicate he is not competent to make a rational decision.

2. Responded to a garage at a residence for a fall victim and found a 71-year-old male lying face up on a concrete floor. Patient was responsive and slightly disoriented upon arrival. Pt. was unable to determine why he fell and does not remember the incident. Chief complaint was pain to the right forehead where we found an approximately 2" laceration. Bleeding was controlled and spinal precautions were taken. Patient denied any other pain until almost at the hospital when he began complaining of pain in his right hip and shoulder. Assessment revealed no obvious deformity or visible trauma.

1. The patient was found prone in the ditch.

2. The right distal femur is protruding through the skin on the lateral aspect of the leg just proximal to the knee.

   You roll the patient over while protecting his spine and find that he is not breathing. The airway is opened with a technique that does not compromise the spine. Blood is found in the airway. You suction his airway and insert an oral airway. You continue to hold the spine and the mask in place while your partner squeezes the bag for ventilations.

3. The patient was rolled to a supine position while maintaining spinal stabilization. Assessment of the ABCs revealed blood in the airway that was suctioned. An OPA was inserted. The patient was not breathing so BVM ventilations were begun using two-rescuer technique with a jaw-thrust maneuver.

   The patient is assessed and prepared for transport. The assessment revealed an abnormal bulge at the back of the patient's neck, a cut on the palm side of the left wrist, and wide scrapes on the right side of the patient's chest, extending from the level of the nipple around the side ending at the armpit with deformity and a crackling sensation noted when touched.

4. The physical examination revealed a deformity on the patient's posterior neck. A laceration was noted on the patient's anterior left wrist and a wide abrasion on the patient's right chest at the nipple level across to the midaxillary line with crepitation.

Note: This case study provides examples of documentation using correct anatomical terms. Accurate documentation can be done in many forms and styles. This is one example.

ANSWERS TO RETRO REVIEW QUESTIONS

1. *Answer:* b. *oxygen (Chapter 6)*
2. *Answer:* c. *lifesaving interventions prevent doing it (Chapter 12)*
3. *Answer:* a. *Scene size-up (Chapter 7)*

ANSWERS TO CHAPTER 15 GENERAL PHARMACOLOGY

ANSWERS TO SHORT ANSWER QUESTIONS

1. *Answer:* *Apply the glucose gel to a tongue depressor and place it between the patient's cheek and gum or under the tongue. Why? First of all, it is quickly absorbed by the mucosa of the mouth, and if the patient experiences a decreased level of responsiveness, it can easily be removed.*

2. *Answer:* *Activated charcoal, oral glucose, oxygen, prescribed inhalers, nitroglycerin, and epinephrine auto-injectors.*

ANSWERS TO MULTIPLE-CHOICE QUESTIONS

1. *Answer:* c. *medications*
2. *Answer:* a. *Viagra*
3. *Answer:* d. *under the patient's tongue*
4. *Answer:* c. *increased heart rates*
5. *Answer:* a. *is unresponsive*

ANSWERS TO SCENARIO QUESTIONS

1. *Answer:* c. *oxygen*
2. *Answer:* b. *No, because his systolic pressure is too low.*
1. *Answer:* d. *Administer glucose sublingually.*
2. *Answer:* b. *Low sugar levels in his bloodstream.*

ANSWERS TO CASE STUDY QUESTIONS

1. Yes, due to her history and level of distress, she should receive oxygen by nonrebreather mask at 15 lpm.

2. You will want to determine whether it is the girl's own inhaler and whether she has used it already for this event. If so, how many times has she used it? Has she experienced any relief after using it?

1. On the basis of the fact that the girl gave herself six doses of the inhaler and experienced no relief, you will want to confirm whether the medication has expired. You will also want to know whether the mother has another inhaler.

2. No. You may only assist a patient with his own medication.

1. You must determine that the nitroglycerin is prescribed to the patient and that he does not have allergies to the medication. Ask him the prescribed dose of the medication and how he takes it. You must also ask whether the patient has taken any of his nitroglycerin already. Nitroglycerin tablets lose their potency quickly when opened. They lose this even more quickly when not kept in a sealed, dark container. Determining the age of the medication may be helpful.

2. Protocols vary as far as the minimum systolic blood pressure required to give nitroglycerin. Protocols usually require a minimum systolic pressure of 100 mmHg but now 110 to120 mmHg is common. Since the patient has a history of hypertension (high blood pressure), his pressure of 122 over 78 may actually be low for him. In this case, caution would be advised. Medical direction will help with this decision. His elevated pulse may add to your concern.

3. For the current history, you need to know the four rights of medication administration and that his signs and symptoms match the indications for the medication (chest pain). His past history will reveal a condition for which the medication is prescribed (cardiac). It is crucial for you to determine whether the patient has taken any medications for erectile dysfunction (Viagra, Levitra, and so on) or had these medications prescribed to him. Advise the doctor of your findings.

4. Doctor _____, this is EMT _____ on _____ ambulance who is en route to your location with a 60-year-old male patient who is complaining of 8/10 crushing substernal chest pain which came on at rest. His vitals are pulse 92 and slightly irregular, respirations 20, blood pressure 122/78, PERL, skin warm and dry. The patient has a history of hypertension and heart attack 5 years ago. He has prescribed nitroglycerin that he has not taken yet. Would you like us to assist him with this medication?

5. There are actually many formats these reports can take. Most importantly, they should contain key information without being too long-winded. The physicians are likely busy in the ED and would like an accurate and complete but to-the-point radio or cell phone report.

ANSWERS TO RETRO REVIEW QUESTIONS

1. *Answer:* b. *The virus does not survive well outside the body.*
2. *Answer:* d. *inertia*
3. *Answer:* c. *Repeaters*

ANSWERS TO CHAPTER 16 RESPIRATORY EMERGENCIES

ANSWERS TO SHORT ANSWER QUESTIONS

1. *Answer:* *Wheezing, increased breathing effort on exhalation, and very rapid breathing without stridor.*
2. *Answer:* *Inadequate breathing is breathing that is not sufficient to support life.*

ANSWERS TO MULTIPLE-CHOICE QUESTIONS

1. *Answer:* a. *moderate*
2. *Answer:* c. *Seesaw breathing*
3. *Answer:* b. *breathing normally*
4. *Answer:* d. *rhonchi*
5. *Answer:* a. *hypoxic drive*

ANSWERS TO SCENARIO QUESTIONS

1. *Answer:* b. *The patient may have developed a hypoxic drive.*
2. *Answer:* c. *Contact on-line medical direction and request instructions.*
3. *Answer:* a. *A COPD patient breathes because oxygen levels are low, whereas a non-COPD patient breathes because carbon dioxide levels are high.*

1. *Answer:* *d.* *in very critical condition*
2. *Answer:* *b.* *No. Unlike an adult patient, this child's decreasing pulse during respiratory difficulty means trouble.*
3. *Answer:* *c.* *Ensure that the child's airway is not obstructed.*
1. *Answer:* *b.* *administer high-concentration oxygen and attempt to calm her.*
2. *Answer:* *d.* *Not until you have determined the nature and extent of her injuries.*
3. *Answer:* *c.* *By making sure that the patient's chest rises and falls.*

ANSWERS TO CASE STUDY QUESTIONS

1. He is standing in the "tripod" position, which is common for conscious patients in moderate to severe distress. You are also likely to see accessory muscle use in his neck, abdomen, and chest.
2. Due to his level of distress and the fact that he does not have his inhaler with him, it is appropriate to place him on 15 lpm by nonrebreather mask.

1. The answer is a simple no. As an EMT-B, you may only assist with the administration of an inhaler if your protocols allow it and if the medication has been prescribed specifically to the patient. There are many unforeseen dangers in sharing prescription medications with friends and family and this practice should be avoided.
2. This patient should remain a high priority for transport due to the severity of his distress. Without his medication, his condition could worsen at a moment's notice. It is best to keep all patients in moderate to severe respiratory distress as high priority for transport just in case their condition takes a turn for the worse.

1. While family members most often do not have medical training, they know when things are bad. Generally, you should listen. Family members know the way the patient normally is and know that unresponsiveness, altered mental status, and seizures are very, very bad things.

   The patient's poor color and obvious difficulty in breathing should help you, in and of itself, to form a general impression of a critical patient requiring immediate emergency care and transportation.
2. Begin with latex gloves and eye protection. Have a face shield or mask readily available in the event the patient spits, sprays, or requires suction. You will not be able to ventilate using a pocket face mask if you are wearing a mask yourself, but the pocket face mask will cover the patient's mouth and nose, preventing substances from spraying.

1. Yes, and this is perhaps the most important determination you can make. In CPR class, you are taught to check and determine whether the patient is breathing. As an EMT-B, you will be checking to see whether the patient is breathing adequately. There is a time between when the patient breathes normally and when he stops breathing. This is a time when providing assisted ventilations may truly be lifesaving by preventing respiratory and cardiac arrest.

   You should listen to the lungs for air movement and watch the chest for expansion (or lack of expansion). This should complete the exam and verify inadequate breathing.
2. No. The patient is breathing inadequately. He is breathing at a rate below 10, the ventilations are extremely labored, and his mental status and color indicate poor perfusion. He requires immediate assisted ventilations.

1. No. While patients with emphysema may have some level of hypoxic drive, this patient needs immediate high-concentration oxygen and assisted ventilations.

2. Yes. Medics might choose to intubate the patient (pass a tube through the nose or mouth of the patient and into the trachea to maximize ventilations and control the airway). EKG monitoring, IV, and medications are also appropriate now—and certainly later if the patient goes into cardiac arrest.

1. Fifteen seconds is the time limit for suctioning (each time). It may be repeated as necessary after reoxygenation.

2. A Yankaur (tonsil-tip or rigid) catheter is most appropriate. In some cases where vomitus is especially thick, you may use the tubing alone while rolling the patient to his side and sweeping the big chunks or thick material out with your gloved hand.

ANSWERS TO RETRO REVIEW QUESTIONS

1. *Answer:* c. *five (Chapter 6)*
2. *Answer:* b. *reassess the vital signs (Chapter 10)*
3. *Answer:* d. *Rollover crashes (Chapter 7)*

ANSWERS TO CHAPTER 17 CARDIAC EMERGENCIES

ANSWERS TO SHORT ANSWER QUESTIONS

1. *Answer : AEDs should not be used on patients under one year of age or when the cardiac arrest was preceded by trauma.*
2. *Answer: The four links are early access to EMS, early CPR, early defibrillation, and early advanced care.*

ANSWERS TO MULTIPLE-CHOICE QUESTIONS

1. *Answer:* c. *Biphasic*
2. *Answer:* b. *less than 100*
3. *Answer:* c. *oxygen*
4. *Answer:* a. *8*
5. *Answer:* d. *VF*

ANSWERS TO SCENARIO QUESTIONS

1. *Answer:* c. *move him out of the stands*
2. *Answer:* b. *As soon as it is available.*
3. *Answer:* a. *Approximately every 60 seconds*
1. *Answer:* a. *begin CPR*
2. *Answer:* d. *A position of comfort.*
3. *Answer:* c. *The AED will indicate "no shock advised."*

ANSWERS TO CASE STUDY QUESTIONS

1. Between his history and the description that the pain is "tightness" and that it comes on with exertion is the possibility the pain could be cardiac in nature. You could go on to determine whether his chest is tender to the touch and whether anything he does makes the pain better or worse. You will also want to rule out trauma by asking him whether he suffered any type of injury recently.

2. Yes, oxygen is definitely indicated for any patient suspected of having cardiac chest pain and should be considered for chest pain of any origin. Given his history and presentation, you should suggest a nonrebreather mask at 15 lpm.

1. You will want to confirm the instructions that his doctor gave him for taking the nitro. Typically, patients are allowed up to three tablets in 15 minutes if no relief is obtained. Once you confirm that he has only taken two and that it has been at least 5 minutes since the last one, you can assist him in taking another. Do so only after confirming his systolic blood pressure is at least 100. This may require contacting medical direction. Your local protocols may vary.

2. It is best to maintain a position of comfort for the patient. Allow the patient to determine the best position. For most patients experiencing chest pain, it will be in the sitting or semiseated position.

1. From the standpoint of her complaint of weakness, the patient does not appear to be a high priority, but see how the case progresses. What you find may change your mind.

2. Patients do not always comprehend what the problem is. The patient tells you that she feels weak, but she is also having some difficulty breathing. While what the patient tells you is very important, your observations are equally important. The respiratory distress with the increased pulse should make you want to look further and suspect that something could be wrong.

1. The pulse remains high and you now see that the respirations are also elevated. Her dyspnea is worsened when she exerts herself. She has some significant risk factors for heart problems (high blood pressure and diabetes) and the greatest factor is that women, diabetic and the elderly, often have heart problems without having the "typical" chest pain. This could be the case here.

2. One easy thing to look for is whether she has any swelling (fluid) in her ankles. You should additionally ask whether she has had to sleep on more pillows recently—also an indication of fluid accumulation from heart problems. Since she has a history of diabetes, if you have a blood–glucose monitor and you are allowed to use it under local protocol, checking her blood–glucose reading would also be prudent.

1. Bringing the AED on more than just calls for cardiac arrest or "man down" is important. If the patient loses a 10 percent chance of survival for each minute the heart is stopped, how much would you lose running back to the ambulance to get the AED? Unknown problems, seizures, chest pain, and respiratory distress are all candidates for bringing the AED.

2. It may not have been a direct cause, but it is not appropriate to have patients who are experiencing difficulty breathing or having chest pain perform any exertion at all. This increases the workload of the heart and respiratory system that are already compromised.

ANSWERS TO RETRO REVIEW QUESTIONS

1. *Answer:*   *b.*   *A reason not to take the prescribed medication. (Chapter 15)*

2. *Answer:*   *a.*   *general impression (Chapter 8)*

3. *Answer:*   *d.*   *three (Chapter 15)*

ANSWERS TO CHAPTER 18
ACUTE ABDOMINAL EMERGENCIES

ANSWERS TO SHORT ANSWER QUESTIONS

1. *Answer:* Referred pain is felt in an area other than where the pain originates. It is usually related to shared nerve pathways.
2. *Answer:* A pregnancy that is developing outside of the uterus.

ANSWERS TO MULTIPLE-CHOICE QUESTIONS

1. *Answer:* b. guarding
2. *Answer:* c. tearing
3. *Answer:* d. internal bleeding
4. *Answer:* b. solid
5. *Answer:* a. visceral

ANSWERS TO SCENARIO QUESTIONS

1. *Answer:* c. "What makes the pain better or worse?"
2. *Answer:* c. hollow
3. *Answer:* d. "Have you had sexual intercourse in the past 12 to 24 hours?"

1. *Answer:* a. myocardial infarction
2. *Answer:* a. a suspected aortic aneurysm
3. *Answer:* c. ask the patient whether he has ever had an abdominal aneurysm

ANSWERS TO CASE STUDY QUESTIONS

1. In all likelihood, the abdominal pain is the most serious. This is due to the fact that the abdomen is very tender, indicating a strong likelihood that underlying organs have been damaged. Damaged organs mean uncontrolled bleeding that must be stopped.
2. The most likely reason for his rigid abdomen is the fact that he is in pain and "guarding" his abdomen. This is often the case with responsive patients with abdominal injuries. Now if this man were unresponsive and still had a rigid abdomen, the likely cause would be internal bleeding. Because we cannot easily differentiate the difference in the field, we must always treat for the worst and assume he has internal bleeding and expedite transport.

1. Considering the mechanism of injury and the fact that he is rapidly getting worse, you will not want to waste time with his orthopedic injuries. You must manage his spine by placing him on a long board and packaging his extremity injuries the best you can as fast as you can. You will most likely not take the time to place a traction splint on this man's right leg.
2. This man has likely suffered major blunt trauma to the abdomen causing serious internal bleeding. Given his signs and symptoms, he is most likely suffering from hemorrhagic shock from internal injuries. The most you can do for this man is provide high-flow oxygen, control all external bleeding, and expedite transport to an appropriate receiving hospital or call for an ALS unit.

1. Patients with severe pain anywhere are generally given a high priority. Additionally, since the pain brought her to the floor and is substantial, bringing her promptly to the hospital would both bring her closer to receiving hospital care and to pain relief.
2. The SAMPLE history would be performed first. This would give you an idea of the type of pain, onset, and the events leading up to it. Additionally,

during the history, the patient can point to or describe painful areas so they may be palpated last.

1. Yes. This should be done respectfully, but it is appropriate to ask these questions as part of the history. In this setting, it may be best to ask in a private situation—rather than when coworkers are around.

2. Ask when her last period was, whether she is overdue for her period, whether her periods are regular, whether she has ever had this pain before associated with her cycle, whether she is or could be pregnant (usually meaning whether she has had intercourse during the last cycle), and so on. Answers to some questions will generate others.

1. While you are not in a position to diagnose, this should be considered a very serious condition (e.g. ectopic pregnancy that is discussed in Chapter 24). Whether it is bad menstrual cramps, an ectopic pregnancy, a ruptured ovarian cyst, or appendicitis, the bottom line is that she is in severe pain and should be transported promptly.

2. The vital signs could indicate many things including shock or pain. As a young, healthy adult, 104 over 64 may be quite normal. *But* remember that blood pressure drops last and she *does* have an increased pulse and respirations with cool, moist skin. Consider this compensated shock—which could decompensate quickly. Pain could be responsible for the changes, but you should never assume the least. You should look at what is the more serious possibility—and that is shock.

ANSWERS TO RETRO REVIEW QUESTIONS

1. *Answer:* c. *Check the lower eyelids. (Chapter 9)*
2. *Answer:* d. *ongoing assessments (Chapter 12)*
3. *Answer:* a. *Activated charcoal (Chapter 15)*

ANSWERS TO CHAPTER 19 DIABETIC EMERGENCIES AND ALTERED MENTAL STATUS

ANSWERS TO SHORT ANSWER QUESTIONS

1. *Answer:* *A condition in which the patient has two or more seizures without regaining full consciousness.*
2. *Answer:* *Diabetes mellitus is caused by a decrease in the body's ability to produce or utilize insulin. As a result, excessive amounts of glucose develop in the blood stream and are spilled over into the urine. High sugar causes an increase in urine output that leads to abnormal thirst.*

ANSWERS TO MULTIPLE-CHOICE QUESTIONS

1. *Answer:* c. *hyperglycemia*
2. *Answer:* a. *failure to take seizure control medication*
3. *Answer:* d. *simple fainting*
4. *Answer:* b. *pancreas*
5. *Answer:* d. *Idiopathic*

ANSWERS TO SCENARIO QUESTIONS

1. *Answer:* b. *become hypoglycemic*
2. *Answer:* c. *Administer oral glucose followed by high-concentration oxygen and transport in the semi-Fowler's position.*

1. *Answer:* b. *transient ischemic attack (TIA)*
2. *Answer:* d. *Cincinnati Prehospital Stroke Scale*
3. *Answer:* b. *expressive*

1. *Answer:* b. *Administer high-concentration oxygen, transport immediately, and request an ALS intercept.*
2. *Answer:* c. *status epilepticus*
3. *Answer:* d. *irregular electrical activity in the brain*

ANSWERS TO CASE STUDY QUESTIONS

1. You will attempt to get a response from this patient by introducing yourself. You will be looking for an appropriate response from her. Because she is awake and looking around, it is safe to assume she is breathing and has a pulse. You will want to confirm that she is breathing with a good tidal volume and that her pulse is within normal limits.

2. You will want to know whether she is aware of what is going on with her or whether she has pain anywhere. You will also want to ask whether she has any medical history that might explain her present condition.

1. Given her altered mental status and the fact that she is a diabetic, she is probably suffering from low blood sugar (hypoglycemia). If left untreated, hypoglycemia will lead to insulin shock and unconsciousness.

2. You should try and give this patient something to eat or drink as long as she can manage her own airway during the process. Oral glucose, if carried on your ambulance, is appropriate here. Place the glucose on a tongue depressor and place it in the side of her mouth between the cheek and gums. If the work site has a break room, some orange juice with a sugar packet or two added will also work. Have her hold the cup or food and take sips or bites on her own. Watch carefully that she does not choke.

1. The components of the initial assessment are always the same. The way you perform them may differ from patient to patient. In this case, you would form a general impression of a man who is conscious but unable to communicate. His airway is clear, but his drool indicates he may need suctioning at any time. Listen for gurgling and observe for buildup of fluids because he may not be able to clear his airway. This would be worsened if he were lying down. Observe breathing effort, rate, and depth. Check a radial pulse. Since he is conscious, he has a pulse but checking the radial pulse will give you a quick idea of the rate. If the radial pulse is absent on both sides and there is a carotid pulse, it would indicate a low blood pressure.

2. If the patient cannot speak but seems to understand, you will need to provide reassurance to the patient as this is a terrifying situation. In order to get answers to questions, you may need to create a system of communication (e.g. the patient blinks his eyes twice for yes).

1. This presentation indicates a neurological condition, possibly stroke. In addition to getting a medical history, obtain the events leading up to her husband's current condition. This would include any headaches, weakness, dizziness, and so on.

2. A neurological examination including the ability to sense and move extremities as well as a prehospital stroke scale. The Cincinnati Prehospital Stroke Scale is one example that examines for facial droop, speech abnormalities, and arm drift.

1. This is definitely altered mental status. It looks like stroke but could actually be a diabetic condition or some other problem, even with the facial droop. Keep an open mind. Maintaining a high transport priority will be important in any scenario. En route you can check his blood glucose if you

are allowed to do so. Asking other questions about use of medications (accidental or intentional overdose?), alcohol ingestion, or other causes of altered mental status is wise. Remember the size-up, examination of the patient's surroundings, and breath odors will also provide clues.

2. This patient is a high priority for transport. His altered mental status and the potential for developing airway problems, unconsciousness, and other neurological symptoms support this decision.

3. Depending on your local protocols and the hospital resources you have in your area, you should transport the patient to a hospital that specializes in the treatment of stroke. This usually requires the availability of a CT scanner (CAT scan) and neurological specialists. If these are not available in your area, you will likely be directed by protocol to transport to the nearest facility for stabilization and treatment. The patient may be transported to a further facility by helicopter or a specialized transport team.

ANSWERS TO RETRO REVIEW QUESTIONS

1. *Answer:* d. *over the brachial artery (Chapter 9)*
2. *Answer:* b. *interfere with the placement of the electrode pad (Chapter 17)*
3. *Answer:* c. *Nasopharyngeal (Chapter 6)*

ANSWERS TO CHAPTER 20 ALLERGIC REACTIONS

ANSWERS TO SHORT ANSWER QUESTIONS

1. *Answer:* *Epinephrine, when administered as a medication, constricts blood vessels and dilates bronchioles.*
2. *Answer:* *The first time an allergen is encountered, the immune system develops antibodies in response. Each subsequent exposure will cause a reaction between the allergen and the antibodies, which results in the allergic reaction.*

ANSWERS TO MULTIPLE-CHOICE QUESTIONS

1. *Answer:* a. *peanuts*
2. *Answer:* d. *hypertension*
3. *Answer:* b. *respiratory distress*
4. *Answer:* c. *Their immune systems are too underdeveloped.*
5. *Answer:* c. *latex*

ANSWERS TO SCENARIO QUESTIONS

1. *Answer:* b. *Send one of the other individuals to retrieve the EpiPen® while you call for EMS and monitor the patient.*
2. *Answer:* a. *hand it to the patient and remind him how to use it*
3. *Answer:* d. *thigh*

1. *Answer:* c. *oxygen*
2. *Answer:* a. *request an ALS intercept*
3. *Answer:* d. *The patient is having respiratory difficulty after exposure to a potential allergen.*

ANSWERS TO CASE STUDY QUESTIONS

1. You will want to confirm whether the girl knows she was stung by a bee. Did she feel a sting and if so, where was the sting on her body? Look at that area for evidence of a possible sting. You will also want to know whether the girl has a known allergy to bees and what happened the last time she was stung.

2. You will want to start her on high-flow oxygen at 15 lpm by nonrebreather mask. Keep her in a position of comfort and obtain a set of baseline vitals.

1. First, it must be within your local protocols to administer. Assuming that it is, you must confirm that the medication is indeed prescribed for the patient and that the expiration date on the medication has not passed.

2. 1. Remove safety cap and place black end of pen against the patient's thigh.
   2. Push the injector firmly against the thigh. Hold in place for 10 seconds.
   3. Remove the injector and record the time.
   4. Handle the pen with caution as it is an exposed sharp and may stick someone else.
   5. Monitor ABCs and vital signs and transport immediately.

1. In addition to the traditional ABCs, signs of shock will be noticeable in the initial assessment if present. These will include poor skin color with rapid pulse and respirations. You do not need a blood pressure reading to determine that the patient is unstable or potentially unstable.

2. In addition to the signs noted above, specifically ask the patient whether she feels any swelling in the airway, face, mouth, tongue, or lips. Ask about respiratory distress, chest tightness, fast heartbeat, or a feeling of impending doom. Feeling dizzy, lightheaded, or weak may also indicate shock.

3. You may note signs of airway swelling (edema), wheezing, stridor (audible without a stethoscope), and hives on the face, neck, or torso.

1. No. Anaphylaxis treatment in the field is based on respiratory compromise, shock, or both. In this case neither is present. Two points are important here. Patients can have anaphylaxis without hives or any outward appearance of the condition. Secondly, it is important to begin treatment early for best effect. In this case, the patient has neither respiratory compromise nor signs of shock. She should be monitored carefully so signs of respiratory compromise or compensated shock are caught early. Nausea and vomiting can be signs of allergic reaction or a side effect of some painkillers. Monitor the patient carefully.

2. The patient should be given oxygen by nonrebreather mask (by cannula if she is frequently vomiting and the mask is getting in the way). She should be placed in a position of comfort that will allow her to vomit without restriction. Be prepared to suction if necessary. If signs of respiratory or cardiac compromise develop, the epinephrine auto-injector should be administered according to local protocol. Treat for shock and notify ALS personnel per protocol.

3. Yes. The potential reaction to medication (or allergic reaction), severe enough so that EMS was called, is a good indication for transport.

ANSWERS TO RETRO REVIEW QUESTIONS

1. *Answer:* *c.* *Every 5 minutes.*
2. *Answer:* *d.* *medium*
3. *Answer:* *b.* *reassessing scene safety*

ANSWERS TO CHAPTER 21
POISONING AND OVERDOSE EMERGENCIES

ANSWERS TO SHORT ANSWER QUESTIONS

1. *Answer:* Because syrup of ipecac (a substance traditionally used to induce vomiting after poison ingestion) normally takes 15 to 20 minutes to work and only empties about a third of the contents of the patient's stomach, its use has largely been abandoned.

2. *Answer:* A depressed level of consciousness, pinpoint pupils, and respiratory depression are three common signs of narcotic overdose and are known as the opiate triad.

ANSWERS TO MULTIPLE-CHOICE QUESTIONS

1. *Answer:* d. illicit drugs
2. *Answer:* a. Volatile chemicals
3. *Answer:* b. Dilution with water or milk.
4. *Answer:* c. leave the scene and remain in a safe place until law enforcement arrives
5. *Answer:* c. surface area

ANSWERS TO SCENARIO QUESTIONS

1. *Answer:* c. narcotic
2. *Answer:* b. track marks
3. *Answer:* a. Latex exam gloves, a mask, and protective eyewear.

1. *Answer:* c. remove her clothing and begin flushing her skin
2. *Answer:* d. Aspiration of the caustic liquid.
3. *Answer:* b. the emergency-care instructions on the bottle of drain cleaner are wrong (Patients who have ingested caustic substances should never be made to vomit, as this can cause further damage to the esophagus and airway when the substance is regurgitated.)

1. *Answer:* b. carbon monoxide poisoning
2. *Answer:* c. move both patients out of the building
3. *Answer:* d. Oxygen

ANSWERS TO CASE STUDY QUESTIONS

1. The initial assessment of this patient will consist of an attempt to speak to the child and confirm that he is breathing adequately and has a good pulse.
2. You might begin by asking the mother whether she actually saw any of the pills in the boy's mouth. You will also want to study the pill container and determine on the basis of the fill date of the prescription how many pills were likely in the bottle when the boy opened it.

1. On the basis of the fact that there were a total of 20 pills to begin with and the prescription states to take one pill twice a day and it has been six days, there should have been eight pills remaining in the bottle.
2. Did the mother take all pills as prescribed? Has she given the child anything else since she called EMS? Is the child allergic to anything? How much does the child weigh?

1. Although the police are present and this is in a "decent" part of town, the presentation of the patient should cause you to keep a level of awareness

as you continue your assessment. In addition to scene safety and resources, the size-up is also a time to make observations about what might have caused this patient's condition.

2. You should prepare yourself, both mentally and with equipment, to begin work on a critically ill patient. You should request ALS if available, be sure you have the proper equipment you need including an AED, oxygen, suction, and a method of moving the patient promptly from the scene as it appears that the patient is a high priority. Additional personnel (e.g. engine company or other EMTs) would also be helpful.

1. The initial assessment identifies and treats life-threats in the ABCs. This patient needs some emergency care in this area. He has a pulse and is not bleeding, so treatment would be focused on providing ventilations to the patient since it appears he is breathing inadequately. Suctioning him as necessary due to his unresponsiveness is also required. The patient may or may not have a gag reflex, but an OPA would be prudent if he accepts it.

2. You will be working hard and fast. Generally, one EMT will get the stretcher and prepare for transport while the second stays and ventilates the patient. Since the patient is breathing inadequately, someone must stay with the patient to ventilate at all times. If there are stairs between you and the patient, you will move down one landing, ventilate a bit, and then move again until you get to the ambulance. In some areas, the police will help in retrieving equipment and/or patient emergency care.

1. In the setting of an altered mental status with the potential for medication involvement, an overdose of a narcotic drug may be indicated. This suspicion is furthered by the unresponsiveness and shallow respirations, also symptoms of drugs that depress the central nervous system.

2. Oxygen administered through a pocket face mask or bag-valve-mask device is the most needed intervention. Others that may be appropriate for altered mental status (oral glucose and activated charcoal) are contraindicated due to the patient's unresponsiveness.

3. Follow your local protocols. This may involve contacting your local medical direction, whether it is at the receiving hospital or through a separate physician. Some systems may prefer you to call the poison-control center directly in cases of poisoning.

Answers to Retro Review Questions

1. *Answer:* c. *hypoglycemia*
2. *Answer:* c. *What do you think caused the pain?*
3. *Answer:* c. *glucose*

ANSWERS TO CHAPTER 22 ENVIRONMENTAL EMERGENCIES

Answers to Short Answer Questions

1. *Answer:* Rapid warming will circulate unoxygenated, acidic, cold blood, and cool the vital central areas of the body, possibly causing cardiac arrest.
2. *Answer:* Rattlesnakes, copperheads, water moccasins, and coral snakes are the only poisonous snakes native to the United States.

Answers to Multiple-choice Questions

1. *Answer:* b. *convection*
2. *Answer:* c. *Microscopic ice crystals can cause serious tissue damage.*
3. *Answer:* a. *hyperthermia*
4. *Answer:* b. *arterial gas embolism*
5. *Answer:* d. *flat-bottomed aluminum boat*

Answers to Scenario Questions

1. *Answer:* b. *Remove all of the patient's clothing, splint his leg, and transport him with all but his lower extremities wrapped in heated blankets.*
2. *Answer:* d. *conduction*
3. *Answer:* a. *Hot packs warming the torso (core)*
1. *Answer:* d. *rinse the affected area with rubbing alcohol*
2. *Answer:* c. *decompression sickness*
3. *Answer:* a. *hyperbaric-trauma-care center*
1. *Answer:* c. *heat stroke*
2. *Answer:* a. *Place him in the air conditioned ambulance; remove his clothes; apply cool packs to his neck, armpits, and groin; keep his skin wet; administer high-concentration oxygen; and transport immediately.*
3. *Answer:* d. *his body is reacting to the loss of salt and fluid*

Answers to Case Study Questions

1. Given the presentation and the environmental conditions, you should suspect heat stroke.
2. Given the likelihood of a heat emergency with this patient, your priority should be to cool him as rapidly as you can.

1. The most likely cause of convulsions in the heat-emergency patient is the overheating of the brain. This is a very serious sign and may be life threatening. There is little you can do to treat the convulsions aside from protecting the patient from injury.
2. You will want to place cold packs around the core of this man's body. Place packs around his neck, under his arms, and over his groin. This will help cool the core temperature. Oxygen is also important for this man, especially since he is convulsing. Place him on 15 lpm by nonrebreather mask.

1. It is difficult to determine and it must be assumed that it could have been the whole time the patient was unaccounted for. With the low temperature and wind chill, it is reasonable to expect the patient to be in serious condition.
2. The initial assessment focuses on the ABCs with a general impression and priority decision. The patient has a patent airway, is breathing adequately, and does not appear to be injured or bleeding. You apply oxygen. You may often think that the assessment steps are strictly performed in order but you can also multitask by having someone get blankets and hot packs while the initial assessment is done. The initial assessment is always the first part of assessment after size-up, but this does not mean others cannot begin taking a history or, in this case, begin to warm the patient while you begin the assessment.

1. The fact that he was outside in that temperature for any amount of time makes it potentially serious. The fact that he is not shivering, combined with his pale skin and marginally low pulse, also lean toward this being

serious. Remember that shivering stops when the body gets into the 90- to 95-degree range. A lack of shivering can actually be a serious sign.

2. The patient's age puts him at a greater risk for hypothermia, as does his history of diabetes. His inability to communicate due to Alzheimer's adds an extra level of complexity to the call.

1. Since that patient is conscious, he would be actively rewarmed. This would include blankets and hot packs around the body's core. He would also be treated gently and not jostled, to prevent further injury or cardiac problems. Oxygen would be continued en route. Vitals signs would be monitored every 5 minutes.

2. Active rewarming uses blankets and heat (e.g. hot packs) to bring up the body temperature and is used when the patient is conscious and mildly to moderately hypothermic. Passive rewarming is done in severe cases of hypothermia when rewarming outside of the hospital could be dangerous. Passive rewarming includes maintaining body heat and preventing further hypothermia using blankets—without external warming devices.

ANSWERS TO RETRO REVIEW QUESTIONS

1. *Answer:* *c.* *unease*
2. *Answer:* *b.* *hypertension*
3. *Answer:* *a.* *stair chair*

ANSWERS TO CHAPTER 23 BEHAVIORAL EMERGENCIES

ANSWERS TO SHORT ANSWER QUESTIONS

1. *Answer:* *Individuals who have made the decision to commit suicide can actually experience an improvement in attitude. This is due to the fact that there is now an "end in sight" to their depression.*
2. *Answer:* *The aggressive or hostile patient may respond inappropriately to people, attempt to hurt himself or others, have a rapid pulse and rapid respirations, speak or move rapidly, and appear anxious, nervous, or "panicky."*

ANSWERS TO MULTIPLE-CHOICE QUESTIONS

1. *Answer:* *b.* *Lack of oxygen*
2. *Answer:* *d.* *All of the above*
3. *Answer:* *c.* *Low blood sugar*

ANSWERS TO SCENARIO QUESTIONS

1. *Answer:* *c.* *indicate to your partner to contact law enforcement*
2. *Answer:* *a.* *Quickly exit the ambulance and run to a safe location.*
1. *Answer:* *b.* *taking an authoritative tone*
2. *Answer:* *d.* *"Why am I too late to help you?"*

ANSWERS TO CASE STUDY QUESTIONS

1. On the basis of the suspicious nature of this call, the report of screaming, and the general reputation of the neighborhood, you decide to get an ETA from dispatch for law enforcement and wait in the ambulance.

1. It is clear the man is distraught over something and emotionally upset. Because he is not violent or threatening anyone, you should try and talk him into allowing you to help. Give the history that he has shared about injuring himself, it is very questionable whether this man is competent enough to refuse emergency care.

1. Given the history and his emotional state of mind, this man is not capable of making competent decisions about his own emergency care. You might proceed by asking the officer to get involved, and if necessary have him restrain the patient before you can transport.

1. Most people would have a similar thought: that this was a psych emergency. The most correct and medically appropriate approach would be considering the patient as having an altered mental status. This is an open-minded approach that takes into account that the patient could be experiencing a diabetic emergency, overdose, head injury, severe intoxication, or another physical problem causing his unusual behavior.

2. This is a challenge because approaching a patient with unusual behavior comes with issues, the most important being your safety and the potential for an unpredictable response to your advances and emergency care. This does not reduce the need for an initial assessment. Since the patient appears conscious, you may be able to observe his respiratory rate and depth, see whether there are any problems with bleeding (blood in the mouth or drooling) and look for outward injuries that could cause bleeding—all from a slight distance.

1. People care is the only thing you have to win over the patient. Nothing in your EMS bag or gear will help you here. Get on the patient's level, take your time, listen, and be honest. Do this safely. Do not enter the patient's personal space unless the patient approves your doing so.

1. In most areas, the police have the authority to take a person to a hospital or psychiatric facility against his will. Many states have mental-hygiene laws that also allow certain physicians (some require signatures of two physicians) to commit a person involuntarily.

2. The police. The police should also carry out the potentially dangerous physical-restraint process although EMTs may help with proper and safe-restraint equipment and preparing the patient for transport.

ANSWERS TO RETRO REVIEW QUESTIONS

1. *Answer:* c. *aneurysm*
2. *Answer:* d. *twelve*
3. *Answer:* b. *anaphylaxis*

ANSWERS TO CHAPTER 24 OBSTETRIC AND GYNECOLOGICAL EMERGENCIES

ANSWERS TO SHORT ANSWER QUESTIONS

1. *Answer:* Because of slowed digestion and delayed gastric emptying, there is a greater risk the patient will vomit and aspirate.

2. *Answer:* If the mother is in a supine position, the combined weight of the uterus and its contents may compress the inferior vena cava, thereby decreasing the volume of blood returning to the heart. This can cause dizziness and a decrease in blood pressure.

ANSWERS TO MULTIPLE-CHOICE QUESTIONS

1. *Answer:* b. *premature placental separation*
2. *Answer:* a. *first*
3. *Answer:* c. *the baby is birthing in the normal, head-first manner*
4. *Answer:* d. *fetal distress*
5. *Answer:* b. *Low blood pressure*

ANSWERS TO SCENARIO QUESTIONS

1. *Answer:* a. *Secured to a long spine board that is tilted to the left.*
2. *Answer:* c. *Reassure her that the baby is well protected in the uterus.*
3. *Answer:* d. *30–35 percent*
1. *Answer:* a. *Take BSI precautions, assure an adequate airway, assess for signs of shock, administer high-concentration oxygen, and transport immediately.*
2. *Answer:* c. *hemorrhagic*
3. *Answer:* b. *It is not possible and should not be attempted.*
1. *Answer:* d. *With this patient's birthing history and current contractions, it is possible that she might deliver the baby into the toilet.*
2. *Answer:* b. *Inserting several gloved fingers into the vagina and keeping the baby from pressing on the cord.*
3. *Answer:* c. *With her head down and her buttocks raised with a pillow.*

ANSWERS TO CASE STUDY QUESTIONS

1. You need to reassure the father that you are there to help and need to do a quick assessment of his girlfriend. You may want to have the park ranger take the man aside and get a history from him. This will allow you to do your job without him as a distraction.

2. You will want to find out whether the three small children in the tent are hers. Finding out about prior labors/births will help you make the stay or go decision.

1. On the basis of the prior history of early deliveries and the fact that she is already crowning, has contractions that are 3 minutes apart, and the extended transport time back to town, you should be prepared for an on-scene delivery.

2. From the beginning of one contraction to the beginning of the next.

1. The quick look at the patient as you approach allows you to form a general impression. In this case, you will see how the patient looks. How is her skin color? Is her skin moist? Does she appear conscious and aware of your presence? Do you see any blood around the patient or room?

2. Yes. It is not the location, it is the amount of blood loss that causes shock. Some places have the potential to lose more blood than others. Conditions within the female reproductive system can cause serious, if not fatal bleeding.

1. Vaginal bleeding is often quantified by the number of sanitary napkins that the patient has soaked through over a given time period. This is often compared by the patient to a normal menstrual cycle. (e.g. using more or less than for the monthly period). Determining blood loss is always challenging and this is no different.

2. The patient should be questioned about her last period and when she would expect her next period. Ask about whether the patient may be pregnant (missed menstrual cycles) and whether this type of event has

ever happened before. Ask the patient about the onset of the bleeding (sudden vs. gradual) and whether it was accompanied by any pain.

3. You should palpate the abdominal quadrants. Palpate areas that are tender or painful last. It is usually not necessary to inspect the vaginal area unless the cause of the bleeding is traumatic and external, which may benefit from direct pressure.

1. EMTs will never insert anything into the vagina and unfortunately internal bleeding cannot be controlled in the field. Treating the patient for shock, including oxygen and the Trendelenberg position, is appropriate.

ANSWERS TO RETRO REVIEW QUESTIONS

1. *Answer:* b. *delirium tremens*
2. *Answer:* c. *tendon*
3. *Answer:* d. *data element*

ANSWERS TO CHAPTER 25 PUTTING IT TOGETHER FOR THE MEDICAL PATIENT

ANSWERS TO SHORT ANSWER QUESTIONS

1. *Answer:* *If unusual circumstances are making the patient's situation difficult to assess, you should contact medical direction.*
2. *Answer:* *Is the patient's airway patent? Is the patient breathing? Does the patient have sufficient circulation? What transport priority is this patient? Are there any interventions that you can perform?*

ANSWERS TO MULTIPLE-CHOICE QUESTIONS

1. *Answer:* b. *Ask the patient to explain the disease.*
2. *Answer:* d. *treatments*
3. *Answer:* c. *Monitor the ABCs and transport.*

ANSWERS TO SCENARIO QUESTIONS

1. *Answer:* d. *Obtain baseline vitals.*
2. *Answer:* a. *Multiply the daily prescription amount by the number of days since the prescription was filled, add that amount to the number of pills currently left in the bottle, and subtract that sum from the originally prescribed quantity of pills.*
3. *Answer:* b. *Try to get the SAMPLE information from the student who knows the patient.*

1. *Answer:* c. *Complete an initial assessment.*
2. *Answer:* a. *Calmly continue to reassure her.*
3. *Answer:* b. *medical direction*

ANSWERS TO CASE STUDY QUESTIONS

1. You will want to determine exactly what happened and whether the patient can tell you what happened. You will want to determine, if possible, why the patient fell and whether she remembers the event.
2. If a patient remembers why he fell, such as tripping over the cat or just stepping wrong, it is referred to as a mechanical fall. It is important to differentiate a mechanical fall from a fall for unknown reasons such as a

patient who may have passed out from some underlying medical problem and injured himself during the fall.

1. Medication name, patient's name, doctor's name, date prescribed, and number of pills along with frequency that the pills should be taken.

2. Given her age, irregular pulse, and the fall, it would be best to treat this patient as unstable and take vitals every 5 minutes.

1. The general impression of this patient is that of a noncritical patient with a medical complaint.

2. Technically, you do not need gloves or goggles unless he spits, vomits, bleeds, or otherwise decides to share his fluids with you. Most providers will wear gloves as a precaution.

1. While it is sometimes helpful to have a more tangible complaint (such as chest pain) to explore, it is not necessary. The signs and symptoms portion of your SAMPLE history would explore weakness as the symptom. You would perform all other portions of the initial assessment, focused history, and ongoing assessment, staying alert for unusual findings. Many patients who experience sepsis (serious infection in the blood), strokes, or heart attacks actually present with weakness as one of the symptoms.

1. It is not wise to assume that a patient who presents with nontangible symptoms has a psychiatric condition or is faking. Cardiac conditions such as a low pulse rate, stroke, and other medical conditions can present as weakness. The general rule in medicine is not to write things off as psychiatric until other causes have been ruled out.

2. Opinions may differ on this. He is oriented and has a good color. There is no apparent distress. Putting oxygen on would not hurt or be wrong but may not be necessary.

ANSWERS TO RETRO REVIEW QUESTIONS

1. *Answer:* c. *lymph*
2. *Answer:* d. *volatile-chemical abuse*
3. *Answer:* a. *Pancreas (it is retroperitoneal)*

ANSWERS TO CHAPTER 26 BLEEDING AND SHOCK

ANSWERS TO SHORT ANSWER QUESTIONS

1. *Answer:* *If a majority of the patient's blood vessels dilate, as in the case of anaphylaxis, there would not be sufficient blood volume in the system to allow for proper perfusion.*

2. *Answer:* *The presence of a mechanism of injury consistent with those known to cause internal bleeding.*

ANSWERS TO MULTIPLE-CHOICE QUESTIONS

1. *Answer:* c. *abnormal lung sounds*
2. *Answer:* a. *capillary bleeding*
3. *Answer:* b. *nose*
4. *Answer:* d. *1,000 cc*
5. *Answer:* c. *50 percent*

ANSWERS TO SCENARIO QUESTIONS

1. *Answer:* b. *administer oxygen with a nonrebreather mask at 15 lp m, place the patient flat on the gurney with his legs raised 8 to 12 inches, keep him warm, and transport immediately*

2. *Answer:* a. *spleen*

3. *Answer:* d. *At the moment of injury.*

1. *Answer:* b. *apply a tourniquet to each leg*

2. *Answer:* a. *administer oxygen at 15 pm with a nonrebreather mask and provide immediate transportation*

3. *Answer:* c. *femoral*

4. *Answer:* d. *a critical-incident-stress debriefing*

1. *Answer:* a. *contact medical direction for advice*

2. *Answer:* c. *check for a distal pulse*

3. *Answer:* d. *the shock position*

ANSWERS TO CASE STUDY QUESTIONS

1. You should realize that a kick from a horse in the patient's abdomen is in itself a likely significant mechanism of injury. You may want to get information from bystanders about whether the patient was thrown or fell, causing further injuries or lost consciousness. You can also check the size of the horse to get an idea of the force that was generated by the animal.

2. You will want to know whether there is a suspected spinal injury before rendering emergency care. This can be determined by asking how he fell and onto what surface. Does he have pain in his neck and did he hit his head or lose consciousness during the fall?

1. Yes. Given the mechanism of injury and his presentation, he is definitely a candidate for oxygen. He should receive high-flow oxygen at 15 lpm by nonrebreather mask.

2. This patient should be treated as an unstable patient because he is showing several signs of shock. You will want to take his vitals every 5 minutes during transport. If he is indeed bleeding internally, you can anticipate that his blood pressure will continue to decrease while his pulse will continue to increase.

1. The man is conscious and sitting up but appears to have a significant blood loss.

2. The size-up should begin with safety, then a BSI determination. Gloves and eyewear at a minimum are appropriate here. You should determine the number of patients and whether any resources are needed. An ALS request or, if you are a significant distance from a hospital, air medical evacuation may be necessary.

1. The patient is sitting up and able to keep his airway clear. His respirations are a bit fast. Oxygen is essential. When checking the pulse, determine whether a radial pulse is present at the wrist. But also get a feel for whether it seems rapid. And while your hand is at the wrist, note the color, temperature, and condition of the skin. Cool, moist skin with a rapid pulse and rapid respirations indicate shock, something that you must recognize early.

2. Yes. It is soaked with blood and preventing you from assessing the wound and effectively controlling bleeding. Remove it carefully in the event that clots have formed and are attached to the towel.

3. The significant blood loss gives this patient a high priority for transport.

1. Regardless of the cause and size of an extremity wound, bleeding is controlled by direct pressure and elevation. If this does not work, a pressure bandage could be applied and the pressure point (in this case brachial) used. A tourniquet may be used on an extremity as a last resort, but the need for a tourniquet is quite rare.

2. As noted in the initial assessment above, look for moist skin with poor color, rapid pulse and rapid respirations, and possibly an increased capillary-refill time (greater than 2 seconds).

ANSWERS TO RETRO REVIEW QUESTIONS

1. *Answer:* c. *vagus nerve*
2. *Answer:* d. *reasonable force*
3. *Answer:* a. *syncope*

ANSWERS TO CHAPTER 27 SOFT-TISSUE INJURIES

ANSWERS TO SHORT ANSWER QUESTIONS

1. *Answer:* *To seal any potentially open neck veins and prevent the introduction of an air embolus into the patient's blood stream.*
2. *Answer:* *An abdominal wound so deep and large that organs protrude through the wound opening.*

ANSWERS TO MULTIPLE-CHOICE QUESTIONS

1. *Answer:* c. *bleeding has been controlled*
2. *Answer:* d. *severity*
3. *Answer:* a. *protection, water balance, temperature regulation, excretion and impact absorption*
4. *Answer:* c. *the burn*
5. *Answer:* a. *Infrared light*

ANSWERS TO SCENARIO QUESTIONS

1. *Answer:* b. *treating for shock*
2. *Answer:* d. *both cardiac tamponade and traumatic asphyxia*
3. *Answer:* c. *the difference between systolic and diastolic readings*

1. *Answer:* b. *28*
2. *Answer:* d. *Spinal injury*
3. *Answer:* c. *full-thickness*

1. *Answer:* b. *Place your gloved hand firmly over the puncture site.*
2. *Answer:* a. *hemopneumothorax*
3. *Answer:* d. *penetrating*

ANSWERS TO CASE STUDY QUESTIONS

1. Given that he is conscious and did not suffer a major mechanism of injury, it would be appropriate to conduct a focused assessment of the injury site.
2. You will want to make certain that the officers have searched the patient for any possible weapons.

1. It appears that this man has a sucking chest wound and air is building up inside his chest cavity (pneumothorax).

2. You will want to listen carefully to this man's breath sounds. It is likely that you will not hear breath sounds on the injured side due to an injured lung.

1. As additional apparatus arrives, be careful your ambulance is not blocked in. If this occurs, you will be unable to transport. Additional patients you discover may need additional ambulances. If the burns are serious, you may require ALS or air medical evacuation for these patients to a burn center.

2. Most likely yes. While you have one patient now, there could be others. Firefighters may become injured or exhausted. Depending on the system in your community, EMS may be a part of fireground rehabilitation, which will require additional resources. Advise the incident or EMS commander that additional resources may be needed.

1. You have observed critical burns. This patient's burns involve the hands and are circumferential; both place this patient's burns in the critical classification. Since this is a fire scene, you suspect that he may have also inhaled smoke and you should be prepared to treat smoke or toxic inhalation. If the burns are still hot, you may need to use sterile saline to stop the burning process. You should be planning prompt transportation to a burn center (if available) and providing early notification so the hospital can be prepared.

2. In addition to the ABC steps discussed throughout your textbook, be alert for signs of smoke inhalation and/or airway burns including singed facial hair, soot around the mouth and nose, coughing, or complaints of throat irritation. Oxygen should be applied by nonrebreather mask. Respiratory effort and level of consciousness should be monitored carefully throughout the call.

1. Four-and-a-half percent. The entire arm is 9 percent, half of that is 4 1/2 percent. The burns appear to be full-thickness burns.

2. Loose clothes may be cut away, but anything stuck to the skin should not be removed. If the wedding ring can be removed, it should be. This is because the metal can continue to hold heat. The body's response to the burns may be to swell. This could cause constriction of tissue and difficulty in removing the ring at a later time. Do it now if possible. If you have gauze pads available, it may be helpful to place them in between the fingers to prevent the tissue sticking together after bandaging.

3. This is dependent on local protocol, but many areas would recommend dressings moistened with sterile saline. Many areas recommend wet dressings if the BSA burned is less than 10 percent. Moistened dressings applied to larger areas may promote hypothermia.

ANSWERS TO RETRO REVIEW QUESTIONS

1. *Answer:* d. *15 to 20*
2. *Answer:* a. *all*
3. *Answer:* c. *ask law enforcement personnel to force the patient to accept treatment*

ANSWERS TO CHAPTER 28 MUSCULOSKELETAL INJURIES

ANSWERS TO SHORT ANSWER QUESTIONS

1. *Answer:* *Two battlefield surgeons during World War I noticed that after a femur fracture the large muscles of the thigh would contract and cause the fractured bone ends to override each other and damage blood vessels. The traction splint prevented this from occurring, thereby reducing the mortality rate from femur fractures by 60 percent.*

2. *Answer:* *Contact medical direction for permission to gently move the lower leg anteriorly to allow for circulation and transport immediately. Follow local protocols.*

ANSWERS TO MULTIPLE-CHOICE QUESTIONS

1. *Answer:* *d. open fracture*
2. *Answer:* *c. pelvic wrap*
3. *Answer:* *a. Pelvic*
4. *Answer:* *d. reassess distal circulation, sensation, and motor function*
5. *Answer:* *b. connective*

ANSWERS TO SCENARIO QUESTIONS

1. *Answer:* *d. utilizing a traction splint*
2. *Answer:* *c. head, spinal, and internal injuries*
3. *Answer:* *b. complete an initial assessment*

1. *Answer:* *c. attempt to realign his foot*
2. *Answer:* *d. immobilize the patient's knee*
3. *Answer:* *a. apply an ice pack*

1. *Answer:* *c. Logroll the patient gently onto his right side.*
2. *Answer:* *a. Place a folded blanket between the patient's legs from groin to ankles and bind his legs together with wide cravats.*
3. *Answer:* *b. proximal femur*

ANSWERS TO CASE STUDY QUESTIONS

1. Given that his ABCs are intact and there is no suspicion of spinal injury, the biggest concern will be for the circulatory status of his lower right leg.

2. You must begin by assessing for the presence of a pulse in the right foot. You can assess the dorsalis pedis or pedal pulse on the top of the foot or you can assess for the posterior tibial pulse behind the medial ankle bone. You will also want to check the foot for sensation and motor function as part of your complete assessment of the injury.

1. Due to the fact that you are unable to locate either pulse in this man's foot, it is going to be necessary to straighten his injury in an attempt to restore circulation.

2. At that point, you will have no choice but to splint the extremity and transport immediately to the nearest receiving hospital.

1. Investigate further. It is common for patients to focus on the most obvious or painful injury and not realize there are injuries somewhere else.

2. Yes. You should determine whether the fall was caused by some accident (slipping or tripping) as opposed to a medical emergency such as syncope, dizziness, or weakness.

1. Your examination of the wrist would include gentle palpation of the area identified by the patient as painful for DCAP-BTLS. You would also check for a radial pulse and the capillary-refill time in the fingers. Ask the patient to wiggle his fingers gently. You should ask about any sensations distal to the injury such as numbness and tingling. There is no need to have the patient squeeze your hand as this could aggravate an injury.

1. The official answer is, "I don't know, but I will treat it like it is." Not every fracture is dramatic and angulated. The wrist joint (where the radius and ulna meet the hand) consists of several small bones in which breaks might not be visible. Additionally, some sprains can be quite serious. Resist asking a question that really cannot be answered without an X ray. Your treatment will not change because of it.

2. Yes. Splint it. Apply cold for pain control and to reduce swelling, and monitor the injury site and distal areas for circulation frequently.

ANSWERS TO RETRO REVIEW QUESTIONS

1. *Answer:* d. *24th*
2. *Answer:* b. *A universal dressing.*
3. *Answer:* c. *elevated pulse*

ANSWERS TO CHAPTER 29 INJURIES TO THE HEAD AND SPINE

ANSWERS TO SHORT ANSWER QUESTIONS

1. *Answer:* *Because you will very rarely ever find obvious spinal deformities.*
2. *Answer:* *A direct brain injury, which is always the result of an open head injury, occurs when the brain tissue itself is lacerated, punctured, or bruised by broken bones or foreign objects.*

ANSWERS TO MULTIPLE-CHOICE QUESTIONS

1. *Answer:* a. *neurogenic shock*
2. *Answer:* c. *overtreat*
3. *Answer:* d. *short spine boards*
4. *Answer:* b. *infant*
5. *Answer:* a. *thoracic*

ANSWERS TO SCENARIO QUESTIONS

1. *Answer:* d. *has a compromised airway*
2. *Answer:* a. *rotated into a lateral recumbent position*
3. *Answer:* c. *apply direct pressure*

1. *Answer:* a. *the patient is secured to the spine board*
2. *Answer:* b. *head*
3. *Answer:* b. *Extremity paralysis*

1. *Answer:* d. *Insert an oropharyngeal airway without hyperextending her neck.*

1. *Answer:* b. *critical*
2. *Answer:* c. *It can help reduce brain-tissue swelling by lowering carbon dioxide levels and raising oxygen levels.*

Answers to Case Study Questions

1. Since the initial assessment appears all right for the time being, you will want to perform a rapid trauma assessment based on the mechanism of injury (fall from height and head injury). You will want to get the open wound on the head dressed appropriately and then focus in on his suspected spinal injuries.

2. Given the nature of his suspected injuries, a long backboard will be the most appropriate immobilization device. You will also want to apply an appropriate size cervical collar before securing him to the board.

   Your rapid trauma assessment reveals only a deformed right forearm but no other obvious injuries. The patient is beginning to regain consciousness as you place the cervical collar around his neck.

1. Given that he has a significant head injury, this man is likely to become combative, making it more difficult to properly immobilize him.

2. Once this man gets secured to the back board, you must pay particular attention to his airway. If he vomits, he will not be able to turn his head or clear his own airway. You must have a suction device ready and be prepared to roll the entire board should he vomit. Taking an additional person in the back of the ambulance to assist during the ride to the hospital is a good idea.

1. Specialists have referred to these events as collisions for years because most are preventable. Therefore, they are not strictly accidents. Collisions caused by inattention, cell-phone use, speeding, and other causes are not truly "accidents."

2. As you approach, look for downed wires, leaking fluids including gasoline, and fire. In any collision, be alert for broken glass and jagged metal that can cause injuries. If the air bag has not been deployed, that could be a danger as well.

1. As you approach, you should have noticed how much "crunch" or damage was caused when the car hit the tree. Once inside the car, you will be alert for damage to the interior caused by the patient's body. This includes damage to the windshield, steering wheel, and dash. Evidence of seat-belt use will also be important.

2. Even though your hands are "tied up" with stabilization, you can ask questions including whether the patient hurts anywhere, whether she remembers the crash, what caused the crash (did she have a medical problem that caused it or did an animal run out in front of her?), does she have any medical problems, and complete the remainder of the SAMPLE history.

1. You would tell them what you know so far. How concise and detailed you are would depend on how serious the patient is. A serious patient would require rapid extrication. You would give a quick synopsis of why you thought the patient was serious. You could be more detailed if the patient did not appear serious. In either event, you would give all of the detailed SAMPLE information after the extrication was in progress or completed.

2. The patient is conscious, alert, and oriented with normal skin color and condition. Her only complaint is neck pain. If the damage to the car is not substantial and the patient has no life-threats (ABCs or shock), the patient would be extricated using a short board or vest-type extrication device with a cervical collar. She would be moved to a long board and to the ambulance stretcher.

ANSWERS TO RETRO REVIEW QUESTIONS

1. *Answer:* b. *treat for shock*
2. *Answer:* d. *run data*
3. *Answer:* a. *latex allergy*

ANSWERS TO CHAPTER 30 PUTTING IT ALL TOGETHER FOR THE TRAUMA PATIENT

ANSWERS TO SHORT ANSWER QUESTIONS

1. *Answer:* A universal splint is the immobilization of the entire patient to a long spine board rather than splinting injured extremities individually.

2. *Answer:* Trauma patients need to be delivered to definitive care as soon as possible because EMS providers are rarely able to stabilize a trauma patient in the field.

ANSWERS TO MULTIPLE-CHOICE QUESTIONS

1. *Answer:* a. *practice*
2. *Answer:* d. *treat immediate life-threats*
3. *Answer:* c. *presents with a deformed thigh and paradoxical chest movement*

ANSWERS TO SCENARIO QUESTIONS

1. *Answer:* c. *the patient has a partially occluded airway*
2. *Answer:* d. *stroke, spinal injury, and/or diabetic emergency*
3. *Answer:* b. *Place the injured arm to the side of his body as you are securing the patient to the backboard.*

1. *Answer:* c. *Seal the patient's open neck wounds with your gloved hands.*
2. *Answer:* d. *complete a rapid trauma assessment*
3. *Answer:* b. *universal splint*

ANSWERS TO CASE STUDY QUESTIONS

1. You will want to try and determine where the patient was seated in the vehicle and whether she was wearing a seat belt. You will also want to quickly inspect the interior of the vehicle to assess the amount of intrusion and whether there were air bags that deployed.

2. Due to the significant MOI, this patient should receive a rapid trauma assessment.

1. The blood pressure seems a little low relative to the rapid pulse rate. The pulse rate is elevated and is significant because the patient is unresponsive. This patient is likely showing signs of shock.

2. This patient should be quickly placed on a long backboard with cervical immobilization and transported rapidly to the nearest hospital. You must initiate high-flow oxygen and bleeding control during the initial assessment.

1. By checking his ABCs. Much of this can be done with conversation, observation of breathing, and a pulse check at the wrist. Your initial impression does not reveal significant distress.

406 Appendix A • *Answers to Chapter Review Questions*

2. In the EMS, you will be faced with many types of calls and situations, even some like this. You may be shocked, find them humorous, or even disgusting. None of your personal feelings for any situation should be visible to the patient. You should treat all patients with dignity and respect.

1. No. Since he has shown you the area around the anus, examining it for blood or discharge is appropriate. This might indicate tears of the rectal mucosa and/or internal bleeding.

2. Place the patient in a position of comfort. Monitor him for changes in levels of pain or discomfort. Look for changes in his condition or shock that could indicate bleeding or internal trauma. Transport and reassuring the patient are sometimes the most significant treatment for cases that are not anywhere in the book.

ANSWERS TO RETRO REVIEW QUESTIONS

1. *Answer:* a. *provide artificial ventilations*
2. *Answer:* c. *torn ligaments*
3. *Answer:* b. *Begin CPR and transport immediately.*

ANSWERS TO CHAPTER 31 INFANTS AND CHILDREN

ANSWERS TO SHORT ANSWER QUESTIONS

1. *Answer:* *Since many pediatric patients are fearful of oxygen masks, it may be more effective to have a rescuer or parent hold an oxygen source (tubing, mask, and so on) about 2 inches from the child's face. The patient will be inhaling the oxygen as it passes by his nose and mouth.*

2. *Answer:* *A shunt is a drainage device that runs from the brain to the abdomen to relieve excess cerebrospinal fluid.*

ANSWERS TO MULTIPLE-CHOICE QUESTIONS

1. *Answer:* c. *meningitis*
2. *Answer:* b. *a physician has informed them of the child's death*
3. *Answer:* c. *Trauma*
4. *Answer:* d. *say anything that would make the patient feel responsible for the event*
5. *Answer:* a. *regression*

ANSWERS TO SCENARIO QUESTIONS

1. *Answer:* d. *insert it with the tip pointing downward using a tongue depressor*
2. *Answer:* d. *5 minutes*
3. *Answer:* a. *secured to a long spine board*

1. *Answer:* c. *Shock*
2. *Answer:* d. *the child's crying*
3. *Answer:* a. *life threatening*

1. *Answer:* b. *is normal*
2. *Answer:* b. *ask her to help calm the child*
3. *Answer:* d. *spleen*

Answers to Case Study Questions

1. It is a good idea to at least examine the child and look for any signs of respiratory difficulty.

2. You will want to observe the child for any signs of respiratory distress and advise the parents to watch the child closely for any signs of difficulty in breathing, such as increased respiratory rate, use of accessory muscles, and drooling. You will also want to examine the abdomen for any signs or symptoms of trauma resulting from the abdominal thrusts.

1. Your first clue that something was not right was the reluctance on the father's part to allow you to see or examine the baby. The presence of bruises on the baby's back and arm are inconsistent with the types of bruises commonly found on toddlers.

2. Most states have identified EMTs as "mandatory reporters" of situations involving suspected abuse or neglect. You should speak to your instructor about the specific laws in your state. In most cases, you should document your findings in an objective prehospital-care report and immediately inform your supervisor of your concerns and/or suspicions. In some states, you may be required to report your suspicions to child-protective services or a law-enforcement officer.

1. You find that the child has good muscle tone and is alert enough to be wary of you and seek refuge with his grandmother. You should additionally look for the patient's skin color (is it pale, gray, or cyanotic?) and work of breathing (use of accessory muscles, retractions, nasal flaring, and grunting).

2. The doorway assessment sets a foundation for the initial assessment and is an excellent start. It provides much of the information you need for the initial assessment. The initial assessment goes into a bit more detail in evaluating mental status, airway, breathing, and circulation. You should check capillary refill. You should begin interventions such as oxygen.

1. The patient will most likely not tolerate a mask. In fact, the stress of fighting with the child to apply a mask could be harmful. Use "blow-by" oxygen held by his grandmother.

2. You will obtain respiratory rate and effort; pulse; skin color, temperature, and condition; and capillary refill.

1. The pulse is at the high end of normal, the capillary refill is normal, and the respirations are slightly above "normal" rates. These are in line with a young patient in some respiratory distress. Equally important is the patient's response to strangers, which is aggressive and appropriate for his age level.

2. They essentially say the same thing. The PAT showed a patient with good muscle tone, appropriate response, good capillary refill, and some labored but adequate breathing. The vitals say the same thing. He needs to be transported but is not in extremis or in respiratory failure. All of these signs should be monitored carefully en route to the hospital.

Answers to Retro Review Questions

1. *Answer:* c. *do not resuscitate order (Chapter 3)*
2. *Answer:* d. *pertinent negative (Chapter 10/11)*
3. *Answer:* c. *Head-on (Chapter 7)*

ANSWERS TO CHAPTER 32
GERIATRIC EMERGENCIES

ANSWERS TO SHORT ANSWER QUESTIONS

1. *Answer:* One of the most serious causes of abdominal pain among elderly patients is an **A**bdominal **A**ortic **A**neurysm (or triple A).

2. *Answer:* Diverticulosis is a condition in which the intestines develop an outpouching or sac in which food can become lodged—which causes an inflammation known as diverticulitis.

ANSWERS TO MULTIPLE-CHOICE QUESTIONS

1. *Answer:* c. Grapefruit juice
2. *Answer:* a. shingles
3. *Answer:* d. An altered mental status may be part of the patient's baseline condition.
4. *Answer:* b. commit suicide
5. *Answer:* c. sudden weakness and no chest pain

ANSWERS TO SCENARIO QUESTIONS

1. *Answer:* c. A hip or proximal femur fracture.
2. *Answer:* d. No, the LVN explained that it is a chronic condition.

1. *Answer:* b. decreased sensitivity to pain
2. *Answer:* a. confabulation

ANSWERS TO CASE STUDY QUESTIONS

1. Given her poor general impression, it is probably a good idea to cover her with a blanket and start her on oxygen at 15 lpm by nonrebreather mask.

2. Since no one saw what happened to her and you cannot rule out a possible fall, you must manage her cervical spine while conducting a rapid trauma assessment.

1. On the basis of the presentation of the leg being shorter and rotated, there is a strong likelihood that she may have dislocated or broken her right hip.

2. You will need to carefully assess the distal extremity to confirm the status of circulation, sensation, and motor function. Most likely the best option for packaging her up for transport will be a long spine board and cervical collar. You will want to place a blanket over the board first and place some kind of pad beneath her head for added comfort on the ride to the hospital.

1. It appears that the patient has an altered mental status and may have fallen.

2. Begin by asking the patient. Complete an initial assessment including mental status. Look for signs of injury or pain when the patient moves, even if he denies injury. A quick head-to-toe exam may be in order if you have even the slightest doubt.

1. The prime concerns would be the numerous medical conditions possible with the elderly. Stroke or TIA would be high on that list. Falling and hitting his head is another potential cause. Other causes are accidental or intentional overdoses, diabetic conditions, and seizures.

2. Altered-mental-status cases are the ultimate detective cases. Perform a SAMPLE history to determine whether he has a history of respiratory, cardiac, diabetic, or central-nervous system (stroke and seizure) problems. Medications will also help out here. Check medication containers and

types. Sleep-inducing and antidepressant medications are both very common in the geriatric population. Your observations of the scene may be very important later on.

ANSWERS TO RETRO REVIEW QUESTIONS

1. *Answer:* b. *high fevers (Chapter 31)*
2. *Answer:* b. *vital signs (Chapter 11)*
3. *Answer:* d. *Elevate the mother's buttocks, administer oxygen, wrap the exposed cord with a sterile towel, insert several gloved fingers into the mother's vagina to keep the baby off the cord, and transport immediately. (Chapter 24)*

ANSWERS TO CHAPTER 33 AMBULANCE OPERATIONS

ANSWERS TO SHORT ANSWER QUESTIONS

1. *Answer:* *The run is not over until the ambulance personnel and equipment are ready for the next response.*
2. *Answer:* *A true emergency is one in which the best information available to you indicates that loss of life and limb is possible.*

ANSWERS TO MULTIPLE-CHOICE QUESTIONS

1. *Answer:* c. *constriction bands*
2. *Answer:* b. *Transmission*
3. *Answer:* d. *thumper*
4. *Answer:* c. *are being escorted by the flight personnel*
5. *Answer:* a. *in front of the wreckage*

ANSWERS TO SCENARIO QUESTIONS

1. *Answer:* b. *Between the oncoming cars and the collision, at the crest of the hill.*
2. *Answer:* d. *approaching vehicles will be traveling at excessive speeds*
3. *Answer:* a. *Set the parking brake and chock the wheels.*
1. *Answer:* d. *Wait with him in the emergency department, ensuring that you are not in the staff's way.*
2. *Answer:* c. *any condition changes that you have noticed*
3. *Answer:* c. *Complete the PCR.*

ANSWERS TO CASE STUDY QUESTIONS

1. There are two primary dangers with this activity. The first is the danger of following too closely and if the lead vehicle has to make an emergency stop, the vehicle following may not have time to stop safely. The second danger is that most motorists who have stopped or pulled to the side for the lead vehicle are not expecting a second vehicle to be close behind. There is a great danger of one of these motorists pulling out into the path of the second vehicle once the lead vehicle has passed.
2. Your partner will not be able to complete a proper inventory during code 3 driving and will likely not be seat belted in. If your partner is not seated next to you during code 3 driving, you are also losing an important second set of eyes that will be needed for safety reasons.

1. In an ideal situation, you would want to pull past the crash scene and park in front of the scene. This will typically provide extra protection from oncoming traffic and afford you an easy exit from the scene.

2. You will want to make certain that you park a safe distance from the scene but not so far that it makes getting equipment difficult. You must also consider wind direction and slope so that you can park upwind and uphill from the crash should there be toxic fumes or leaking materials from the vehicles.

1. It appears that the bag containing the straps and collars was not in your ambulance when you started the shift. If you look back on calls, you may find that the equipment was used recently and was lost, misplaced, or not returned.

2. By realizing the importance of keeping an ambulance stocked completely and by returning equipment in a usable condition after you yourself use it. You should also check the rig as soon as possible after the start of your shift to prevent surprises such as this.

1. Call for another ambulance or improvise. Your using a rolled towel or thin blanket as a makeshift collar and head block and taping the patient to the board instead of strapping would accomplish the same purpose although it is much more difficult and certainly not as pretty when you get to the hospital. If the patient were critically injured, waiting for another ambulance would certainly harm the patient. It could be worse: Imagine not having your AED when faced with a cardiac-arrest patient.

1. No. Your rig would be inadequately prepared for a similar event.

ANSWERS TO RETRO REVIEW QUESTIONS

1. *Answer:* b. *hypoglycemia (Chapter 19)*
2. *Answer:* c. *have witnesses sign statements attesting to the refusal (Chapter 3)*
3. *Answer:* a. *about as effective as the CPR performed by a lay person who has been trained (Chapter 8)*

ANSWERS TO CHAPTER 34 GAINING ACCESS AND RESCUE OPERATIONS

ANSWERS TO SHORT ANSWER QUESTIONS

1. *Answer:* *Flares can spew molten phosphorus, which can cause full-thickness burns to the holder's skin.*
2. *Answer:* *During rescue operations, such as extrications, the EMT-B should wear protective headgear, eye protection, hand protection, and body protection.*

ANSWERS TO MULTIPLE-CHOICE QUESTIONS

1. *Answer:* c. *deployed air bags*
2. *Answer:* d. *remove the ground cable from the battery*
3. *Answer:* c. *Because it is your job to keep the patient safe and to prevent further injuries.*
4. *Answer:* d. *Loaded*
5. *Answer:* b. *laminated*

ANSWERS TO SCENARIO QUESTIONS

1. *Answer:* a. *catalytic converters*
2. *Answer:* b. *A:B:C dry-chemical*
3. *Answer:* d. *Wait for the fire department to arrive and prepare to treat him if he survives.*
1. *Answer:* c. *Instruct the patient not to move while awaiting the rescue squad.*
2. *Answer:* a. *reassurance*
3. *Answer:* d. *Build a box crib with 4 x 4s under the car.*
1. *Answer:* c. *ground gradient*
2. *Answer:* b. *Turn around and hop on one foot to a safe place.*

ANSWERS TO CASE STUDY QUESTIONS

1. You might try to get the semiresponsive patient to unlock the doors; otherwise you will most likely have to break a window to gain entry.

2. Your first choice will be a window that is not adjacent to one of the vehicle's occupants. Breaking a window next to an occupant may spray pieces of glass onto the patient.

1. You can place a blanket or salvage cover over the opening of the window and down onto the seat of the car. That way when you climb in, you will not come into direct contact with broken glass. You may want to don heavy protective gloves while you make your entry into the vehicle.

2. This patient is a candidate for rapid extrication. Every effort must be made to get this patient out of the vehicle quickly if she is going to have any chance for survival.

1. The immediate hazards are the unstable vehicle on its side and the traffic traveling around the crash scene. Additionally, there may be broken glass or sharp metal that is dangerous.

2. No. Not until the vehicle is stabilized. You should not enter or approach the vehicle until it is stabilized. There is a great risk of injury to you and further injury to the patients if it moves or flips onto either side.

3. The fire department can stabilize the vehicle and carry out any rescue techniques to gain access. The police will be necessary for crash investigation and traffic control. Additional ambulances should be summoned on the basis of the number and severity of the patients you find. When you cannot get to patients, assume the worst (that they are seriously injured) and get additional ambulances accordingly.

1. You should be wearing protective clothing, either fire or EMS turnout gear, and eye and hand protection.

2. Ideally, this should be a joint decision between fire and EMS personnel on the scene. You will need to decide the priority and method of extrication (e.g. rapid or with a short board) on the basis of the patient's condition. The fire service personnel will contribute their expertise in extrication to meet those goals. While it does not always happen that way, each contributing his input and working together gets to a prompt, safe, and effective result.

ANSWERS TO RETRO REVIEW QUESTIONS

1. *Answer:* c. *Reassess as much of the patient's back as you can touch without moving the patient. (Chapter 10)*
2. *Answer:* b. *hypotension (Chapter 15/17)*
3. *Answer:* c. *call for air rescue (Chapter 10/33)*

ANSWERS TO CHAPTER 35 SPECIAL OPERATIONS

ANSWERS TO SHORT ANSWER QUESTIONS

1. *Answer:* In a singular-command situation, one agency controls all of the resources and operations during an incident. Unified command, on the other hand, means that each agency (police, fire, EMS, and so on) works independently yet cooperates on the incident objective.

2. *Answer:* Hazardous materials incidents will most likely take place in factories, along railroads, and on local, state, and federal highways.

ANSWERS TO MULTIPLE-CHOICE QUESTIONS

1. *Answer:* c. six
2. *Answer:* d. First Responder Operations
3. *Answer:* b. staging officer
4. *Answer:* c. triage
5. *Answer:* a. brightly colored vests

ANSWERS TO SCENARIO QUESTIONS

1. *Answer:* c. use your unit's binoculars and initially survey the scene from where you are
2. *Answer:* b. yellow
3. *Answer:* a. Use your unit's PA system and direct all individuals who can walk to leave the train.
1. *Answer:* c. incident commander
2. *Answer:* b. "Dispatch, this is Unit 75. We are on scene with a three-car MVA. I've got one severely entrapped "delayed" patient and four additional "immediate" patients. Dispatch a rescue squad and five paramedic ambulances. I will now be called Thompson Road Command, and I need police for traffic control."
3. *Answer:* a. singular
1. *Answer:* d. Have dispatch contact the factory and ask somebody to meet you outside.
2. *Answer:* c. upwind and on the same level as the factory
3. *Answer:* b. consult your ERG2000

ANSWERS TO CASE STUDY QUESTIONS

1. You will want to report your findings to the dispatcher and position your vehicle a safe distance upwind and uphill from the incident.
2. You will want to let them know of the hazmat potential because of the large tanker truck as well as the overturned railcars. You must request a specialized hazmat team as well as fire-suppression resources.

1. See Emergency Response Guide.
2. See Emergency Response Guide.

1. The scene size-up is crucial on this call. Requesting additional ambulances is one part of the size-up. Dealing with the building as a second scene is another. Are patients in the building? Is the building safe structurally? The

fire department should be notified to deal with this and the potential need for extrication.

2. At this point, it is difficult to tell. You do not know whether the people outside the van are patients or bystanders or whether any more are inside the van out of sight. As a general rule, it is best to estimate high early as it is better to cancel ambulances you do not need than to have too few.

3. Notify the dispatcher that you have an MCI. Priority 3 patients may be able to double up or ultimately refuse treatment so another six ambulances are needed. The dispatcher will call neighboring agencies for mutual-aid station coverage and will have them available for response to the scene if needed.

1. The treatment officer ensures patients are triaged and treated according to their triage priority. This officer matches patients with ambulances and equipment. In a small-scale MCI, there may be additional roles (e.g. secondary triage).

2. No patient should leave the scene without the transporting crew speaking with the transport officer. This officer logs patient names and hospital destinations. In large incidents, the transportation officer (or an aide) contacts hospitals to check on availability for different types of patients. Patients are distributed to hospitals on the basis of priority, hospital capabilities, and patient load.

ANSWERS TO RETRO REVIEW QUESTIONS

1. *Answer:* c. *A detailed physical exam. (Chapter 10)*
2. *Answer:* d. *remove the positive battery cable first (Chapter 34)*
3. *Answer:* b. *apply a bulky pressure dressing to the stump, wrap the attached foot with a sterile dressing, and treat for shock as you transport immediately (Chapter 27)*

ANSWERS TO CHAPTER 36 TERRORISM AND EMS

ANSWERS TO SHORT ANSWER QUESTIONS

1. *Answer:* *Strategies are broad, general plans designed to achieve a desired outcome, whereas tactics are specific actions taken to accomplish assigned tasks.*

2. *Answer:* *April 19 is the anniversary of both the destruction of the Branch Davidian compound in Waco, Texas, and the bombing of the Alfred P. Murrah Federal Building in Oklahoma City. That date has become a rallying point for antigovernment extremists and a potential date for future "attacks."*

ANSWERS TO MULTIPLE-CHOICE QUESTIONS

1. *Answer:* b. *technological hazards*
2. *Answer:* c. **O***ccupancy,* **T***ype,* **T***iming, and* **O***n-scene.*
3. *Answer:* a. *respirable*
4. *Answer:* d. *emergency responders*
5. *Answer:* b. *firearms*

ANSWERS TO SCENARIO QUESTIONS

1. *Answer:* d. *Move your ambulance a good distance away while relaying the entire situation to dispatch and set up an incident-command post.*
2. *Answer:* a. *evaluate the OTTO signs*
3. *Answer:* c. *chemical weapon*
1. *Answer:* c. *allow law enforcement to clear the scene*
2. *Answer:* c. *suicide bombing*
3. *Answer:* d. *search them for weapons*
1. *Answer:* c. *the dispersion of radiological materials*
2. *Answer:* d. *secondary devices*
3. *Answer:* b. *psychological*

ANSWERS TO CASE STUDY QUESTIONS

1. The fact that some type of explosion has occurred at a highly publicized event where large numbers of people are gathered is a strong indication that it could be a terrorist event.
2. There are likely to be blast injuries if the explosion was large enough. Burns and open wounds will also be likely. If panic has overcome the crowd, you may also see injuries caused by the rush of the crowd as it attempts to exit the arena. Broken bones and possible tramplings are a strong possibility.

1. You must take into consideration the proximity to the primary event and of course wind direction. Any chemicals that may have been released by the blast will follow wind currents.
2. You must be extra alert for any sign of a possible secondary device or threat. Many terrorists will detonate a secondary device after EMS has arrived at the scene to inflict injury and death to those attempting to assist at such an incident.

1. Yes. Terrorism involves a deliberate, illegal act that is designed to intimidate. Terrorism may be small or large scale, by a wide range of methods, and by both domestic and international sources.
2. This event is etiological—one that is designed to cause disease. Although it has not been tested and confirmed as positively containing anthrax, it has also caused a significant psychological impact. In the CBRNE classification, this would be a potential biological weapon.

1. The patients should be decontaminated before you come into contact with them.

1. After decontamination, you will wear a respirator, face/eye protection, protection from secretions and splashing, and gloves.
2. Decontaminated patients may be brought to a hospital but only if the hospital is involved well in advance and was allowed to make preparations. In some cases, the public-health authorities may be involved and they may coordinate treatment of patients such as this.

ANSWERS TO RETRO REVIEW QUESTIONS

1. *Answer:* a. *the patient is in cardiac arrest*
2. *Answer:* c. *The patient's ongoing vital signs.*
3. *Answer:* d. *any substance that can harm the body*

ANSWERS TO CHAPTER 37 ADVANCED AIRWAY MANAGEMENT

ANSWERS TO SHORT ANSWER QUESTIONS

1. *Answer:* The NG tube is commonly used to decompress the stomach and proximal bowel of excess air.
2. *Answer:* Since infants and children have small chests, sounds are easily transmitted from one area to another. The best indicator is symmetrical chest rise and fall during ventilation.

ANSWERS TO MULTIPLE-CHOICE QUESTIONS

1. *Answer:* c. suction catheter
2. *Answer:* b. gastric distention
3. *Answer:* a. vallecula
4. *Answer:* d. esophageal intubation
5. *Answer:* b. two

ANSWERS TO SCENARIO QUESTIONS

1. *Answer:* b. intubate orally
2. *Answer:* d. performed an esophageal intubation
3. *Answer:* c. cricoid pressure

1. *Answer:* b. begin rescue breathing
2. *Answer:* d. The patient's pulse will slow.
3. *Answer:* a. 7.5

ANSWERS TO CASE STUDY QUESTIONS

1. In general, a size 8.0 or 8.5 tube will be appropriate for an adult male.
2. You will ask the firefighter to begin providing ventilations every 2 seconds in an effort to hyperventilate the patient. You will also want to get all of the equipment prepared and handy, including a suction device.

1. Ask the firefighter to apply gentle cricoid pressure in an effort to push the vocal cords posterior and into view.
2. By placing the BVM onto the end of the ET tube and asking the firefighter to ventilate every 2 seconds. Using a stethoscope, you can listen for equal breath sounds bilaterally and confirm the absence of gurgling over the epigastrium.

1. He is scared, may be in denial, and may not have any medical training. You might sometimes feel frustrated that this information was not conveyed to the dispatcher, that CPR was not done sooner, or that he just did not get how serious things were. In this case, a marriage of 50 years may be coming to an end and this is quite traumatic to the husband, and he should be treated with great respect, compassion, and understanding. Even if he does not seem to "get it."
2. Defibrillation would come before intubation.

1. The choices are not good. Keep suctioning and cause hypoxia or stop suctioning, blow the vomit into the lungs, and cause fatal aspiration pneumonia. It is important to realize that you are often dealt difficult decisions. In this case, you will probably have to continue suctioning. Do

so aggressively and quickly. Hopefully, the patient will give you a break long enough to ventilate a bit.

2. It could be the large pasta lunch she had. It could also be the fact that ventilations are being given too forcefully or quickly, forcing air into the stomach. This will likely cause vomiting. The second cause is preventable. Slow, full breaths are the rule for a reason.

1. Many systems have protocols for how many intubation attempts may be made. The choices when your tries are unsuccessful are to go with another device (e.g. Combitube) or to use BLS techniques.

ANSWERS TO RETRO REVIEW QUESTIONS

1. *Answer:*   d.   *All of the above. (Chapter 35)*
2. *Answer:*   c.   *Tell your partner to quickly hop on one foot back to the ambulance.*
3. *Answer:*   b.   *the Cincinnati Stroke Scale*

Index

automatic transport ventilators (ATVs), 351
automaticity, 26
AVPU, 59
AVPU scale, 260

B

backboard, 30, 75, 92, 112, 205, 267, 308
back injuries, 34
bag valve mask, 195
bandages, 239
basal cell carcinoma, 240
baseline vital signs, 66, 70, 82, 83, 275
baseline vitals, 68, 74, 156, 177
basic anatomical differences, 279
basophils, 230
bazmats, 322
behavioral emergency, 202, 204
    common signs and symptoms of, 203
    emergency care for, 203
bilateral, 350
biological agents, 337
    absorption, 337
    exposure to, 337
    inhalation, 337
    injection, 337
bipolar, 249
black widow, 192
bleeding, 227
    arterial, 227
    capillary, 227
    venous, 227
blood, 27, 41
    platelets, 27
    red blood cells, 27
    white blood cells, 27, 229
blood loss, 227, 228, 234, 247, 248, 280
blood pressure, 22, 27, 66–68, 70, 91
    high, 22
    low, 229
bodily fluids, 8
body heat, 189
body mechanics, 33
body substance isolation. See BSI
body surface area (BSA), 244, 279, 281
brachial pulse, 66
bradycardia, 135, 180
brain, 259, 348
brainstem, 348
breathing difficulty, 5, 13, 75, 124, 178, 243
breech presentation, 210, 211
bronchi, 348
bronchial, 220
bronchioles, 126, 127, 165, 167, 168
bronchoconstriction, 168
brown recluse, 192
BSI, 8, 13, 42, 50, 79, 130, 146, 179, 211, 224, 227, 239, 260, 350
burnout, 9

burns, 75, 189, 238, 239, 244, 272, 281, 282
    agent/source, 238
    depth, 238
BVM, 353, 355

C

calcium, 252
capillary refill, 67, 92, 281, 287
cardiac, 247
cardiac arrest, 59, 131, 136–138, 157, 192, 239, 262, 281, 303, 304, 349, 350, 354
cardiac asthma, 220, 221
cardiac compromise, 135, 136, 138, 272
cardiac problems, 136
    See also cardiac compromise
cardiogenic, 272
cardiovascular system, 26
    blood vessels, 26
    heart, 26
carina, 348
carrying devices, 33, 34
    See also spine board; stair chair; stretcher
cartilage, 248
catalytic converter, 313, 314
catheter, 131
central nervous system, 179, 259
central pulse, 27
central rewarming, 190
centroroides exilcauda scorpion, 193
cephalic presentation, 210
cervical collar, 75, 260–262, 267, 308
chain of survival, 136, 137
CHEM-TEL, 324
CHEM-TEL hotline, 340
CHEMTREC, 324
CHEMTREC hotline, 340
chest injuries, 238
    cardiac tamponade, 238
    complications, 238
    forms, 238
chest pain, 22, 115, 136, 141
chief complaint, 58, 74, 76, 83, 92, 100, 104, 220, 292, 296
child abuse, 282
    signs of physical abuse, 282
    signs of sexual abuse, 282
chin-lift maneuver, 41, 42, 59
chronic bronchitis, 115, 126
circulatory system, 67, 227
clothes drag, 34
code 3 driving, 307
cold zone, 323, 324
    rehab sector, 323
command name, 326
communication, 2, 33, 100, 101, 301, 323, 326
    interpersonal, 99, 100
    radio/cellular, 99
    verbal, 99

National Registry of Emergency Medical
    Technicians (NREMT), 2
nature of illness (NOI), 50
nausea, 166, 213
near-drowning, 190, 192
negligence, 18, 108
nerve agents, 252
nervous system, 27, 176, 259
    autonomic, 27, 259
    central, 259
    peripheral, 27, 259
neutrophils, 230
NG, 351
nitroglycerin, 22, 23, 67, 83, 120, 135, 136
noisy breathing, 124
nonmelanoma, 240
nonrebreather mask, 5, 42, 70, 79, 120, 125, 141,
    146, 156, 166, 190, 217, 243, 244

O

objective statements, 108
obstetrics, 210, 217
occlusive dressing, 238
Occupational Safety and Health Administration
    (OSHA), 322
one-person moves, 34
ongoing assessments, 91, 92, 94, 100, 146, 177,
    178, 203, 303, 311, 350
open wounds, 76, 237, 239, 260, 313, 324
OPQRST, 71, 82, 83
    mnemonic, 146
    questions, 125
organ donors, 19
organophosphate poisoning, 181
organophosphates, 180, 181, 252
oropharyngeal airway (OPA), 42, 60, 79, 260, 280,
    353
oropharyngeal suctioning, 349
oropharynx, 348, 349
orotracheal suctioning, 351
OTTO mnemonic, 336
overdose, 47, 115, 176, 179, 184, 190, 297
oxygen, 86, 87, 141, 156, 190, 216, 229, 280, 281,
    287
oxygen cylinder, 42
oxygen saturation, 67, 71, 125, 224
oxygen therapy, 42, 198, 233

P

palpation, 67, 68, 74, 146, 256
pancreas, 27, 154
PASG, 228, 250
passive rewarming, 190, 199
patella, 26, 251
patent airway, 40, 190, 221, 237, 239, 348
pathogens, 8
patient advocacy, 2, 5, 311

patient airway, 166
patient assessment, 2, 5, 50, 67, 146, 156
patient restraint, 204
pediatric patients, 262, 279
    anatomical differences, 279
    common causes of shock in, 279, 280
    intubation, 350
    other medical emergencies, 281
    signs of respiratory distress, 279, 281
    signs of shock in, 279, 280
    special concerns, 279, 280
pelvic wrap, 250
pelvis, 26, 76, 238, 250, 260
    ilium, 26
    ischium, 26
penetrating trauma, 228
penetrations. *See* punctures
perfusion, 27, 59, 138, 227, 228, 230, 272
    See also hypoperfusion
peritoneum, 247
    parietal, 145
    visceral, 145
peritonitis, 147
personal protective equipment (PPE), 8, 10, 50,
    179, 312, 324
    gowns, 8
    masks, 8
    protective gloves, 8
pertinent negatives, 108
pertinent subjective information, 108
physiology, 25, 27, 204, 349
piggyback carry, 34
placenta, 210–212
placenta previa, 212
platelets, 230
PMS, 249, 261
pneumatic antishock garments, 250
pneumonia, 8
pocket face mask, 42, 124
poison, 176, 177
    absorbed, 177, 178, 336
    activated charcoal, 177
    dilution, 177, 325, 338
    ingested, 177, 194, 336
    inhaled, 177, 336
    injected, 177, 192, 193
poisoning, 176, 178, 180, 181, 193, 281
poisonous snakes, 193
polyuria, 155
positional asphyxia, 204, 205
positional terms, 26
posttraumatic stress disorder (PTSD), 9
potassium, 252
power grip, 33
power lift, 33
pre-eclampsia, 213
pregnancy, 210, 212, 213
    emergencies in complications of, 212
    HELLP syndrome, 213